REFLECTIONS ON
RENAL FUNCTION

REFLECTIONS ON RENAL FUNCTION

JAMES R. ROBINSON
MD, PhD, ScD, FRSNZ, FRACP
Emeritus Professor of Physiology
University of Otago Medical School
Dunedin
New Zealand

SECOND EDITION

BLACKWELL SCIENTIFIC PUBLICATIONS
OXFORD LONDON EDINBURGH
BOSTON PALO ALTO MELBOURNE

© 1988 by
Blackwell Scientific Publications
Editorial offices:
Osney Mead, Oxford OX2 0EL
  (*Orders*: Tel. 0865 240201)
8 John Street, London WC1N 2ES
23 Ainslie Place, Edinburgh EH3 6AJ
Three Cambridge Center, Suite 208
  Cambridge, Massachusetts 02142, USA
667 Lytton Avenue, Palo Alto
  California 94301, USA
107 Barry Street, Carlton
  Victoria 3053, Australia

First published 1954
Second edition 1988

Set by Setrite Typesetters Ltd, Hong Kong
Printed and bound in Great Britain by
Redwood Burn Ltd, Trowbridge

DISTRIBUTORS

USA
  Year Book Medical Publishers
  200 North LaSalle Street
  Chicago, Illinois 60601
  (*Orders*: Tel. 312 726−9733)

Canada
  The C.V. Mosby Company
  5240 Finch Avenue East
  Scarborough, Ontario
  (*Orders*: Tel. 416−298−1588)

Australia
  Blackwell Scientific Publications
  (Australia) Pty Ltd
  107 Barry Street
  Carlton, Victoria 3053
  (*Orders*: Tel. (03) 347 0300)

British Library
Cataloguing in Publication Data

Robinson, James R.
  Reflections on renal function — 2nd ed.
  1. Kidneys
  I. Title
  612'.463   QP249
  ISBN 0−632−02102−0

Contents

Preface

The original Reflections on Renal Function appeared 33 years ago. A great deal has changed since then, but the aims of the book have not. Though longer than its predecessor, it is still more a commentary on the physiology of the kidneys as this is presented in a very extensive and sometimes contradictory literature, rather than a treatise. I have described without going into too much detail, something of what we think the kidney does, how we think it does it, and why we think so. Some large and detailed comprehensive treatises exist; these are excellent sources of information and evaluation, but they are expensive and somewhat unwieldy.

'Notes and impressions of a kidney-watcher' might be a fitting subtitle, with due apologies to Lewis Thomas; for I have not, like the giants of the recent past, Homer Smith and Robert Pitts, spent a lifetime in the forefront of renal research. It was a great privilege and delight to meet them and their ilk on many occasions, but for most of my life I have been a watcher quite literally from afar.

I have again tried to provide an introduction for newcomers, including students, a guide to visitors from other specialities and a commentary which may interest those already familiar with the field. I have retained 'Reflections' in the title because it still gives a fair indication of the rather personal way in which the subject is treated. I have sometimes expressed results from other species in human terms or magnitudes, and emphasized the kidneys' contributions to keeping people alive and well. The treatment is admittedly uneven. The nature of glomerular filtration, its often neglected variations, and the regulation of the volumes of body fluids, are discussed at greater length than matters in which I was less keenly interested or about which I was more ignorant. Some sections may seem little more than lecture notes; but they are supported by references to more detailed information or opinions based on richer experience. Metabolic aspects of renal function have received rather summary treatment; there is more about what the tubular epithelium does than about how it does it, and not very much about the molecular and cellular mechanisms of epithelial transport. In other sections, which are more like letters to a friend, I have tried to tell a coherent story rather than to present a plethora of conflicting views. The aim to keep to a moderate compass imposed restrictions on how much could be discussed. It would have been far easier to write a hundred pages on tubuloglomerular feedback than the half dozen I allowed myself in the interests of balance.

Hence far more has been left out than put in! I have ambled along a mile or so of a beach, picked up a few dozen pebbles and shells here and there that caught my fancy, and arranged them in a pattern that pleased me. I hope that others will find my pebbles interesting and be tempted to go after the many more that I left behind. And I humbly apologize to all those whose favourite pebbles failed to catch my eye, or seemed too large to pick up. My ignorance will be only too obvious to experts on all aspects of renal physiology. But if their favourite topics had been dealt with adequately, the book would have been vastly longer, and possibly no better balanced.

The choice of references was not easy. Reviewers in the *Annual Review of Physiology* have cited more than 9000 publications since the first *Reflections* appeared. If all relevant articles were included, the bibliography would be far longer than the intentionally fairly brief text. I have recognized some early workers who established facts or proposed principles, and then used reviews for access to many later publications confirming, denying or filling in details of what went before. In the list of references the sections of the text to which each chiefly relates are given in square brackets. This may make the bibliography useful both as a supplementary and as an author index, as it is in Homer Smith's (1951) classic. My debt to Homer Smith is obvious; his book is a rich quarry which yielded a big haul of solid rock! Editorial reviews in the *American Journal* of *Physiology* and in *Kidney International* were also invaluable, and will appeal to all who want to keep up with the advance of renal physiology.

The urge to produce a new version of the book written so long ago came in the first instance from the publisher. Without Per Saugman's interest and encouragement neither this version nor its predecessor would have been written. His urging was reinforced by my fellow members of the Executive Committee of the International Society of Nephrology a decade ago. I made the excuses then that *Reflections* could not be written without time to reflect; and that I would not have time before I retired. So it became a retirement project; and then it nearly foundered, for one of the consequences of retirement was the loss of a superb departmental secretary. My portable typewriter was a poor substitute, and the need for frequent updating was quite daunting until my daughter persuaded me that I should get a computer for my 70th birthday. After that, what had been developing into an impossible chore became a pleasure; my wife put up with the addiction, and the task was completed.

J.R.R.
Dunedin, New Zealand

Abbreviations

ACTH	adrenocorticotrophic hormone	PCV	packed cell volume (haematocrit)
ADH	antidiuretic hormone	pd	potential difference
ANF	atrial natriuretic factor	PG	prostaglandin
ANP	atrial natriuretic peptide	pI	isoelectric point
AT	angiotensin	PPG	phosphate-dependent glutaminase
ATP	adenosine triphosphate		
ATPase	adenosine triphosphatase	PSP	phenol sulphone phthalein
AVP	arginine vasopressin	PTH	parathyroid hormone
DEAE	diethylaminoethyl	RAP	renal arterial plasma
ECF	extracellular fluid	RBF	renal blood flow
ECFV	volume of extracellular fluid	RL	renal lymph
		RNG	renal gluconeogenesis
ERPF	effective renal plasma flow	RPF	renal plasma flow
FF	filtration fraction	RQ	respiratory quotient
FFA	free fatty acids	RVP	renal venous plasma
GFR	glomerular filtration rate	SNFF	single nephron filtration fraction
GH	growth hormone		
GNG	gluconeogenesis	SNGFR	single nephron filtration rate
GTB	gomerulotubular balance		
ICF	intracellular fluid	SOH	supraopticohypophyseal
JGA	juxtaglomerular apparatus	TBW	total body water
LDH	lactic dehydrogenase	TEA	tetraethylammonium
LMWP	low-molecular-weight protein	TGFB	tubuloglomerular feedback
		Tm	tubular maximum transport rate
NMN	N-methylnicotinamide		
PAH	p-aminohippurate	Tm_g	Tm for glucose
		TSH	thyroid stimulating hormone

CHAPTER 1
Introduction

1.1 THE KIDNEYS' FUNCTIONS

The functions of the kidneys are essential for life. A person without kidneys or support systems as a substitute can live perhaps a couple of weeks. During that time no urine is produced, and the concentrations of nitrogenous waste products in the blood increase. Each human kidney ordinarily makes less than a litre of urine in 24 hours, though it receives about 900 litres of arterial blood. The total volume of blood flowing through the two kidneys is close to 1250 ml/min, about a quarter of the resting cardiac output for 300 g of renal tissue! Urine may be produced as slowly as 0.5 ml/min when it is most concentrated, and as quickly as 20 ml/min when it is dilute and watery. But no more than about 20 ml of the water that enters the kidneys in 1250 ml of arterial blood normally leaves in the urine. About 2 ml is returned to the blood through lymphatics and the rest directly by the renal veins.

The urine consists mainly of water. In it are dissolved end-products of metabolism, foreign substances including drugs and products of their detoxication, and hormones and their metabolites. But it would do the kidneys less than justice to state merely that they 'purify the blood' by excreting waste products in the urine. They also excrete varying quantities of many normal constituents of the body, and so help to regulate the metabolic balances of these substances. They can be excreted rapidly when present in excess, but when they are scarce the kidney can conserve them, and they largely disappear from the urine. By suitably alternating excretion and retention of solutes and water the kidneys regulate the volumes and the compositions (including pH and osmolality) of the body's principal fluids. One of their most important functions is to secrete about 180 litres of extracellular fluid (ECF) into the blood every day.

Although most of what appears in the urine was formerly present in the blood, the kidneys' activity is not limited to transferring things from the blood to the urine. Some solutes are generated within the kidneys and added to the urine, or to the blood, or to both. Renal cells manufacture large amounts of hydrogen ions, which they add to the urine, and corresponding amounts of bicarbonate ions, which they add to the plasma. They make ammonium, which leaves in both blood and urine (most leaves by the renal veins unless the urine is strongly acid). The kidneys also secrete hormones. Some, like prostaglandins (PGs) and kallikrein, appear to exert local effects within the kidney which are not yet well defined. Others are exported in the

I

blood; notably erythropoietin, which stimulates the bone marrow to produce erythrocytes, and active metabolites of vitamin D, which promote the intestinal absorption of calcium and its deposition in the skeleton.

Erythropoietin is a rather stable, acidic glycoprotein of molecular weight about 34 000 (in man), which is formed predominantly in the kidney. Its precise composition and cells of origin — whether tubular epithelial or glomerular mesangial, remain to be determined. The kidney holds no more than minimal stores, but production can somehow be increased many-fold in a few hours in response to a reduction in the partial pressure of oxygen. A detailed review by Jelkman (1986) with about 800 references leaves many questions unanswered. The biologically active, hormonal form of vitamin D_3, 1,25-dihydroxyvitamin D_3, is produced exclusively in the kidney by an enzyme (25-(OH)-cholecalciferol-1α-hydroxylase) in the mitochondria of proximal tubular cells (Guder & Ross, 1984; Kumar, 1986). Parathormone (PTH) stimulates the activity of this enzyme, as do low concentrations of calcium and phosphate. One of the kidneys' most important humoral agents, renin, is not a hormone in its own right, but an enzyme which generates angiotensin (AT) from a precursor in the plasma (See Sections 1.3 and 7.4.3).

1.2 RENAL STRUCTURE AS A BACKGROUND FOR FUNCTION

Many textbooks contain useful accounts of the structure of the kidneys. Pitts (1974) gave a clear outline of the salient features, and Tisher (1976) a more elaborate description with ultrastructural details. The meagre account that follows is no more than a ground plan to illustrate the parts which will be mentioned most frequently. Each human kidney has more than a million more or less similar units (the nephrons), arranged in parallel between the vascular system and the renal pelvis which collects the urine. Figure 1.1 shows diagrammatically a couple of typical nephrons against a longitudinal section of one of the eight to 10 conical pyramids which have their bases in the cortex and project into the pelvis. The boundaries of the cortex and of the medulla and its zones (recognizable on the cut surface by differences of colour and texture) are indicated.

Each nephron commences with a glomerulus, which is a globular tuft of capillary loops, about 100 μm in diameter, surrounded by Bowman's capsule which leads into a proximal tubule. This consists of a convoluted portion (proximal convoluted tubule) nearest to the glomerulus, and a straight portion (pars recta or proximal straight tubule). Proximal tubules are about 14 mm long, 65 μm in external diameter. They have columnar cells with large nuclei, a prominent luminal brush border and abundant, conspicuous mitochondria at right angles to the basement membrane in the convoluted portion, fewer and less regularly arranged in the straight portion. The proximal straight

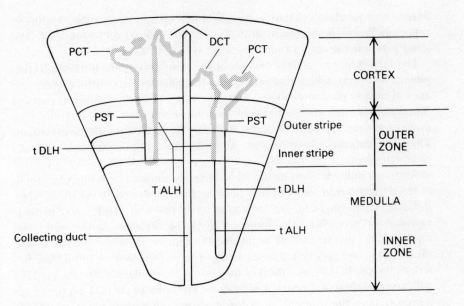

Fig. 1.1 The principal features of typical nephrons.
PCT   = proximal convoluted tubule
PST   = proximal straight tubule
DCT   = distal convoluted tubule
tDLH = thin descending limb of loop of Henle
tALH = thin ascending limb of loop of Henle
TALH = thick ascending limb of loop of Henle.

tubules run radially away from the surface of the kidney into the medulla, to continue beyond the junction between the outer and inner stripes of the outer zone as the thin, descending limbs of loops of Henle. These are 14 to 22 μm in diameter, with thin, flat epithelial cells and they differ in length from nephron to nephron. More or less deeply in the medulla they become a little thicker and then abruptly turn through 180° to become ascending limbs. Between the inner and the outer zones of the medulla the epithelium becomes columnar and the tube continues as the thick ascending limb of the loop of Henle. This continues towards the surface of the kidney until it passes between the afferent and efferent arterioles of its own glomerulus of origin, and then turns away to become the distal convoluted tubule. This segment is characterized by tall columnar cells, without brush borders, but with basal striations due to mitochondria arranged close together at right angles to the basement membrane. Thus the proximal and distal tubules lie near to their corresponding glomeruli in the renal cortex, while the loops of Henle plunge down into the medulla, where they make hairpin bends. The distal tubules, 2 to 9 mm long and up to 50 μm in external diameter, end in collecting tubules which descend again into the medulla but do not return. Each drains about a dozen distal tubules, and they successively join up into larger tubes, ending in collecting ducts about 200 μm in diameter, of which 40 or 50 open into the renal pelvis at the apex of each pyramid (Oliver, 1968).

The final stages in the elaboration of the urine take place in the collecting tubules and ducts, which share important functions with the distal tubules and are not merely passive conduits. They are often loosely regarded as parts of the nephrons, though they are far less numerous than the nephrons they drain, and they are derived embryologically from the ureteric diverticulum. They have cubical cells with spherical nuclei, sharp boundaries and relatively clear cytoplasm.

Although individual nephrons are sufficiently similar that we tend to think of renal functions in terms of one giant nephron, they are not all alike. They differ most strikingly in the lengths of their loops of Henle, and in their vascular arrangements. The loops of Henle of nephrons in the outer two thirds of the cortex (cortical nephrons) are shorter, do not descend far into the medulla, and may lack thin segments. The loops belonging to juxtamedullary nephrons, in the inner third of the cortex, plunge deeply into the medulla and have long thin segments. The efferent arterioles of cortical nephrons are narrower than the afferent, and divide at once to deliver blood which has been through the glomerular capillaries to a plexus of peritubular capillaries among the convoluted tubules. Juxtamedullary glomeruli are usually larger in diameter (in other animals if not in man; Lameire *et al.*, 1977), their efferent arterioles are substantially wider than those of cortical nephrons and than their own afferent arterioles, and, besides peritubular capillaries, they supply venous channels (descending vasa recta) which run parallel to the loops of Henle down into the medulla. There the descending vasa recta supply a network of capillaries deep in the medulla from which blood is collected by ascending vasa recta which bring it back towards the junction between cortex and medulla to be discharged into veins (Fourman & Moffat, 1971). The vasa recta carry the entire blood supply to the loops of Henle and the collecting ducts in the deep medulla and the renal papilla. Although they are wider than capillaries, the vasa recta have thin walls. Presumably they, as well as the capillary network they perfuse, favour ready exchange by diffusion between the blood and the contents of the thin limbs of Henle's loops. The proportion of juxtamedullary to cortical nephrons differs from one species to another. Human kidneys have about one long-looped nephron in seven, rats have one in four and all the nephrons of some desert-dwelling rodents have long loops.

1.3 INKLINGS OF RENAL FUNCTION

Although Galen showed that the kidneys make the urine (Fulton, 1966), no-one could begin to understand how this was done before William Bowman (1842) established that the 'renal corpuscles' were drained by the tubules.

Bowman's proposal that the glomeruli secreted the water, and possibly the inorganic salts, while the cells lining the tubules secreted the characteristic organic compounds in the urine was too vitalistic for Ludwig (1844), who proposed a purely physical theory. According to this, the glomeruli produced a solution by filtration, not by secretion, containing everything that was dissolved in the plasma except the proteins, and could themselves excrete all the constituents of the urine. The tubules then had to reabsorb most of the water, and all the useful solutes not destined to be excreted, but Ludwig regarded this too as a purely physical process, driven by the osmotic action of plasma that had become concentrated by losing filtrate in the glomeruli. Such a view was only tenable because nothing was known then about the magnitudes of osmotic pressures. Hoppe (1859) argued that Ludwig's endosmotic mechanism could not produce urines more concentrated than the blood; he had observed that dogs' urine took up water from serum across a membrane of pig's bladder, and deduced that the urine must be more concentrated than the blood. Ludwig's conception of glomerular function was close to ours today, but we regard the tubular reabsorption that has to follow it as a secretory process, carried out by living cells, which cannot be explained by a simple physical mechanism. We also appreciate that the epithelial cells lining the tubules can transfer organic and inorganic solutes between the tubular fluid and the blood in both directions and we recognize a division of labour between successive segments which makes the cells lining the tubule act like an assembly line, modifying the product as it passes along.

An important morphological feature of mammalian kidneys is that the tubular assembly line is not straight. It changes direction twice; where the ascending limbs of the loops of Henle turn back towards the cortex, and where the collecting tubules turn away from the kidney's surface to go down through the depths of the medulla. The first turnabout, aided by a relatively slow flow of blood through the vascular channels in the medulla, allows solutes removed without water from tubular fluid in the ascending limbs to be parked for a time in the deep medulla, instead of passing directly into blood leaving the kidney. These solutes become concentrated in the medulla as they are delayed there while water passes onward round the loops. The second turnabout brings the collecting ducts back through the region where solutes have been parked in enhanced concentration, so that the urine can be concentrated and reduced in volume by osmotic removal of water when the collecting ducts are sufficiently permeable.

The glomerular capillaries look like an apparatus for producing a protein-free filtrate from the plasma, while the lining of the tubules has the characters of a secreting epithelium. Even the thin segments of the loops show selective permeablity, quite unlike the walls of capillaries, and the collecting ducts are able to transport ions like hydrogen, sodium and potassium against steep gradients. The mammalian kidney has therefore features of two distinct (but closely integrated) kinds of organ; one vascular, the other secretory. The vascular organ is the aggregate of glomerular capillary tufts, perfused with blood at a high pressure, each projecting outside the body proper into the closed end of a renal tubule which is an extension, through the lower urinary tract, of the external environment. The tubular lumen is surrounded by the body but strictly outside it, like the lumen of the alimentary tract. The vascular organ excretes, at least temporarily, water and all the dissolved constituents of the blood at rates proportional to their concentrations in the plasma. The secretory organ is the aggregate of tubular cells, organized as a well controlled frontier between the body and that part of the external environment that fills the tubular lumina. These frontier cells recover a large part of the water and solutes that were temporarily excreted by the vascular organ, leaving a fraction behind to be permanently excreted in the urine, together with some solutes extracted from the blood by the cells, and other substances they have themselves manufactured.

The vascular organ is indiscriminately excretory, and it carries out its function using energy made available by the heart muscle, stored in the elastic fibres of the aorta and the renal arteries and transmitted and applied as the potential energy represented by the hydrostatic pressure of the arterial blood. Thus the vascular organ uses energy from outside the kidney, whereas the secretory organ uses energy released by metabolism within the tubular cells for its more complex and discriminating functions. These include some specialized tasks of excretion and synthesis, but most importantly the major conervative functions of the kidney. The 180 litres or so of ECF which the renal tubules secrete into the blood each day through the renal veins may be compared with about 2 litres of ingested fluid and 8 litres from digestive secretions which are absorbed from the alimentary tract and delivered through the portal vein. However, although the secretory organ is essentially metabolic in function and energy supply, it is not wholly responsible for the kidney's endocrine functions; for renin, the first renal 'hormone' to be discovered, turned out to be a product of the glomeruli. Cook & Pickering (1959) in Oxford perfused kidneys of freshly killed rabbits with magnetic oxide of iron suspended in gum acacia. The oxide particles lodged in glomeruli, so that these could be separated from tubular tissue with an electromagnet after disrupting slices of the renal cortex by pushing them through a fine stainless steel sieve; and predominantly (95%) glomerular fractions always exhibited far more renin activity than predominantly tubular fractions. Renin is now known to be manufactured in modified arteriolar smooth muscle cells. To this extent it is therefore a product of the vascular organ, which is appropriate, for renin is partly responsible, through AT and aldosterone, for maintaining blood pressure and blood volume (Section 7.4.3).

1.4 DIRECTION OF TRANSPORT AND SOME DEFINITIONS

The process of secretion, implying transport across an epithelial layer against gradients or in the absence of apparent driving forces, can occur in either direction. There is general agreement to refer to transport from tubular lumen to blood as reabsorption, but peptides which are removed from the glomerular filtrate and then broken down in the tubular cells are said to be reabsorbed, although they are not returned to the blood. Moreover, most of the bicarbonate which is 'reabsorbed' and added to the plasma is actually generated in the tubular cells, while the corresponding filtered bicarbonate is converted to carbonic acid in the lumen. The common feature of all these is transport in the direction from lumen to blood.

Transport in the opposite direction has sometimes been referred to as tubular excretion, but this can lead to confusion with eventual excretion from the body in the fully elaborated urine. Substances may be excreted by filtration from the glomerular capillaries with or without the assistance of epithelial transport from blood to tubular fluid. But some or all of what enters the tubules by filtration or cellular transport may be reabsorbed downstream and so fail to be excreted. For example, glucose filtered through the glomeruli is normally wholly reabsorbed, and none is excreted in the urine. Most of the hydrogen ions which are added to the tubular fluid combine there with bases and do not appear in the urine. These hydrogen ions are secreted into the tubular fluid but they are not excreted. Incidentally, they are not derived from the plasma but generated in the epithelial cells at the same time as bicarbonate ions which are added to the plasma. Secretion by the epithelial cells includes the synthesis of substances which may be added to the tubular urine, or to the blood, or to both, so that the definition of tubular secretion should include transport into the lumen of substances formed in the cells as well as of solutes derived from the plasma.

To minimize confusion, it is convenient to describe transport towards the plasma as tubular reabsorption (even though not all substances traverse the whole distance between tubular fluid and plasma), to describe transport towards the lumen as tubular secretion and to reserve the term renal excretion to indicate removal from the body in the urine.

Thus:

(TUBULAR) REABSORPTION = transfer from tubular fluid or cells towards the plasma

(TUBULAR) SECRETION = transfer into tubular fluid through or from tubular cells

(RENAL) EXCRETION = removal from the body in the urine

These definitions are summarized diagrammatically in Fig. 1.2. It is important to note that the activities depicted in Fig. 1.2 are not confined to the

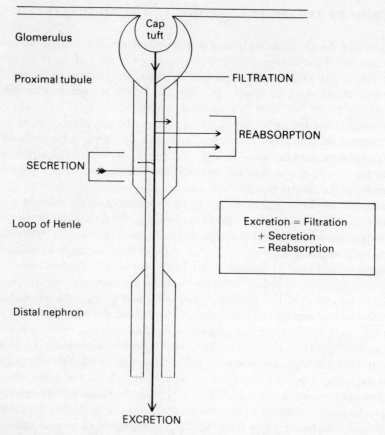

Glomerulus

Cap tuft

Proximal tubule

FILTRATION

REABSORPTION

SECRETION

Excretion = Filtration
+ Secretion
− Reabsorption

Loop of Henle

Distal nephron

EXCRETION

Fig. 1.2 Diagram to illustrate the definitions of the principal processes of transport in the nephron.

proximal tubules. A great deal of reabsorption occurs from the loops of Henle, especially the ascending limbs. Moreover, the distal segments of the nephron and the collecting system are capable of reabsorbing and secreting ions against steep gradients.

CHAPTER 2
The renal circulation

2.1 INTRODUCTION

The total flow of blood through the renal arteries can be measured without regard to the kidneys' functions, and the regulation of their share of the cardiac output can be considered in the context of the vascular system as a whole. But most measurements of the rate of the renal circulation employ indirect methods which depend upon the excretion of substances in the urine; and the distribution of blood within the kidneys depends upon vascular arrangements which are also important for understanding how they perform their functions.

2.2 THE KIDNEYS' BLOOD SUPPLY

2.2.1 Introduction

The renal arteries are short, wide, primary branches of the abdominal aorta, able to deliver a rapid flow of blood with a minimal loss of pressure. Mammalian kidneys receive 3 to 5 ml of blood for each gram of tissue (Aukland, 1976). In a man weighing 70 kg, 300 g of renal tissue (less than 0.5% of the body's mass) takes between a fifth and a quarter of the heart's resting output. Even though renal cortical tissue is among the most rapidly metabolizing (Krebs, 1950), the blood supplied is so much more than is required to carry the oxygen the kidneys consume that the renal circulation is almost an arteriovenous shunt. Claude Bernard (1859) devoted a whole, fascinating lecture to the question of why the renal venous blood is so red. Since venous blood from salivary glands was dark when they were resting but became red when they were stimulated to secrete, while the kidneys' venous blood became dark under unfavourable conditions when they produced no urine, he offered the logical suggestion that their venous blood is normally red because they secrete all the time, and not intermittently like many other glands. A century later it seems better to attribute the small arteriovenous difference to the rapid arterial inflow. The abundant blood supply reflects the services the kidneys render to and through the blood, rather than their own metabolic needs.

2.2.2 Methods of measuring renal blood flow

Methods are characterized as direct when a measuring device is connected in series with a renal artery or vein, and as semidirect when they are made on blood flowing in a renal vessel without dividing it. Indirect methods, which are based on rates of excretion, are only applicable when the kidneys are producing urine.

Cushny (1926) credited Landergren and Tigerstedt with the first direct measurement in dogs in 1893; they used a modified Ludwig Stromuhr in the renal artery, and Cushny remarked that the kidney did not secrete. Barcroft & Brodie (1905) used a graduated tube, which they introduced into the renal vein and could alternately allow to fill and empty into the vena cava by pulling on loops of string. This avoided interrupting the arterial supply to the kidney and cutting the nerves around the renal artery, but the dogs were eviscerated, anaesthetized with chloroform, and probably in a state of surgical shock. Starling (1898, in Schäfer's great textbook) praised Roy's 'oncometer' with which changes in the volume of an organ enclosed in a rigid box could be measured precisely. Brodie & Russell (1905) arranged to occlude the renal vein suddenly inside the box, and measured the initial rate of swelling of the kidney before pressure built up in the veins. This should have been equal to the rate of arterial inflow. Although they did not interrupt the continuity of the renal circulation, their results agreed with those of Barcroft & Brodie (1905) and were also probably low because of the surgical handling required to fit the oncometer round the kidney and its vessels. These, and other similarly drastic early experiments served at least to establish that the renal blood flow (RBF) was not less than 1 to 3 ml/min per g of kidney; and it could be expected to be even larger in intact animals.

The introduction of semidirect methods represented a substantial advance. The thermostromuhr (Rein, 1929) could be placed round the renal artery at a preliminary operation, after which the animal was allowed to recover, with electrical leads brought out through the incision. Blood was heated by passing a high-frequency current between two electrodes placed athwart the vessel, which did not have to be opened. The rise in temperature measured by a thermojunction applied closely to the wall of the vessel downstream varied inversely with the flow of blood. But with a short, wide vessel, the flow profile usually precludes complete mixing and makes absolute measurements unreliable; surprisingly large errors may arise from incidental variations in the initial temperature of the blood (Barcroft & Loughridge, 1938). Subsequent refinements included the use of an electrically heated wire which is inserted into the vessel and acquires a temperature related inversely to the flow past it; thermodilution methods in which a bolus of cold saline is injected upstream from a temperature sensor (White et al. 1967); and electromagnetic and ultrasonic flowmeters which do not require the wall of the vessel to be penetrated. Such methods avoid drastic surgery close to the time of measurement and can be applied to conscious, healthy animals. Their chief limitation (apart from the need to link the animal to the recording apparatus) is that it is difficult or impossible to calibrate the equipment under the precise conditions of its use. These techniques can give good indications of changes in one animal, but they cannot so readily yield absolute measurements for comparison between different animals.

Though they are applied to large vessels, these semidirect methods do not measure flow as such, but some other quantity such as a change in temperature, which is related to the flow. They have been called 'admixture methods' (Kramer *et al.*, 1963), and they have found less application to the kidney than to other organs because they were largely supplanted by indirect methods developed by Homer Smith and his colleagues. Smith was primarily a zoologist, but he attracted clinicians into his laboratory, and his methods were quickly applied to human subjects and to patients in hospitals all over the world. (See Chasis & Goldring, 1965, for a fascinating profile of this remarkable pioneer of nephrology.)

2.2.3 Indirect measurement of renal blood flow

The direct and the admixture methods require measurements on blood only, and they can be applied to any organ. For organs with substantial and measurable exchanges between blood and another phase, the law of conservation of matter can be applied in the form of the Fick principle to determine blood flow by less invasive indirect methods. The classical application employs the exchange of oxygen or carbon dioxide across the pulmonary alveolar membrane, together with differences between arterial and venous blood, to calculate the flow through the lungs as a good approximation to cardiac output. Urine is simpler to collect than respiratory gases, and the rate of excretion of a substance which is transferred from blood to urine without being created, stored or destroyed in the kidneys can be divided by the difference between its concentrations in arterial and in renal venous blood to calculate the flow of blood through the kidneys.

Blood passes through the kidneys too rapidly for substances used for indirect measurements of flow to be removed from the erythrocytes, even if they enter these in the general circulation. Consequently excretion is effectively from plasma to urine, and calculations based on Fick's principle yield the volume of plasma passing through the kidneys in a given time (the renal plasma flow, RPF). The renal blood flow can be calculated from this if the haematocrit is known. By analogy with the familiar Fick equation for cardiac output,

$$RPF = \frac{V \cdot [X]_U}{[X]_{RAP} - [X]_{RVP}} \tag{2.1}$$

where RPF denotes renal plasma flow; V denotes the rate of production of urine ('minute volume' when expressed in ml/min); and the square brackets indicate concentrations of X in urine (U), renal arterial plasma (RAP) and renal venous plasma (RVP). Since the ratio of the urinary concentration to the difference between the arterial and venous concentrations is dimensionless, RPF has the same units as V.

This formula would be strictly valid only if the arterial inflow and the venous outflow of blood were the same, and if the whole of the substance X that disappeared from the plasma appeared in the urine. In fact, solutes and water leave the kidneys in the renal lymph as well as in venous blood and urine; and the venous outflow is less than the arterial inflow to the kidney by the sum of the flows of urine and renal lymph. A more detailed balance sheet for a substance X that is delivered in renal arterial plasma and leaves the kidneys in urine, lymph and venous blood is set out in equation (2.2).

$$RPF \cdot [X]_{RAP} = V \cdot [X]_U + L \cdot [X]_{RL} + (RPF - V - L) \cdot [X]_{RVP} \quad (2.2)$$

Square brackets again denote concentrations in RAP, U, renal lymph (RL) and RVP. Inflow of renal arterial plasma is denoted by RPF; fluid leaves the kidneys in urine, lymph and venous blood at rates V, L and $(RPF - V - L)$ respectively.

Collecting terms,

$$RPF \cdot ([X]_{RAP} - [X]_{RVP}) = V \cdot ([X]_U - [X]_{RVP}) + L \cdot ([X]_{RL} - [X]_{RVP}) \quad (2.3)$$

so that

$$RPF = \frac{V \cdot ([X]_U - [X]_{RVP})}{[X]_{RAP} - [X]_{RVP}} + \frac{L \cdot ([X]_{RL} - [X]_{RVP})}{[X]_{RAP} - [X]_{RVP}} \quad (2.4)$$

The first term on the right contains quantities which are not too difficult to measure, but the rate of flow of lymph from the kidneys and its composition are not readily determined. Fortunately, the second term is usually of minor importance. The flow of lymph measured in dogs is of the same order as the flow of urine, usually less. The concentrations of constituents of the urine in renal lymph are similar to their concentrations in the plasma, and for test solutes which are rapidly excreted these are usually two orders of magnitude smaller than their concentrations in the urine (Mayerson, 1963; Keyl et al., 1965; cf. Bull & Metaxas, 1962, who derived a slightly different formula for renal venous plasma outflow instead of arterial plasma inflow). The multiplier of L in equation (2.4) is therefore usually not greater than 1.0, and the lymphatic term can be neglected without serious loss of accuracy, leaving a simpler, approximate expression first proposed by Wolf (1941; cf. Wolf, 1950, p. 65):

$$RPF = \frac{V \cdot ([X]_U - [X]_{RVP})}{[X]_{RAP} - [X]_{RVP}} \quad (2.5)$$

Equation (2.5) corresponds to the familiar Fick expression (2.1) with allowances for the differences between arterial and venous flow and for loss of solute via the renal vein. If the *extraction* of X; E_X is defined as the fraction of the solute in the renal arterial plasma that is removed by the kidneys, or the ratio of the arteriovenous difference to the concentration in arterial plasma, i.e. if

$$E_X = \frac{[X]_{RAP} - [X]_{RVP}}{[X]_{RAP}} \qquad (2.6)$$

the denominator of (2.5) can be replaced by $E_X . [X]_{RAP}$, giving

$$RPF = \frac{V . ([X]_U - [X]_{RVP})}{E_X . [X]_{RAP}} \qquad (2.7)$$

Finally, for any substances which are completely removed from the renal arterial blood and quantitatively excreted in the urine after one passage through the kidneys, $[X]_{RVP} = O$, $E_X = 1.00$, and equation (2.7) takes the still simpler form

$$RPF = \frac{V . [X]_U}{[X]_{RAP}} \qquad (2.8)$$

which states that for such substances the rate of delivery to the kidneys, $RPF . [X]_{RAP}$, is equal to the rate of exretion in the urine, $V . [X]_U$, and this offers a relatively simple method for measuring RPF. Note that urine collected from the bladder ordinarily comes from both kidneys; hence $V . [X]_U$ is the combined rate of excretion from both kidneys and the calculated value of RPF is the total plasma flow to both kidneys.

2.2.3.1 A DIGRESSION ON RENAL CLEARANCES

The expression on the right of equation (2.8) keeps turning up, although apart from the very special circumstances of the last paragraph it is not numerically equal to the RPF. Since the concentrations cancel, it has the dimensions of a volume per unit time; but what is this volume? The numerator of the expression is the urinary minute volume multiplied by the concentration in the urine, that is, the rate at which a substance is excreted; the amount excreted in 1 minute — 'something you could hold in your hand' as Homer Smith used to say. Dividing this amount by $[X]_{RAP}$, the concentration in the arterial plasma, gives the volume of plasma from which the amount of solute excreted in 1 minute could have been obtained. Hence $V . [X]_U/[X]_{RAP}$ is the smallest volume of plasma from which the solute X would have to be cleared each minute to account for its rate of excretion $V . [X]_U$. Accordingly $V . [X]_U/[X]_{RAP}$ has been called the *renal plasma clearance* of X, denoted by C_X. Values of C_X measured experimentally for a wide variety of substances range from zero to the RPF, which sets an upper limit to the rate at which the kidneys can excrete a substance they transfer from the blood and do not themselves generate. A given clearance value does not of course mean that the kidneys actually clear all the solute X from the first C_X ml of plasma they receive each minute and let the rest go by; nor indeed does the value of C_X generally bear any particular relation to the volume of plasma that flows through the kidneys (except that it cannot be greater than this). To this extent the clearance is an abstraction, and C_X represents a virtual, rather than an actual, volume of plasma that could be collected in a measuring cylinder. When many substances are being excreted simultaneously (as they always are during the production of the urine) they mostly have quite different individual clearances, but there is only one rate at which plasma flows through the kidneys. Their different clearances indicate the proportions in which different substances are extracted from the plasma and excreted; physiologists therefore measure clearances to discover how the kidneys handle different substances.

Möller, *et al.* (1929) introduced the notion of renal clearance (in the shorthand form $C = UV/B$, with U and B standing for concentrations in urine and blood, and V for the urinary minute volume) for clinical assessments of the kidneys' capacity to excrete urea. Patients whose blood urea concentration is neither rising nor falling must, like healthy people, excrete just as much urea each day as they produce, so that the rate of excretion by itself tells little about the efficiency of the kidneys. But kidneys with impaired function need a greater concentration of urea in the blood to maintain the same rate of excretion, and so the clearance is lower. The clearance can be regarded as a rate of excretion 'corrected' for the concentration present in the blood; this is useful for comparing renal function between different individuals, and it is a better indication than the blood urea concentration alone of improvement or deterioration during the course of disease in one person at different times. Urea diffuses very freely between plasma and erythrocytes, but other solutes diffuse less freely, and Homer Smith and his followers therefore exploited plasma rather than whole blood clearances as a powerful tool for investigating how the kidneys function, particularly for distinguishing the contributions of the glomeruli and the renal tubules (Section 3.4).

2.2.3.2 MEASUREMENT OF RENAL PLASMA FLOW

One great advantage of equation (2.8) is that it does not require sampling of renal venous blood, or even of arterial blood. Mixed venous blood provides a close approximation to the arterial blood delivered to the kidneys, and concentrations determined by analysing plasma from mixed venous blood may be used in the clearance formula. The question remains whether substances exist for which equation (2.8) is true, or at least nearly enough true to be useful. Soon after it was discovered how to measure the rate of glomerular filtration (GFR, Section 3.3.2) it became clear that some foreign substances are excreted far more rapidly than could be accounted for by glomerular activity alone. These substances must be added to the urine by the tubular epithelium, and it was apparent that their large clearances could hardly be much less than the RPF, which sets a theoretical upper limit to the clearance of any substance not synthesized in the kidneys. The most promising such substances (see Smith, 1951 for detailed discussion) were diodone (3, 4-di-iodo-4-pyridone-acetic acid, iodopyracet, or diodrast, used by radiologists as a radio-opaque contrast medium which appeared rapidly in the urine after intra-venous injection) and derivatives of hippuric acid such as ortho-iodohippurate (hippuran) and para-aminohippurate (PAH). Para-aminohippurate came to be used most because it gave the same results as diodone but was less toxic and easier to determine chemically. Diodone later returned to favour, together with hippuran, because these can be labelled with radioactive iodine, so that smaller doses can be used and the chemical determinations can be replaced by scintillation counting.

To decide whether such compounds are excreted so completely that equation (2.8) can be used instead of equation (2.7), the extraction E_X must be determined, and this requires sampling renal venous blood as well as arterial or mixed venous blood and urine. In dogs the renal vein can be exposed at operation and directly punctured, or it can be brought under the skin for easy access after explanting the kidney at a preliminary operation. In human subjects and patients, blood can be obtained safely through a flexible catheter introduced through a vein in the arm, passed through the right atrium into the vena cava, and then steered under fluoroscopic control into a renal vein. Plasma taken from renal venous blood while diodone or PAH is being excreted usually has about 10% of the arterial concentration. Smith (1951, 1956) collected results from several laboratories and concluded that $E_{diodone}$ and E_{PAH} could be accepted as identical and equal to 0.9, despite some results as low as 0.8 for diodone in explanted kidneys of dogs.

In the absence of a substance whose clearance is precisely equal to total RPF, highly accurate measurements can only be made by sampling renal venous blood and using equation (2.5) or equation (2.7); but two approximate procedures are often followed to avoid catheterizing the renal vein.

1   It is assumed that, provided the concentration in the plasma is low so that secretory processes are not saturated, all PAH from plasma that is exposed to secreting tissue appears in the urine. The clearance of PAH is then equal to the flow of plasma presented to the secretory apparatus, and this has been called the *effective renal plasma flow*, ERPF. The effective must necessarily be less than the total plasma flow because the renal arteries perfuse nonsecreting structures like the capsule, walls of large vessels, and hilar and perirenal fat. Smith (1956) suggested that the ERPF is a quantity in its own right which is precisely measured by the clearance of PAH. But a value of 0.9 for E_{PAH} would imply that 10% of the total RPF was ineffective, and it seems unlikely that so much of the kidneys' blood bypasses secretory tissue (though this convenient fiction saves countless patients from transcardiac catheterization and yields adequate results for clinical purposes). It is reasonable to admit that PAH is largely but not completely extracted from blood passing through

the kidneys, and to regard the clearance of PAH as a useful approximation to the total RPF.

2   It is assumed that E_{PAH} always has the value 0.9 found on occasions when it has actually been measured, and that $[PAH]_{RVP}$ is small enough to neglect in the numerator of equation (2.7). It is usually two orders of magnitude smaller than $[PAH]_U$. Equation (2.7) then becomes

$$\text{RPF} = \frac{V \cdot [PAH]_U}{0.9 \, [PAH]_{RAP}} = \frac{C_{PAH}}{0.9} \qquad (2.9)$$

which states that since 90% of incoming PAH is excreted, the clearance of PAH is 90% of the total RPF. The generalized form of equation (2.9), RPF $= C_X/E_X$, can only be safely used when E_X is close to 1.0, as it is for PAH and diodone. Equation (2.5) or equation (2.7) must be used whenever E_X is small; and failure to do this for urea (E between 0.03 and 0.06) or for inulin (E about 0.2) may lead to errors of 4 to 14% in RPF (Smith, 1951).

Regardless of how renal clearances are to be interpreted, some precautions are necessary to obtain reliable measurements. Because of 'dead space' in the kidneys and lower urinary tract, several minutes elapse before a new substance presented in a constant concentration in the arterial blood emerges in the urine at a constant rate. During the 'dead space delay', which is of the order of 5 minutes and includes equilibration of concentrations across membranes as well as transit of fluids (Bradley & Wheeler, 1958), concentrations and rates of excretion are changing, and cannot be used to calculate meaningful clearances. For reliable results a steady state must be attained in which the rate of urinary flow and the concentrations in plasma and urine have become stable. In practice it takes about 30 minutes to reach 'equilibrium' between bladder urine and arterial plasma, and blood samples should be taken 6 minutes before the midpoints of the timed collections of urine which will provide corresponding values of urinary flows and concentrations. Establishing a suitable steady state and maintaining it over, say, three consecutive collecting periods of at least 10 minutes each, requires continuous intravenous infusion of water and the substance whose clearance is being determined (Smith, 1956). Unless the subject can empty the bladder completely it may be necessary to collect the urine through an indwelling catheter. The risks of infection must be frankly considered, and rigorous aseptic precautions taken if it is decided to do this.

2.2.3.3 COMPARISON OF INDIRECT WITH DIRECT METHODS

The older direct methods of measuring RBF are not acceptable for clinical work or human experiments, but confidence in the less traumatic and more convenient indirect methods rests partly on comparisons with direct measurements made under the same conditions. Plasma flows derived from measured clearances are converted to whole blood flows (RBF) by using the packed cell volume (PCV, or haematocrit) of the blood entering the kidneys. When the

PCV is expressed in ml per ml; RBF = RPF/(1 − PCV). Good comparisons were made and reviewed by Selkurt (1946, 1963) and by Bálint (1961). Under favourable conditions the two methods agreed reasonably well, but when the perfusing blood pressure was low or renal function otherwise impaired, the indirect methods often greatly understimated RBF; and when no urine was produced they could not be used at all, although blood continued to flow through the nonfunctioning kidneys. Conn et al. (1953) adapted the nitrous oxide uptake technique introduced by Kety and Schmidt for measuring cerebral blood flow with the hope of applying it to the kidneys of anuric patients. Their method agreed well with a bubble flowmeter in dogs during ischaemia and hypotension, and also agreed closely with PAH clearance under normal conditions (Conn et al., 1953).

The indirect methods can only yield average values for RBF over the considerable periods of time required to make clearance measurements, but it appears safe to conclude that these are as accurate as direct measurements, provided that the kidneys are healthy and producing urine steadily at a normal rate. Single determinations may then be expected to come within 5 or 10% of the actual circulation rate, and the disturbance to the animal caused by direct measurements is likely to produce greater alterations than this. As renal function becomes increasingly impaired by disease or inadequate perfusion of the kidneys, the indirect measurements become less and less trustworthy; they tend, however, to overestimate the departure from normality rather than to obscure it. For clinical purposes they are being increasingly replaced by renographic techniques (Strauss et al., 1979) which provide immediately available visual records of the approximate volume and localization of blood flowing through the kidneys. For example, the flow through the two kidneys separately can be estimated by scanning the abdomen with a gamma camera after injecting ^{123}I-hippuran (McKay et al., 1981).

2.2.4 The magnitude of the renal blood flow

The rate of the renal circulation is usually greater in larger than in smaller animals. In general, particularly within a species, it varies with the surface area rather than with the mass of the body. Homer Smith (1951, p. 544) collected more than 200 values for clearances of diodone and PAH from different laboratories, expressed them per $1.73\,m^2$ of body surface, and proposed that normal human RPF averaged 600 ml/min for women and 655 ml/min for men. The range of variation was better illustrated in a table (Smith, 1956, p. 32) giving means and standard deviations for clearance of PAH in a smaller number of subjects as 592 ± 153 ml/min for women and 654 ± 163 ml/min for men. Taking 630 ml/min as an average for both sexes, and 0.9 for the extraction of PAH, the total RPF for a normal adult with 1.73^2 of body surface is 700 ml/min. With a PCV of 0.44 the 'normal' RBF is 700/(1 − 0.44) = 700/0.56 = 1250 ml/min; about a quarter of the basal cardiac output. A smaller renal fraction of cardiac output (15%, Wade & Bishop, 1962) was found when RPF and cardiac output were measured simultaneously, because the procedure increases cardiac output, and the 'resting' cardiac output is no longer basal; but Wade and Bishop agreed with Homer Smith's (1951) opinion that the human kidneys get about a fifth of the cardiac output at rest. This is less than the fraction of one quarter mentioned above, but the figures for 'renal blood flow' in the tables given by Smith (1951, 1956) and by Wade & Bishop (1962) are actually effective renal blood flows based on clearances of PAH uncorrected for extraction. Between a quarter and a fifth of the resting cardiac output is a large share for a pair of organs responsible for 6 to 8% of the body's consumption of oxygen. The renal arteriovenous difference averages about 1.3 ml/dl and blood from the renal vein is usually still 90% saturated with oxygen (Wade & Bishop, 1962).

The kidneys of laboratory animals also receive an abundant supply of blood. Smith (1951, p. 568) compared the renal clearances of PAH in rat, rabbit, dog and man; on the basis of body mass the rat had the largest RPF (22 ml/min per kg) and man the smallest (10 ml/min per kg) with rabbit and dog between. Man came highest, per 1.73 m^2 of body surface, with 600 ml/min followed by rabbit (512), dog (460) and rat (253). But all four had similar plasma flows of 2 to 3 ml/min per g of kidney. The mass of kidney tissue might therefore provide the best basis for comparing RPF in different animals — if it could be determined during life!

The kidney is remarkable in that when it is perfused at normal pressures the arteriovenous difference for oxygen remains constant, and does not vary inversely with RBF. Most of the kidney's oxygen is used to provide energy for reabsorbing a large amount of sodium (25 000 mmol each day normally in man) which is filtered by the glomeruli at a rate roughly proportional to the RPF. A major component of the oxygen consumption is therefore proportional to the blood flow (Kramer & Deetjen, 1960). When perfusion pressures are too low for filtration to occur, this component is not called for, the 'basal' oxygen consumption not involved with reabsorption of sodium is constant, and the arteriovenous difference varies inversely with blood flow in the nonfiltering kidney as in other organs (Lassen *et al.*, 1961).

Just as a greater absolute rate of blood flow is found in the larger kidneys of larger animals, so within a species RBF increases with size during early postnatal growth. Rapid changes occur in the immediate postnatal period when the young animal commences its independent existence and its own kidneys have to take over from the maternal organism the task of maintaining the constant internal environment necessary for independent life. Both the clearances and the extraction rates of diodone and PAH are low in the very young (McCance, 1948, 1950). But maturation is rapid, and the RPF of human infants (per 1.73 m^2 of body surface) reaches the lower limits of the normal range for adults between 6 months and 1 year of age (Smith, 1951, p. 501). Thereafter the renal circulation rate maintains a normal adult relation to body surface until a slow decline sets in over the latter half of the span of life.

The kidneys of laboratory animals become increasingly scarred and fibrotic with advancing age even when obvious disease is absent, and Oliver (1939) described degenerative changes in the kidneys of old men without known renal disease. The vessels were usually involved, and declining function appeared to depend upon failure of the circulation rather than primarily upon loss of parenchyma. Davies & Shock (1950) discovered a progressive fall in diodone clearance with increasing age in a group of 70 men between 24 and 89 years old. From the third until the ninth decade the effective plasma flow per $1.73 \, m^2$ of body surface fell steadily from 600 to 300 ml/min.

Primary diseases of the kidney are often accompanied by progressive destruction of renal tissue, usually more rapid and severe than with normal ageing. Reduction in the circulation may not keep pace with loss of tissue in strict proportion, because compensatory hypertrophy of surviving nephrons can occur rapidly. For example, Krohn et al. (1966) reported an average increase of 40% in plasma flow within about 2 weeks in the remaining kidneys of 29 donors of healthy kidneys for transplantation. Changes in circulation are less easy to demonstrate when damage by disease is extensive and severe, because loss of secreting tissue may greatly depress the extraction of PAH and diodone so that their clearances underestimate the residual blood flow. Progressive destruction of nephrons with the advance of disease must however be one of the most important causes of chronic reduction in the overall rate of circulation through the kidneys.

In short: bodily size, age and the amount of renal tissue are the major factors which determine the magnitude of the RBF at rest. The next sections outline some factors which alter the rate of flow, and its physiological control.

2.2.5 Variations in the blood supply of the kidneys

The kidneys receive an exceptionally rich sympathetic innervation, principally adrenergic, and vasoconstrictor to preglomerular vessels in the cortex (Mitchell, 1950; Selkurt, 1963). Cholinergic fibres have also been described (Stein, 1976); they do not have secretomotor nerves like many other glands, for they never rest. The bulk of their oxygen-requiring work is a continual reabsorption of filtered sodium, chloride and water; and no large variations in blood supply are required to meet ordinary fluctuations in activity. The basal rate of blood flow is maximal; but it is not surprising that the kidneys should be well supplied with vasoconstrictor nerves which can be activated when some of their rich blood supply needs to be shared with other organs.

There is normally no more than minimal vasoconstrictor tone when the body is at rest (Anderson et al., 1981). Apart from abnormal circumstances such as anaesthesia and shock, RBF is not increased by denervation, and kidneys which have been transplanted into other persons have rates of circulation within the normal range (Bricker et al., 1956). Homer Smith (1956) defined a man as physiologically resting only when he is 'physically and mentally at ease in the recumbent position in a comfortable bed'. This is the basal condition in which the kidneys' extrinsic nerves exert minimal constrictor tone. Hence most variations of the renal circulation rate are reductions, accompanying departures from the ideal state of bodily rest. These physiological reductions in RBF are not usually dramatic. But the reported stability of the renal circulation may have been partly artefactual, because clearance methods used for measuring RPF are not easy to carry out during strenuous physical activity; they are most reliable under conditions which are least liable to induce changes.

Dramatic increases in renal circulation rate were observed in human subjects by Smith (1951) when the flow approximately doubled during pyrexial reactions to contaminated inulin during pioneering clearance studies. Hepatic flow was also doubled during pyrexial episodes (Bradley et al., 1945). Denervation of the kidneys did not prevent a similar pyrexial increase in RBF in dogs, so that this could not be attributed to a reduction in pre-existing vasomotor tone (Hiatt, 1942). The most likely cause is a direct action on smooth muscle throughout the body, reducing peripheral resistance, because the cardiac output increased but not the blood pressure. Less dramatic physiological increases in RBF occur in dogs on diets rich in protein (Smith, 1939–40) and when the volume of extracellular fluid (ECFV) or of circulating blood is increased (Bálint, 1961). An associated increase in the GFR may partly underlie the brisk saline diuresis which follows infusions of saline (Baldwin et al., 1950a; cf. Smith, 1951).

Some circumstances in which sympathetic tone is increased and RBF reduced will be mentioned briefly:

1 Change of posture. Homer Smith's ideally resting subject was horizontal. Selkurt (1963) quoted reductions in PAH clearance in normal young men on sitting up (9%) and on standing (15%). Passive change to the erect posture on a tilting table imposes a greater circulatory stress than standing up, and RPF may be reduced by 50% even before fainting occurs and while arterial blood pressure is still maintained above the resting level (Smith, 1939–40). So long as blood pressure remains high, arterial baroreceptors are presumably active, and the renal vasoconstriction may be related to a smaller volume of blood in the large thoracic veins and the heart. Reductions in RBF of up to 30% have followed trapping of blood in the legs beyond cuffs inflated round the thighs (Bálint, 1961).

2 Muscular exertion. Clearance studies are less easy to carry out in exercising than in resting subjects; some of the more satisfactory human studies showed little effect of light exercise, though strenuous exercise reduced the renal circulation to about half, and maximal exercise to a quarter of rates at rest (Wade & Bishop, 1962; Selkurt, 1963). Because dogs seemed less affected than men by running on treadmills, Thurau (1964) suggested that the reduction in RBF might be partly postural and not related to the exercise as such. However, when recumbent subjects worked on stationary bicycles in bed, pedalling hard enough to double cardiac output lowered the RBF by 20%

without a change in posture (Bucht *et al.*, 1953; Castenfors, 1967a, b). Renal blood flow seems to be reduced in proportion to the severity of exercise, regardless of posture, because of a general increase in vasomotor activity which is more effective in men than in dogs (Rowell, 1974).

3 Haemorrhage, shock and hypoxia. Renal blood flow is grossly diminished in severe traumatic shock, especially if large amounts of blood have been lost (Selkurt, 1963). Severe hypoxia may also lead to intense renal vasoconstriction, though clearance methods are unreliable under these conditions and deficient extraction of diodone or PAH may cause the actual plasma flow to be underestimated. Anuria occuring during shock does not necessarily mean that renal perfusion has ceased, but it makes measurements by clearance techniques impossible. Oliguria is less severe in man than in dogs, and results of clearance measurements in man agree with those of direct measurements in dogs (Bálint, 1961).

4 Pain and distress. Pain produced by pressure or immersion of a hand or a foot in ice can reduce RBF by as much as a half; and fright and anxiety without actual pain can be equally effective. A patient's RPF fell about 50% when he suddenly became alarmed by a misunderstanding during investigation, and the effect persisted for at least half an hour after the alarm had been dispelled (Smith, 1956, p. 166). Renal blood flow measured with an electro-magnetic flowmeter in conscious dogs was quite unchanged by compression of both carotid arteries, which increased the blood pressure by 40 to 50 mmHg; but it was transiently reduced 40% by clapping the hands or firing a pistol (Gross & Kirchheim, 1980). Traffic in the sympathetic nerves to the kidney was increased 60% by compressing the carotids and 500% by the pistol-shot.

5 Diving. In diving mammals and birds the dramatic circulatory changes which accompany submersion include intense renal vasoconstriction. Seals show a 10-fold reduction in heart rate but maintain their blood pressure by a greatly increased total peripheral resistance. The circulation of blood is almost confined to the heart, lungs and brain; the muscles work anaerobically, and the dive can be prolonged until the most essential tissues have used up the available oxygen. During simulated dives by conscious Weddell seals, cardiac output fell from 40 to 5 l/min and RBF from 4000 to 300 ml/min (Zapol *et al.*, 1979). When the head of a duck was put under water, the percentages of cardiac output received by the heart, head, eye, and adrenal and thyroid glands increased, while the kidneys experienced the greatest decrease (Schmidt-Nielsen, 1975). Similar changes occur in rabbits following irritation of the nasal passages by noxious fumes (Korner, 1971).

6 Some vasoconstrictor agents. Many of the responses just described depend upon humoral as well as neurogenic vasoconstriction. Noradrenaline and angiotensin II (AT II) (Section 2.2.7) are well known as powerful renal vasoconstrictors, with the peculiarity that in moderate doses they reduce RBF while largely preserving glomerular filtration — in whole animals, in isolated perfused kidneys and in single accessible nephrons (Brenner *et al.*, 1976a).

They are discussed in Section 3.3.4.3 (11) as agents which, in large doses, may acutely reduce GFR.

7 Some diseases, not of the kidneys.

(a) Cardiac failure. Substantial reductions in RBF in cardiac patients were first demonstrated by Merrill (1946). Wade & Bishop (1962) tabulated averages from a series of investigations showing (effective) RBFs (per m^2, not per 1.73 m^2) of 231 ml/min for 109 patients with congestive failure compared with 422 ml/min for 124 patients who were not in failure. These are about one third and two thirds of a normal average of 660 ml/min per m^2.

The modest effects of light exercise and postural change in normal individuals are greatly exaggerated in patients with congestive cardiac failure, whose RBF is already less than normal at rest, and who suffer far greater reductions when they are up and about (Merrill & Cargill, 1948; Wade & Bishop, 1962). In patients with mitral stenosis this may happen within 1 or 2 minutes of starting to exercise, and be as quickly reversed when exercise ceases, suggesting that the change is mediated by the renal vasomotor nerves (Bishop *et al.*, 1958).

(b) Chronic bronchitis with emphysema and retention of carbon dioxide may lead to intense renal vasoconstriction. A similarly intense renal vasoconstriction which followed asphyxia in rabbits, and could be prevented by denervating the kidneys, was attributed to a central action of carbon dioxide (Franklin *et al.*, 1951).

(c) Anaemia. In chronic severe anaemia when cardiac output is increased and blood pressure is low, overall peripheral resistance is less than normal, but RPF is usually reduced (Wade & Bishop, 1962). Because of the low PCV, this implies a substantially greater reduction in RBF. Whitaker (1956) reported anaemic patients, some with PCVs as low as 10%, whose average RBF of 365 ml/min per m^2 increased to 633 ml/min per m^2 after their anaemia had been corrected. Cardiac output was less after treatment, and the blood pressure was greater, so that the total peripheral resistance had increased. While anaemia was severe there was renal vasoconstriction with vasodilatation elsewhere, and some of the kidneys' rich supply of blood was diverted to organs with dilated vessels, as happens during exercise.

8 Diseases of the kidneys. Chronic diseases with extensive destruction of nephrons naturally cause chronically low rates of RBF. In severe chronic renal failure, the uptake of PAH by the tubular epithelium may also be impaired. When allowance is made for the resulting depression of E_{PAH}, it may turn out that the total RBF is not reduced in proportion to the destruction of tissue, and surviving nephrons may be hyperaemic in advanced uraemia (Depner & Gulyassy, 1979). In acute renal failure from any of a multitude of causes, oliguria or complete anuria may preclude measurements of RPF by clearance techniques. Brun *et al.* (1955), however, used radioactive krypton to measure the renal circulation in four anuric patients who were in shock following severe poisoning with barbiturates. Values of E_{PAH} were sometimes less than 0.10 during the anuric phase, making C_{PAH} an unsatisfactory index of ERPF; but RBF measured with ^{85}Kr was about 20% of normal, and the kidneys' oxygen consumption was reduced roughly in proportion to 25%.

Persistence of a sufficient flow of blood to meet the need for oxygen is probably essential for the subsequent recovery of renal function. When aerobic cells like those in the renal cortex do not receive enough oxygen to operate their sodium pumps, they take up ECF and swell grossly (Robinson, 1960, 1975a). Although the 'no-reflow phenomenon' (Leaf, 1970) is no longer regarded as important in the kidney, Frega et al. (1980b) showed that if a rat's kidney was first flushed with 10% polyethylene glycol (PEG 6000) so that its cells did not swell while the circulation was interrupted, histological evidence of damage was minimized and function was well preserved after the circulation was restored.

2.2.6 Extrinsic control of renal blood flow

In the normal absence of vasoconstrictor tone, no reflex increases in RBF can be expected; but it is widely believed that the kidneys' vasoconstrictor nerves are included in any general increase in sympathetic activity. A study of 35 patients by Lauson et al. (1944) established that after haemorrhage or severe trauma leading to shock, RBF was reduced even while blood pressure was maintained, and was reduced disproportionately when blood pressure was low; implying that renal vascular resistance increased more than total peripheral resistance. This selective renal vasoconstriction is, however, less striking than that which occurs during exercise; then renal vascular resistance is increased, while total peripheral resistance is greatly reduced, principally because of great vasodilatation in the active muscles, where locally acting vasodilator metabolites override the effects of vasoconstrictor impulses.

Though classical studies reviewed by Bálint (1961) suggested that pressor reflexes from the arterial baroreceptors affect the renal circulation, there is surprisingly little clear evidence linking renal vasoconstrictor activity with the reflexes which control systemic arterial pressure. Heymans et al. (1933) reported that reducing blood pressure in the arterial baroreceptors caused the kidney to shrink, even though systemic arterial pressure was increased. It is, however, difficult to infer blood flow from the volume of the kidney, and clearance measurements indicated that the RBF might be increased or remain unchanged after carotid occlusion. Moreover, stimulation of the isolated carotid sinus by an increase in perfusion pressure usually reduced, and never increased, the flow through the kidney (Heymans & Neill, 1958). Direct measurements with a thermostromuhr in the renal vein confirmed the relatively small effect of baroreceptor reflexes on the kidneys (Hartman et al., 1937). Although the renal venous outflow was reduced 50% when 10% of carbon dioxide was added to the inspired gas, compression of the carotids, which increased the systemic arterial pressure, hardly affected the RBF; and electrical stimulation of the sinus nerve, which lowered arterial blood pressure from 110 to 70 mmHg, reduced the RBF by only about 10%, while the flow through the brachial artery was doubled (Opitz & Smyth, 1937).

Ullrich & Marsh (1963) suggested that vasoconstrictor reflexes spare the kidneys at first. Thus when cardiac output in dogs was reduced by orthostasis or by constricting the pulmonary artery (Berne & Levy, 1950), RPF was reduced less than cardiac output, and the renal vascular resistance increased far less than the total peripheral resistance. Abel & Murphy (1962) measured regional blood flows with thermoelectric flowmeters in dogs during progressive loss of blood. After small losses, renal vascular resistance increased about half as much as iliac or mesenteric, although after losses of more than 20 ml of blood per kg the renal resistance increased more than the iliac but still less than the mesenteric. Korner (1967), in a short survey of the autonomic control of the renal circulation, pointed out that with a blood supply far greater than is required by their needs for oxygen, and with the low basal tone of their resistance vessels, the kidneys appear to be ideal target organs for vasoconstriction during reflex control of the circulation. Yet reflexes from the arterial baroreceptors produce only slight renal vasoconstriction. The arterial chemoreceptors can call forth far more intense renal vasoconstriction when they are strongly stimulated by severe hypoxia (Korner, 1963).

Among receptors whose activity affects the renal circulation, Korner (1967) included the mechanoreceptors on the low-pressure side of the circulation, in the chambers of the heart and the great intrathoracic veins (Gauer & Henry, 1963). These low-pressure baroreceptors are affected by much smaller pressures than those required to stretch the arterial walls, and they may be expected to monitor changes in the volume and distribution of the blood rather than in arterial pressure. Their possible importance in controlling the excretion of sodium to adjust the volumes of blood and ECF is considered in Section 7.4.

Bradley (1951) had already suggested that RBF might depend upon the volume and distribution of blood as well as upon arterial pressure, because it is reduced by orthostasis, by loss of blood, or when cardiac output fails to satisfy the body's needs in quantity (congestive cardiac failure) or in quality (anaemia). Roddie & Shepherd (1958) urged that the low-pressure baroreceptors might be more important than the more familiar arterial baroreceptors in controlling sympathetic tone in resting muscle, and it would not be inappropriate if their afferent input controlled the circulation to the kidneys as well as the hormones which affect tubular reabsorption of sodium. The failure of some observers to demonstrate an increase in RBF when central blood volume was increased by immersing men in water up to their necks (Epstein, 1978) is consistent with an absence of basal constrictor tone; immersion should mitigate the effects of assuming the erect posture. It is also not inconsistent with reductions in RBF when the central blood volume is diminished.

Of the receptors whose afferent discharges affect the renal circulation —

arterial baroreceptors, low-pressure (venous and cardiac) mechanoreceptors, and arterial chemoreceptors, the low-pressure mechanoreceptors may be of the greatest physiological importance. In healthy people alterations in the distribution and volume of circulating blood often occur while arterial blood pressure remains normal and there is no threat of anxoia. Korner (1967, 1971) concluded that vasoconstriction in the renal vascular bed is evoked rather weakly from the arterial baroreceptors alone; quite strongly from the arterial chemoreceptors with severe hypoxia, more strongly from the low-pressure baroreceptors, especially when these work with the arterial barore-ceptors after haemorrhage, and very strongly from nasopharyngeal receptors, as well as in the 'diving response'. Korner also established that the sympathetic vasomotor nerves were more important than circulating catecholamines.

The control of the renal circulation is not wholly extrinsic, however. Section 2.2.7 is a digression on intrinsic mechanisms which need to be introduced before the attempt to sketch an outline of integrated control in Section 2.2.8.

2.2.7 Intrinsic control (autoregulation) of renal blood flow

The discovery that the flow of blood through the kidneys is not much affected by the perfusing pressure is very old. Burton-Opitz & Lucas (1911), who studied dogs with a stromuhr in the left renal vein, wrote 'when the systemic blood pressure rises in consequence of central stimulation of the vagus or sciatic nerve, the kidney endeavours to preserve a normal blood supply...by a tonic setting of its vascular channels'. Hartman et al. (1937), who used Rein's new thermostromuhr, were surprised that the kidney was so remarkably autonomous in spite of its rich sympathetic innervation. Less traumatic indirect methods confirmed these early conclusions. For example, an increase of 43% in systemic arterial pressure following compression of the carotid arteries led to an increase of only 3 to 5% in the clearance of PAH in unanaesthetized rabbits (Forster & Maes, 1947). Increases of about 5% in RBF for a 50% increase in arterial blood pressure are typical for unanaesthetized animals in good condition. This relative constancy of blood flow despite variations in per-fusing pressure has been attributed to 'autoregulation of the renal circulation'.

Since experimental errors in measuring RBF are likely to be at least 5 to 10%, there is a temptation to report no significant increase in flow and to claim that autoregulation is well-nigh perfect. But the same data which show 'no significant increase' may not exclude an increase of 5% (Winton, 1956a, b); and physiological controlling mechanisms require some change in the controlled variable to activate them. An increase of 1% in blood flow for each 10% increase in pressure may therefore be of great physiological impor-tance even though the change does not reach statistical significance in a particular experiment.

Pioneering observations quoted by Winton (1959) showed that autoregula-tion was best seen in intact kidneys supplied with blood in situ, but was still present in kidneys which were denervated, isolated and even perfused with oxygenated solutions containing no erythrocytes (Table 2.1). The dependence on metabolism indicates a biological rather than a purely mechanical process.

Forster & Maes (1947) showed that GFR as well as the RBF, exhibited autoregulation when arterial pressure was increased between about 80 and 120 mmHg; and this was in denervated kidneys, so that the mechanisms must be intrinsic. The apparent absence of an increase in mean filtration pressure implied that the increase in vascular resistance which restricts the RBF must be preglomerular. If the increased resistance is due to vasoconstriction, this must be predominantly of the glomerular afferent arterioles, for constriction of the efferent vessels would increase filtration pressure and GFR. Pappen-heimer & Kinter (1956) proposed that the increased vascular resistance was not due to vasoconstriction, but to an increased viscosity of the blood as the PCV was increased by plasma skimming at higher perfusion pressures. This hypothesis received sympathetic consideration (e.g. Winton, 1956a); but it became untenable as a complete explanation when it was shown that auto-regulation could be preserved by adding cell-free plasma to an artificial perfusing solution (Waugh & Shanks, 1960), and that drugs which paralyse vascular smooth muscle abolished autoregulation even when the blood con-tained a normal proportion of erythrocytes (Thurau & Kramer, 1959). A further possibility, that the vessels were compressed by greater interstitial pressure, seemed to be supported by claims (e.g. Bounous et al., 1960) that autoregulation in the isolated kidney was abolished by removing the capsule. But decapsulation need not abolish autoregulation (Gilmore, 1964); and even with the renal capsule present, pressures in tubules and peritubular capillaries

Table 2.1 Effect on flow of a 50% increase in arterial perfusion pressure

Experimental arrangement	Change in flow
Flow through glass tube	+ 50%
Flow through isolated hind limb of dog[a]	+ 60%
Renal blood flow, unanaesthetized rabbit, denervated kidney[b]	+ 3 to 5%
Renal blood flow, unanaesthetized dog[c]	+ 3 to 5%
Blood flow through kidney perfused from anaesthetized dog[d]	+ 8%
Flow through isolated kidney perfused with defibrinated blood[e]	+ 20%
Flow through kidney perfused with dextran solution[d]	+ 22%
Same after 4 to 10 minutes' arrest of circulation[d]	+ 34%
Flow through isolated kidney perfused with blood cooled to 3 to 12°C[e]	+ 35%
Flow through kidney perfused with dextran–procaine solution[d]	+ 59%
Flow through kidney perfused with oxygenated light oil[d]	+ 69%

References: a Whittaker & Winton (1933)
            b Forster & Maes (1947)
            c Sellwood & Verney (1955)
            d Waugh (1958)
            e Winton (1953).

of rats did not increase with blood pressure unless the vascular smooth muscle was paralysed with papaverine; this permitted pressures to increase, but at the same time abolished autoregulation (Thurau & Wober, 1962). Moreover RBF in dogs actually increased substantially when intrarenal pressure was increased by obstructing the ureter or by osmotic diuretics (Thurau & Henne, 1964).

Thurau (1964) emphasized that drugs like papaverine do not increase the flow of blood through the kidneys when the perfusing pressure is below the range (about 80 to 160 mmHg) in which autoregulation occurs. At these low pressures there should be no vascular tone for the drugs to abolish, and flow through the relaxed vessels parallels the perfusing pressure. When this becomes greater than 80 to 90 mmHg, vascular tone appears and further increases in pressure are quickly countered by corresponding increases in vascular resistance which annul the increases in flow. For example, a sudden increase in arterial pressure from 100 to 200 mmHg at first increased the flow of blood through a dog's kidney, denervated and perfused *in situ*, by 100%. The flow then fell back to its initial rate in about 10 seconds, and later settled to a steady rate 15% greater. After the vascular smooth muscle was paralysed with papaverine, the same increase in pressure always led to the same initial increase in blood flow, but the subsequent decrease to the initial rate was abolished (Thurau & Kramer, 1959). The fact that the peak flow under normal conditions was precisely equal to the sustained flow when vascular muscle was paralysed left little for other than muscular factors to explain.

Bayliss had observed in 1902 that when arterial blood pressure was suddenly increased in dogs, the kidneys swelled immediately and then shrank back to their previous volume in 20 to 30 seconds although the blood pressure was still high. Bayliss was aware that other smooth muscle was stimulated by stretching it, and proposed that the initial stretching when blood pressure was raised stimulated the kidney's vessels directly to increase their tone. But how, on such a myogenic theory, can the vessel wall adjust its tone to maintain, not a constant radius, but a constant flow? To keep the flow constant, the calibre of the vessel must be reduced by about 19% when the pressure is doubled, for, by Poiseuille's law, the resistance varies inversely with the fourth power of the radius of a cylindrical tube. It then follows from Laplace's law that because of the smaller calibre, the tension in the vessel's wall needs to be increased somewhat less than in proportion to the pressure. Keeping tension in the wall strictly proportional to the transmural distending pressure would actually lead to a reduction in flow with increasing pressure (Thurau, 1966). Burton (1965) stated that constriction of vessels in response to stretching of their walls would not control flow, but would lead to instability through positive feedback; and that Bayliss was aware of this. Hence, although the increased vascular resistance underlying autoregulation of renal blood flow is most likely myogenic in origin, its control requires something more than a simple response to stretch.

Since autoregulation of blood flow does not occur when pressures are too low for glomerular filtration to continue, events downstream presumably assist the glomerular vessels to control blood flow and filtration in each individual nephron (Thurau, 1964). No sensor of glomerular flow as such is known; but the thick ascending limb of the loop of Henle makes contact with the vascular pole of its own glomerulus before going on to become the distal convoluted tubule. The taller, more closely packed epithelial cells here form the macula densa, and as early as 1937 Goormaghtigh had suggested that the juxtaglomerular apparatus (JGA) might sense the physicochemical state of the tubular fluid and somehow regulate the glomerular circulation accordingly. The macular cells look relatively unfitted for reabsorption; they form a patch permeable to water in a tubule which is remarkably impermeable, and in man they have a total surface area of around $60\,cm^2$, more than half of which is probably available to sample the tubular fluid (Bohle *et al.*, 1982). Their antiluminal surfaces are apposed to the juxtaglomerular complex and to granular, myoepithelioid cells in the walls of the efferent and afferent glomerular arterioles. They also make contact with extraglomerular mesangial (lacis) cells which are continuous with the glomerular mesangium (Barajas, 1981).

Because most of the filtered sodium is reabsorbed from the proximal tubule and the loop of Henle, the fluid that reaches the macula densa is hyposmolal and has a low concentration of sodium. Guyton (1963) theorized that changes in volume of the macular cells with the osmolarity of the tubular fluid could control the glomerular circulation by releasing a vasoconstrictor, possibly renin, which was known to be made by the myoepithelioid cells and stored in their granules. Thurau (1963) meanwhile proposed that the JGA might increase the tone of the glomerular vessels if the concentration of sodium in the fluid bathing the macula densa became excessive, as it would do in any nephron which filtered too much sodium for its proximal tubule and loop to reabsorb. Thurau & Schnermann (1965) tested this by means of micropuncture techniques (Windhager, 1968). They injected 150 mM sodium chloride into individual distal tubules of rats, backwards towards the macula densa, and saw the proximal tubules of the injected nephrons collapse within 25 seconds while neighbouring proximal tubules were unaffected. Because this dramatic demonstration of a tubuloglomerular feedback (TGFB) was almost uniformly successful in rats on a diet low in sodium and with kidneys rich in renin, whereas it often failed in sodium-replete rats with kidneys showing low renin activity, they too proposed renin as a mediator between the macula densa and the glomerular afferent arterioles. Later refinements revealed graded alterations in proximal tubular flow or single nephron filtration rate (SNGFR, to which glomerular blood flow is roughly proportional) in addition to the crude on–off effect. Sodium bromide acted like the chloride, but choline chloride and mannitol were ineffective and the response was blocked by diuretics like amiloride, which presumably hindered the entry of sodium into the macular cells (Thurau & Mason, 1974).

A vast amount of work on whole kidneys and on single nephrons, reviewed in detail by Navar (1978a) and by Wright & Briggs (1979), largely confirmed that increasing flow out of the proximal tubule through the loop of Henle into the distal tubule can lead to reduction in one or more of: glomerular blood flow, glomerular capillary pressure, GFR, proximal tubular flow, and the 'stop-flow pressure' that builds up in proximal tubules which are blocked mechanically. However, since arterial blood pressure was kept constant in many of these experiments, they cannot establish that the same mechanism would counteract increases in perfusion pressure. It has none the less been widely accepted that TGFB contributes to the autoregulation of glomerular blood flow and filtration, though it cannot be the sole mechanism.

Not all agree that sodium is the essential component of the tubular fluid which affects the macula densa. Wright (1981) found the feedback effect of sodium chloride was enhanced by making the lumen of the distal tubule more negative, which would assist the movement of chloride ions but hinder that of sodium ions across the macula densa. This suggested that the effective stimulus might be the rate of which chloride ions crossed the macular membrane. Briggs (1981) tested many salts by retrograde injection into the distal tubule. Chloride was the most effective anion for operating the feedback, and could only be replaced by bromide. Sodium was a more effective accompanying cation than Cs^+, NH_4^+, K^+, choline, Li^+, Ca^{2+} or Mg^{2+} (in descending order), but was ineffective when partnered by SCN^-, F^-, HCO_3^-, NO_3^- or iodide. There has been considerable debate about whether the effective stimulus might be osmolality as such (Bell, 1982) or concentration-dependent transport of sodium chloride (Schnermann & Briggs, 1982). Retrograde microperfusions of hypotonic (40 to 80 mosm) solutions of sodium chloride, sodium isethionate and choline chloride were equally effective in eliciting feedback responses in rats, suggesting that the macular receptor had no specific ionic requirement (Bell & Navar, 1982). Electrolyte-free solutions can operate the feedback in dogs (Navar, 1978a) and in rats (Bell et al., 1980), but they might do this by affecting the concentration of sodium chloride in the distal tubular fluid.

There is general agreement that the autoregulation of RBF and glomerular filtration depends upon constriction of the glomerular afferent arterioles, but it is less likely that renin is the mediator between the glomerulus and the distal tubule. Renin was discovered by Tigerstedt and Bergmann in 1898, and was not at first well received (Gibbons et al., 1984). It appeared to be a renal hormone released to boost arterial blood pressure if the kidney's blood flow was inadequate. It turned out to be a proteolytic enzyme which had no pressor activity of its own, but which acts on an α-2-globulin (renin substrate, angiotensinogen) in the plasma to release a decapeptide, AT I, from which a converting enzyme forms the active octapeptide AT II. This is a potent vasoconstrictor. It also stimulates thirst by a central action, and stimulates cells in the zona glomerulosa of the adrenal cortex to secrete aldosterone (Peart, 1978). The circumstances which cause renin to be released into the blood will be outlined in Section 7.4.3 on the regulation of the rate of excretion of sodium by the kidneys.

The converting enzyme is present in the kidney as well as renin, and Frega *et al.* (1980a) perfused isolated kidneys from rats on open circuit with a solution which contained no precursor or AT. When renin substrate was added, the flow of renal perfusate was reduced from 25 to 14 ml/min, but GFR was doubled from 0.3 to 0.6 ml/min. Such rates are typical for kidneys perfused with saline solutions containing no haemoglobin (Ross, 1978), and the changes indicated a preferential constriction of the glomerular *efferent* arterioles, which is the normal action of AT II produced in the kidneys (Levens *et al.*, 1981). Both effects were promptly reversed by Sar^4-Ala^8-AT II, an analogue which specifically blocks the peripheral actions of AT II. In so far as autoregulation of blood flow and glomerular filtration depends upon constriction of glomerular *afferent* arterioles, this first demonstration that renin can initiate the formation of AT II within the kidney makes it unlikely to be a mediator of autoregulation, though it could well modulate TGFB (Navar & Rosivall, 1984).

In summary: it has been established that imposed changes in the volume or composition of fluid entering the distal tubule are often followed by compensatory alterations in glomerular blood flow (GBF), capillary pressure or rate of filtration in punctured superficial nephrons of rats and dogs. Other nephrons have similar juxtaglomerular anatomy, and the same may be true for neighbouring unpunctured nephrons, for inaccessible nephrons in the same kidneys, and for nephrons in the intact kidneys of these and other species. Müller-Suur *et al.* (1982) seem to have been the first to demonstrate TGFB in juxtamedullary nephrons of rats.

The precise alteration in the tubular fluid which operates the feedback and the link between the distal nephron and the glomerular vessels are uncertain. This feedback mechanism could help to keep the blood supply of each glomerulus adequate but not too great for the reabsorptive capacity of the attached tubule. The question of whether it restrains GBF and filtration continually, under normal conditions, or only in emergencies when filtration might become excessive or reabsorption inadequate, will be deferred to Section 3.3.5.2 on the intrinsic control of glomerular filtration. Meanwhile, because nephrons are perfused in parallel, and RBF is the sum of all the individual glomerular flows, this mechanism could contribute to the autoregulation of blood flow in the whole kidney and it might provide the fine tuning required for the myogenic mechanism to keep the flow of blood stable. See also a recent evaluation of possible mechanisms subserving autoregulation by Knox & Spielman (1983).

A modest consensus expressed in carefully chosen words that beg few questions was 'that the major fraction of renal autoregulatory adjustments in resistance is mediated by the distal tubuloglomerular feedback mechanism that responds to some component of distal tubular flow and transmits signals to the afferent arteriolar segment of the same nephron' (Navar *et al.*, 1982).

2.2.8 Integrated control of renal blood flow

Intrinsic and extrinsic controls of RBF normally work together, for extrinsic controls impinge on a vascular resistance that is already subject to autoregulation. In the intact mammal, afferent discharges from the arterial baroreceptors reflexly keep systemic arterial blood pressure relatively constant and assure the supply of blood to the heart and brain. So long as arterial pressure is held constant, the kidneys need no autoregulatory mechanism to protect their own circulation against variations in perfusing pressure, but the baroreceptor reflexes are sometimes set to maintain elevated pressures, as may happen during exercise.

The kidneys are not wholly autonomous. Autoregulation does not mean that their blood flow does not alter, only that alterations in arterial pressure do not of themselves cause comparable changes in RBF. Zerbst & Brechmann (1965) showed that in isolated kidneys from rabbits, increased extrinsic tone, produced artificially by stimulating the sympathetic nerves, reduced the RBF but at the same time made it more dependent upon the perfusing pressure. Renal blood flow can also be substantially reduced reflexly *in vivo* by sufficiently strong excitation of the kidneys' autonomic nerves; for example, from both arterial and cardiac baroreceptors together when human subjects assume the erect posture or lose blood (Korner, 1974), from arterial chemoreceptors stimulated by hypoxia (Korner, 1963), from trigeminal nerve endings in the nasopharynx (Korner, 1971) as well as from higher centres with alarm (Smith, 1956; Gross & Kirchheim, 1980) and in the diving response (Schmidt-Nielsen, 1975). Apart from these examples, the effects of extrinsic controls are remarkably modest, possibly because, despite the rich innervation of the kidneys' vessels, they respond less than other vascular beds to maximal stimulation (Korner, 1974).

The baroreceptor reflexes seem to accord the kidneys some priority for blood, and to treat their vessels gently. Winton (1937) remarked that the renal circulation's independence of blood pressure applies 'particularly to the large changes which are brought about by carotid sinus reflexes'. Nearly 40 years later Kirchheim (1976) concluded that these reflexes act mainly on resting muscle, while the renal and mesenteric circulations, which between them have 45% of the total peripheral resistance, are controlled almost entirely by autoregulatory mechanisms. Gross & Kirchheim (1980; cf. Gross *et al.*, 1981) confirmed that although baroreceptor reflexes elicited by compressing the carotid arteries in conscious dogs increased arterial pressure from 40 to 50 mmHg, and also increased the sympathetic discharge to the kidneys, RBF did not change. In so far as the increase in vascular resistance which prevented an increase in blood flow might have been purely autoregulatory, the chief effect of the increased sympathetic discharge was probably to release more renin into the blood rather than to increase vascular tone directly.

If the kidneys' intrinsic mechanisms prevent them from stealing blood from the rest of the body when systemic arterial pressure is raised, the extrinsic controls can be operated to borrow from the kidneys for other organs. With less than 100 ml of contained blood between them, the kidneys are not blood reservoirs; they have flow to lend, not volume to give up. Closing down the renal circulation would not immediately increase the return of blood to the heart, but it would allow the cardiac output to be reduced by nearly one litre per minute without reducing the flow to other sites. This could reduce the work of the heart, or provide more blood flow to go elsewhere when cardiac output cannot be further increased, as during maximal exercise, or when cardiac output is restricted by disease or by a deficient volume of blood. These are the principal circumstances in which RBF is substantially reduced.

2.2.8.1 A NOTE ON CENTRAL CONTROL

Reflex alterations in renal vascular tone can be initiated from arterial and cardiac baroreceptors, from arterial chemoreceptors, and from nasopharyngeal receptors innervated by the trigeminal nerve. The relative participation of the various receptors in different circumstances was summarized in a table by Korner (1974). These afferent sources project onto the classical medullary and pontine centres, which are inhibited by the traffic from the baroreceptors and strongly stimulated by chemoreceptor activity and impulses from trigeminal nerve endings.

Pappenheimer (1960) summed up what was then known about central control in pessimistic terms: the renal circulation is very sensitive to electrical stimulation of the sympathetic nerves and also to adrenaline; the sympathetic supply is profuse, but usually inactive, even when intestinal vessels supplied from the same nerve plexus show constrictor tone. However, strong sympathetic vasoconstriction can occur; for example, with haemorrhage, shock, pain, exercise, postural stresses and also from purely psychic factors. The view that almost the whole mechanism for reflex control of the cardiovascular system resides in the classical pontomedullary centres is inadequate. The dramatic changes with fright and in the diving response indicate that 'higher centres' strongly influence the sympathetic outflow to the kidneys. The response to hypoxia is incomplete in thalamic, and more severely impaired in decerebrate preparations (Korner, 1971). Some suprabulbar links with the hypothalamus, limbic region and fronto-orbital cortex are being uncovered (Korner, 1971; 1974); but no 'centre' controlling the renal circulation has been identified. One experimental difficulty is that anaesthetics interrupt many suprabulbar circuits (Kirchheim, 1976).

In summary: autoregulation plays a major role in controlling the kidneys' blood supply, and allows baroreceptor reflexes to act mainly on the rest of the cardiovscular system; but extrinsic mechanisms can divert more or less of the flow away from the kidneys on occasion. The overriding central control is still elusive 30 years after Homer Smith (1951) concluded that 'the physiological control of the renal circulation is a complete mystery'.

2.3 DISTRIBUTION OF BLOOD FLOW WITHIN THE KIDNEY

2.3.1 Introduction

The renal tubules are supplied with blood that has passed through glomeruli, and the medulla has no glomeruli. Efferent arterioles from juxtamedullary glomeruli supply blood both to a capillary plexus in the outer medulla and to the vasa recta which perfuse the inner medulla. Juxtamedullary are larger than cortical glomeruli, but fewer, so that the renal medulla may be expected to be less generously supplied with blood than the cortex.

Trueta *et al*. (1947; cf. Daniel *et al*., 1952) claimed that the cortical blood supply could be diverted through the juxtamedullary glomeruli and the medullary circulation by strong electrical stimulation of the central end of a cut sciatic nerve, or during shock following prolonged anaesthesia and the application of a tourniquet to a hind limb. The surface of the kidney then became pale, and high speed radiography after injecting radio-opaque thorotrast into the renal artery showed little flow through the outer two thirds of the cortex, while the juxtamedullary vessels appeared dilated. The drastic stimuli that were required to activate it raised doubts about a physiological role for this 'Oxford Shunt', and further work (reviewed by Smith, 1951; Bálint, 1961; Selkurt, 1963; and Thurau, 1964) established only that such powerful stimuli greatly reduced cortical blood flow while the medullary circulation continued. This made the ratio of medullary to cortical flow greater without adding the normal cortical flow to the medullary. But the pioneering work of Trueta and his colleagues did establish that the distribution of blood flow within the kidney was not homogeneous, that the medullary circulation was distinct, and that it was much slower than the cortical, as shown by shadows of thorotrast persisting in the medulla long after the cortex and the renal veins had emptied (Daniel *et al*., 1951).

2.3.2 Measurement of regional blood flow

Quantitative estimates of the rates of cortical and medullary blood flow began a decade later. Kramer *et al*. (1960) placed a small electric lamp in the renal medulla, a reflectometer under the capsule, and a photocell on the surface of the papilla in anaesthetized dogs, and timed the transit of Evans blue injected rapidly into the renal artery. Mean times of 28 seconds through vasa recta in the inner medulla, and 2.5 seconds through the cortex, indicated medullary and cortical blood flows of 22 and 440 ml/min per 100 g of tissue. Improved placing of lamps and photocells (Deetjen et al., 1964) resolved the medulla into outer and inner circulatory zones, with average transit times of 1.25, 5.15 and 22.4 seconds, corresponding to flows of 458, 112 and 29 ml/min per 100 g of tissue in cortex, outer medulla and inner medulla respectively. Taking these regions to contribute 70%, 20% and 10% of the kidney's mass gave the regional rates of flow per 100 g of kidney as 321, 22.4 and 2.9 ml/min respectively.

Meanwhile Thorburn et al. (1963) obtained similar results in unanaesthetized dogs by timing the washing out of an inert gas that had been introduced into the kidney. Radioactive ^{85}Kr was dissolved in saline and injected into the renal artery through a catheter put in place beforehand. The decline in radioactivity as blood washed out the tracer was recorded from a gamma counter placed against the animal's side over the kidney, and was resolved into four exponential components. By freezing, slicing and autoradiography to localize ^{85}Kr remaining in kidneys removed at selected times, these components were identified with cortex, outer medullary zone (including juxtamedullary cortex), inner medulla, and hilar and perirenal fat. The corresponding mean rates of blood flow derived from the declining radioactivity were 462, 132, 17 and 24 ml/min per 100 g of tissue. Cortex, outer medulla and inner medulla were taken to be 75%, 15% and 10% of the kidney's mass, giving regional blood flows per 100 g of kidney as 354, 10 and 2.0 ml/min respectively.

The results for cortical and outer medullary flow were remarkably similar to those deduced from transit of Evans blue. Both techniques indicated that the circulation through the inner medulla was slow and comparable to the flow of urine, but the washout of inert gas gave a lower estimate than the transit of the dye. This difference might have been artefactual because the regions had been defined in different ways, but there are other reasons to expect such a discrepancy.

Vasa recta in the outer medullary zone of the dog's kidney are collected together in medullary bundles surrounded by wider areas containing tubules and peritubular capillaries (Thorburn et al., 1963). Countercurrent exchange between descending and ascending vessels in these bundles should make them act as 'diffusion traps', tending to isolate the interstitial fluid and the contents of vessels and of tubules with permeable walls, in the inner medulla. Autoradiographs showed that ^{85}Kr took several minutes to get into the inner medulla from the renal artery, whereas the hilar fat took it up in a few seconds, as quickly as the cortex (and then retained it for up to an hour, presumably because of the high solubility of krypton in fat). Radioactivity had gone from the outer cortex in 2 minutes and from the outer medulla and juxtamedullary cortex in 6 minutes, but the renal papilla still contained ^{85}Kr 15 minutes after it had gone from the outer medulla. To the extent that this long retention was caused by entrainment in the 'diffusion trap', the rate at which the tracer gas was washed out would underestimate the flow of blood through the inner medulla.

Aukland *et al.* (1964; Aukland & Berliner, 1964) sought to circumvent the unequal rates of penetration of a tracer into different regions by allowing the kidneys to become uniformly saturated with hydrogen supplied to anaesthetized dogs at a concentration of 5% in the inspired gas. They then switched to an inspired gas mixture containing no hydrogen, and measured its disappearance from different regions of the kidney with polarographic microelectrodes. Blood flows derived from the washing of hydrogen out of the cortex agreed well with flow from the renal vein. But it took an hour to establish a uniform concentration of hydrogen in the inner medulla, and the subsequent slow removal depended greatly upon the flow of urine, becoming 15 times faster when V was increased from 0.1 to 5 ml/min. If urine becomes an important vehicle for the removal of hydrogen, the rate at which the gas is washed out must overestimate the inner medullary blood flow during diuresis. The risk of overestimating inner medullary blood flow during diuresis and underestimating it at other times makes the technique generally unreliable, and particularly unsuitable for investigating possible relations between inner medullary blood flow and diuresis.

If inert gases recirculate in the countercurrent system while the blood flows through, so that their rates of disappearence underestimate inner medullary blood flow, rates determined with Evans blue might be more reliable. Evans blue, however, is strongly bound to albumin (Allen & Orahovats, 1951), and could be delayed in the medulla by extravascular circulation of plasma albumin (Barger & Herd, 1973). Blood cells should not be subject to such a delay, and erythrocytes labelled with ^{51}Cr were washed out about 25% faster than ^{131}I-albumin when isolated kidneys equilibrated with both tracers were perfused with unlabelled blood (Ochwadt, 1963). Oxygen leaves the blood vessels even more freely than albumin, and there is a discrepancy between the passage of oxygen and the passage of erythrocytes through the kidney. After the renal artery was suddenly supplied with blood having a higher tension of oxygen and containing erythrocytes labelled with methaemoglobin, labelled cells took about 3.5 seconds to appear in the renal vein, but the renal venous oxygen tension increased 1 or 2 seconds earlier (Levy & Sauceda, 1959). This would be expected if oxygen diffused across from descending to ascending vasa recta in the medullary bundles while cells travelled further into the medulla before returning in venous channels. Such a short path partially bypassing the inner medulla should lead to a progressive reduction in oxygen tension with increasing depth, reflected in a declining oxygen tension in tubular fluid passing through the hypoxic region in the collecting ducts. This could account for the low tensions of oxygen in the urine of men and dogs (up to 40 mmHg when breathing air and 50 mmHg when breathing pure oxygen), which are always much less than the partial pressure of oxygen in renal venous blood (Sarre, 1938; Rennie *et al.*, 1958; Ullrich, 1959).

Attempts have been made to avoid difficulties arising from diffusion by adding to the arterial blood: (1) radioactively labelled microspheres 15 mμ in diameter; (2) frogs' erythrocytes, elliptical, 18 mμ by 10 mμ and recognizably nucleated; or (3) antibodies against glomerular basement membranes. These should all be caught by the glomeruli and indicate the pattern of flowing blood that carried them there. But the particles may not remain uniformly distributed in the moving blood, and the antibodies may not be completely and specifically extracted on one passage (Stein, 1976). Since the kidney has to be removed to localize the tracers by histological methods or autoradiography, these techniques cannot be used to measure changes in one animal during life. Moreover, they depend upon capture by glomeruli and cannot therefore give any information about flow within the medulla. Such methods are quite unacceptable for clinical use, but the renographic techniques (Strauss *et al.*, 1979), being introduced to visualize the flow of blood, can be regarded as successors to the inert gas methods which give useful if nonquantitative information about the distribution of blood flow within human kidneys.

Claims that the circulation can be shifted between cortical and juxtamedullary nephrons to control the balance of sodium and water will be mentioned in section 7.4.4 among possible 'third factors' controlling the excretion of sodium. Reports of redistribution of the flow of blood as such are contradictory. Aukland (1980a,b), who had devoted a great deal of attention to the measurement of regional blood flow, reviewed advances in technique, found no method sufficiently reliable to establish redistribution within the kidney, and sadly echoed the conclusion of Leaf & Cotran (1976) that, despite a large amount of published work from many highly reputable laboratories, 'confusion reigns in this important field of renal physiology'.

2.3.3 Summary

It is established that most, probably more than 90%, of the kidney's large blood supply circulates through the cortex. The outer medulla gets about 7% and the inner medulla about 1% of the dog's total RBF. This smaller flow is not due to a lack of vascular channels, for these occupy about one fifth of the tissue, as in the cortex (Thurau, 1964). More likely, the great resistance of the long path, especially through the narrower descending vasa recta, slows the circulation through the inner medulla. This slow flow of blood is important for the mechanism by which the urine is made concentrated (Section 5.5.3), and it does not commit the medulla to anaerobic metabolism (Bernanke & Epstein, 1965; Cohen 1979). Although its circulation rate is strikingly less than that in the cortex, medullary tissue still receives 15 times as much blood as resting muscle, half as much as the brain, and 30% as much as the heart under basal conditions (Thurau, 1964). The rich blood supply of the renal cortex, suited to the filtering function of the kidney's vascular organ rather than to the metabolic needs of the secretory organ, is quite as remarkable as the relatively poorer blood supply of the medulla. Despite earlier doubts (Thurau, 1964), it has been accepted (Aukland, 1976; Korner, 1971) that the medullary circulation is autoregulated, albeit less perfectly than the cortical.

CHAPTER 3
Glomerular function

3.1 INTRODUCTION

The structure and blood supply of the glomeruli suggest that they should produce an ultrafiltrate of the plasma, though the process is usually called glomerular filtration. This is the first step towards producing the urine, and a knowledge of its rate is essential for analysing the activities of the tubules which operate on the filtrate downstream. It is no exaggeration to say that the measurement of GFR was the beginning of our quantitative understanding of renal function. This chapter deals with the nature and mechanism of glomerular function; the measurement, variations and regulation of the rate of filtration; and finally its implications for the urinary function of the kidney.

3.2 THE GLOMERULUS AS AN ULTRAFILTER

3.2.1 Introduction

Only a decade after Johannes Müller denied that the glomeruli were connected to the tubules or had anything to do with elaborating the urine (Smith, 1964), William Bowman (1842), Assistant Surgeon to the King's College Hospital and Demonstrator in Anatomy at King's College in London, proved by wonderfully skilful dissection and a new technique of injection that, in many animals, without exception the capsule which invests the glomerular capillaries (now known as Bowman's capsule) is 'in truth, the basement membrane of the uriniferous tubules expanded over the tuft of vessels', and drains Bowman's space into the proximal renal tubule. Bowman thought that the glomeruli secreted water to carry urinary solutes secreted by the tubules out into the urine, and when Nussbaum (1878) ligated the renal artery in frogs, the kidneys appropriately ceased to produce urine, even though the tubules were still supplied with blood by the renal portal vein. Ludwig (1844) attached great significance to Bowman's observation that the glomerular afferent arterioles arise from interlobular vessels which come fairly directly from the renal artery and are commonly wider than the efferent arterioles. He rejected the idea of secretion as vitalistic, and argued that the great pressure of the blood in the glomerular capillaries would drive water and most solutes out of the plasma into Bowman's space as a protein-free filtrate. Ludwig's hypothesis was largely neglected until Bayliss (1915) accepted that the evidence for ultrafiltration was 'overwhelming', and Cushny (1917) incorporated it into his 'modern theory' (Richards, 1922).

Bowman's statement that the glomerular capillaries were 'uncovered by any structure' had to be modified as newer techniques revealed the complexity of the barrier between plasma in the capillary lumen and fluid in Bowman's capsule; but the glomerulus still looks like an ultrafilter. The capillaries confine the blood at a high pressure within a thin membrane which in man has about the same total area as the whole external surface of the body. Ultrafiltration should occur if the hydrostatic pressure in the glomerular capillaries is greater than the sum of the pressure in Bowman's capsule and the colloid osmotic pressure due to the proteins in the plasma. Verney & Starling (1922) showed that isolated kidneys of dogs, perfused by a heart-lung preparation, only produced urine if the perfusing pressure was about 20 mmHg greater than the colloid osmotic pressure of the plasma; however, the pressure inside the glomerular capillaries was not measured until a great deal later.

3.2.2 Glomerular capillary pressure

Each renal artery divides successively into interlobar, arcuate, and interlobular arteries. Nearly all the glomerular afferent arterioles come off interlobular arteries (Fourman & Moffatt, 1971); they are therefore only fifth-order branches of the aorta and they should supply all the glomeruli in parallel with blood at the same high pressure. Hayman (1972) estimated that pressures in glomerular capillaries in frogs averaged about 54% of the pressure in the aorta; this was the pressure he had to apply through a pipette inserted into Bowman's capsule in order to collapse half of the capillaries in the glomerular tuft after he blocked the proximal tubule by compressing it with a glass rod.

The first estimates in mammals were informed guesses. Winton (1956b) and Wirz (1956a) both argued that the pressure in the glomerular capillaries should be a little less than the arterial pressure at the lower end of the autoregulatory range in which glomerular blood flow and filtration did not increase with rising perfusion pressure. They proposed 75 mmHg, about two thirds of the pressure in the aorta, for glomerular capillary pressure in dogs; and Thurau (1964) suggested about 70 mmHg for rats. The first attempts at actual measurement were made by Gertz *et al.* (1966), who punctured proximal tubules in rats and obstructed them by injecting viscous oil. Intratubular pressures on the glomerular side of the blocks rose rapidly for about a minute and reached a steady 'stop-flow pressure', which averaged 63 mmHg when the arterial pressure was between 90 and 160 mmHg, but fell in parallel with arterial pressure when this was lowered below 90 mmHg. Adding 25 mmHg (an overestimate) for the colloid osmotic pressure presumed to be opposing filtration gave 88 mmHg as the hydrostatic pressure in the glomerular capillaries. On the basis of this and other estimates prior to 1970, Renkin & Gilmore (1973) concluded that glomerular capillary pressures were of the order of 80 mmHg in rats, 70 mmHg in dogs and 15 mmHg in amphibia.

Brenner *et al.* (1971a) made the first direct measurements, on rats of a mutant Wistar strain which turned up in Thurau's laboratory in Munich and had glomeruli on the surface of the kidneys allowing their vessels to be punctured with micropipettes passed through Bowman's space. Pressures were measured with a new 'servo-null' technique (Wiederhielm *et al.*, 1964) in which a servo system operated by changes in electrical resistance applied and continuously records the pressure required to keep the interface between the fluid whose pressure is being measured and a 1 or 2 M NaCl solution just inside the tip of a micropipette inserted into the fluid. The tip may be as small as 1 μm in diameter, and the system has great sensitivity and small inertia. Pressures in 12 glomerular capillaries of seven anaesthetized Munich Wistar rats were pulsatile, and averaged 60 cm of water, about 45 mmHg, which was only 40% of the pressure in the aorta. This surprisingly low result was soon confirmed (Brenner *et al.*, 1972a). Proximal tubular stop-flow pressures measured by the same servo-null technique, with 20 mmHg added for colloid osmotic pressure, gave estimates of glomerular capillary pressure which usually agreed closely with direct measurements, but were greater in plasma-expanded animals unless fluid was removed from the blocked tubules (Blantz *et al.*, 1972). The stop-flow method never indicated lower reslts than direct measurement; but it was liable to overestimate glomerular capillary pressure, possibly because of vasodilatation due to rising tubular pressures or interruption of distal delivery and TGFB (Navar *et al.*, 1977). This might have contributed to the early high estimates of capillary pressure.

Maddox *et al.* (1974) reported glomerular pressures averaging 48.5 mmHg in nine male squirrel monkeys (*Saimiri sciureus*, a small primate about three times as big as a rat which has kidneys with superficial glomeruli); they also mentioned finding similarly low pressures in occasional superficial glomeruli in Sprague–Dawley rats. Scandinavian workers however published glomerular capillary pressures around 63 mmHg, measured by Brenner's technique, in Sprague–Dawley rats (Källskog *et al.*, 1975; Aukland *et al.*, 1977). Most of the early results for a local Wistar strain (Mø) were between 54 and 63 mmHg, only five out of 68 being 45 mmHg or less. but 2 years later, rats of the same strain had numerous superficial glomeruli and low capillary pressures like those of Munich Wistar rats (Tønder & Aukland, 1979). These low pressures were not confined to the superficial glomeruli; directly measured capillary pressures in deeper glomeruli exposed by cutting a lens-shaped slice 1 or 2 mm thick out of the cortex were not obviously different from pressures in superficial glomeruli punctured through the capsule. Hence rats of some Wistar strains with numerous superficial glomeruli probably do have lower glomerular capillary pressures than other laboratory rats upon which a great deal of work has been published. Sprague–Dawley rats have superficial glomeruli when they are very young, but soon lose them. They may grow to be 50% heavier than mutant Munich Wistar rats, and their kidneys become 25% heavier. The mutants lack circulating growth hormone (GH), and might be regarded as stunted and immature (Harris *et al.*, 1974), but with filtration fractions (FFs) up to 0.4 (Baylis *et al.*, 1977), compared with 0.3 in other rats, 0.2 to 0.3 in dogs and 0.2 in man, their smaller kidneys appear unusually efficient in converting so large a fraction of their plasma into filtrate! Which of all these rats are to be regarded as 'typical'? Smith (1951) remarked that most of the commonly used white rats had been bred for 139 generations, and that if a sibling pair of human individuals had been similarly 'inbred or narrowly cross-bred for 139 generations (at 25 years to a generation since 1525 BC) few students of physiology would expect them to react in a manner comparable to...mongrel individuals' in a present-day population.

The servo-null method has been used to measure stop-flow pressures in dogs (Ott *et al.*, 1976). Preliminary measurements on Munich rats to check techniques gave glomerular capillary pressures averaging 47 mmHg derived from stop-flow pressures and 44 mmHg measured directly; but stop-flow pressures in 14 dogs indicated glomerular capillary pressures averaging 65 mmHg. Some lower pressures have been reported; 60 mmHg during plasma expansion (which increased glomerular capillary pressure in Munich rats; Brenner *et al.*, 1974), and 53 mmHg when arterial pressure was lowered to 87 mmHg to minimize artefacts due to proximal tubular obstruction (Navar *et al.*, 1977; Thomas *et al.*, 1979). Marchand (1978) was not deterred by the absence of superficial glomleruli and punctured 52 glomeruli beneath the renal surface in 16 dogs. Glomerular capillary pressures measured directly by the servo-null technique averaged 57 ± 3 mmHg, in agreement with 58 ± 2 mmHg from stop-flow pressures.

So, finally, there are no measurements in man, but known parameters resemble those for dogs (Arendshorst & Gottschalk, 1985). Dogs and most rats probably have glomerular capillary pressures around 60 mmHg. Munich and some other Wistar rats, and squirrel monkeys, have superficial glomeruli and capillary pressures around 45 mmHg. The small standard errors for groups of measurements at random puncture sites suggest that a very small gradient is sufficient to maintain flow along the capillaries (Brenner *et al.*, 1972a). In some Munich rats and squirrel monkeys, pressure at the ends of the afferent arterioles is probably about 40% of mean aortic pressure, and only falls 1 or 2% along the glomerular capillary bed (Maddox *et al.*, 1974). Hence vascular resistance in the glomerular capillary bed must be very small, as Smith (1951, p. 585) expected from the large number of capillaries and the slow flow of blood in each. The idea goes back to Bowman (1842), who remarked that each afferent arteriole 'suddenly opens into an essemblage of vessels of far greater aggregate capacity than itself, and from which there is but one narrow exit. Hence must arise...a very abrupt retardation in the velocity of the current of blood'. The slow flow and the small gradient have the important corollary that blood is exposed to the glomerular filtering surface for a considerable time at a relatively uniform pressure.

3.2.3 Effective pressure for ultrafiltration

At any point along a glomerular capillary the head of pressure available to produce ultrafiltration (i.e. the effective filtration pressure) is

$$\Delta P_F = (P_{GC} - P_{BC}) - (\pi_{GC} - \pi_{BC}) \tag{3.1}$$

where P_{GC} and P_{BC} are hydrostatic pressures and π_{GC} and π_{BC} are the colloid osmotic (or oncotic) pressures in glomerular capillaries and Bowman's space respectively.

3.2.3.1 THE PROTEIN CONTENT OF CAPSULAR FLUID

The first samples of capsular fluid obtained from frogs were practically free from protein by tests sensitive to about 1% of the concentration in the plasma (Richards, 1938). Although this early conclusion was partly biassed by rejecting samples which contained substantial amounts of protein as likely to have been contaminated by blood from damaged capillaries, later work supported it. Pioneering work on rats and guinea pigs yielded few samples of protein-free fluid from their smaller and less accessible glomeruli, but samples from proximal tubules within 1 mm of the glomeruli were practically free from protein (Walker & Oliver, 1941; Walker et al., 1941). Seventeen out of 41 samples showed no protein by tests sensitive to 80 mg/dl, and eight showed no protein by tests sensitive to 30 mg/dl. Of the 16 samples giving positive tests for protein, nine contained less than 80 mg/dl and only two contained more than 200 mg/dl. More sensitive radioimmunossay (Gaizutis et al., 1972) and micro-electrophoretic techniques (Oken & Flamenbaum, 1971; Eisenbach et al., 1975) gave concentrations of albumin which were always less than 4 and often less than 1 mg/dl. Glomerular fluid from four Munich rats (Brenner et al., 1971a) and four squirrel monkeys (Maddox et al., 1974) contained up to 200 mg/dl of protein; their average oncotic pressures were 0.3 mmHg in the rats and less than 1 mmHg in the monkeys. Almost all samples of early proximal tubular fluid from dogs contained less than 10 mg/dl of protein; the concentration did not depend upon the site of puncture and hence was probably representative of glomerular fluid (Windhager, 1968).

Thus no-one can claim to have shown that protein is totally absent from the glomerular filtrate, but the concentration is small. Since the plasma contains 6000 mg/dl or more, it is reasonable as a first approximation to ignore π_{BC} and to replace equation 3.1 by

$$\Delta P_F = P_{GC} - P_{BC} - \pi_{GC} \tag{3.2}$$

3.2.3.2 PRESSURE IN BOWMAN'S CAPSULE

Winton (1956b) expected the capsular pressure in dogs to be about 20 mmHg, and pressures of that order have been recorded in proximal tubules (Ott *et al.*, 1976; Navar *et al.*, 1977; Marchand, 1978). Windhager (1968) quoted a range from 12.5 to 14.8 mmHg for proximal tubular pressure in rats but more recent measurements with the servo-null technique have been lower, for example 10.9 mmHg (SE ± 0.5 for 62 measurements) in Sprague–Dawley rats (Falchuk & Berliner, 1971). Brenner's group found proximal tubular pressures around 10 to 11 mmHg in Munich rats (Brenner *et al.*, 1974; Baylis *et al.*, 1977); others reported pressures up to 14 mmHg (Blantz *et al.*, 1972). Maddox *et al.* (1974) recorded pressures of 13 mmHg in proximal tubules of squirrel monkeys.

Direct measurements (e.g. 11 mmHg for Sprague–Dawley rats and 13 mmHg for the Scandinavian Wistar strain by Aukland *et al.*, 1977) suggested that pressures are not more than 1 or 2 mmHg greater in Bowman's space than in proximal tubules. Despite reports of 13.5 mmHg in proximal tubules and 16 mmHg in Bowman's space of Sprague–Dawley rats (Källskog *et al.*, 1975) it seems fair to assume that P_{BC} is generally less than 15 mHg in rats and squirrel monkeys, but is 5 to 10 mmHg greater than this in dogs. It follows that there should always be sufficient pressure to effect filtration at least at the arteriolar ends of glomerular capillaries. Representative values for Munich rats are: P_{GC}, 45 mmHg; P_{BC}, 10 mmHg; π_{GC}, 20 mmHg at afferent arteriolar ends of capillaries where the concentration of protein is 6 g/dl (Brenner *et al.*, 1976b,c). Thence $\triangle P_F = 45 - 10 - 20 = 15$ mmHg. The mean effective filtration pressure would become 7.5 mmHg if the plasma lost enough protein-free filtrate to increase its oncotic pressure to 35 mmHg and reduce $\triangle P_F$ to zero. The magnitude of π_{GC} requires further consideration.

3.2.3.3 COLLOID OSMOTIC (ONCOTIC) PRESSURE IN GLOMERULAR CAPILLARIES

The colloid osmotic pressure is the effective osmotic pressure of plasma separated from an ultrafiltrate by a membrane having the capillary wall's selective permeability to solutes with smaller molecules than proteins. In physical terms it is the pressure that is just large enough to prevent re-uptake of ultrafiltrate by osmosis; larger pressures would cause more ultrafiltrate to leave the plasma. The English physiologist EH Starling called it the oncotic (swelling) pressure. He was the first to appreciate its physiological importance and, in 1899, to measure it; his result, 25 mmHg, is still an acceptable order of magnitude for human plasma. About two thirds of this is the osmotic pressure the proteins would exert if they carried no electrical charge. The other third is contributed by the small excess of diffusible ions required for a Gibbs–Donnan membrane equilibrium because the proteins at any physiological pH are non-penetrating polyvalent anions. This 'Donnan excess' becomes very large in salt-free solutions and is very small in high concentrations of salts, but it is not much affected by variations in the ionic strength of the plasma that are compatible with life (Hitchcock, 1945). The oncotic

Table 3.1 Protein content and oncotic pressure of plasma

	Protein g/dl	Albumin/globulin ratio	Oncotic pressure mmHg
Man[a]	7.0	2	28 ± 1
Squirrel monkey[b]	6.8	1	24.4 ± 1.4
Dog[a]	6.0	0.6	18 ± 3
Rat[a]	5.5	1.4	18 ± 1
Munich Wistar rat[c]	5.8		19.4 ± 0.5

References: a Navar, 1978b
            b Maddox et al. 1974
            c Brenner et al. 1972a.

pressure therefore depends mainly upon the total concentration of proteins and the proportion of albumin to globulin, these being the major fractions in the plasma (Table 3.1).

As ultrafiltrate leaves the plasma and the proteins become more concentrated, the oncotic pressure increases; the increase is not linear, and because it could not be calculated theoretically Landis & Pappenheimer (1963) developed the empirical equation

$$\pi_{plas} = 2.1c + 0.16c^2 + 0.009c^3 \qquad (3.3)$$

for predicting the oncotic pressure of plasma containing c g/dl of protein. Measurements with a membrane osmometer confirmed that predictions from this formula were accurate for rats' plasma with c from 3 to 10 g/dl (Brenner et al., 1972a).

A simpler formula without a cubic term

$$\pi = 1.736c + 0.281c^2 \qquad (3.4)$$

gives almost identical results (Blantz et al., 1974), and Maddox et al. (1974) modified Landis and Pappenheimer's original nomogram to predict the increase in oncotic pressure with progressive removal of ultrafiltrate from plasmas with initial concentrations of protein from 4 to 8 g/dl. An initial oncotic pressure of 20 mmHg would increase to 35 mmHg when the plasma had lost 0.3 of its volume of ultrafiltrate. Hence if the pressures were 45 mmHg in the glomerular capillaries and 15 mmHg in Bowman's capsule, the effective filtration pressure $\triangle P_F$ would fall to zero, and filtration would cease when 30% of the plasma had been filtered; there would then be filtration equilibrium in the terminal portions of the glomerular capillaries. This possibility was not seriously entertained until the first direct measurements yielded unexpectedly low values for glomerular capillary pressures. It was then quickly accepted, and generalized — perhaps too enthusiastically, because equilibrium is not always reached in Munich Wistar rats, and may never normally be reached in many other animals (Arendshorst & Gottschalk, 1985).

Deen *et al.* (1973) avoided filtration equilibrium in Munich Wistar rats in order to employ all the available filtering surface to measure glomerular permeability. When 5% of the rats' body weight of isoncotic plasma was infused to increase the animals' blood volume, glomerular plasma flow was trebled and filtration rate more than doubled. The proportion of plasma converted to ultrafiltrate fell from 0.33 to 0.25, and the smaller increase in oncotic pressure left about 5 mmHg of effective filtration pressure at the efferent ends of the glomerular capillaries (Brenner *et al.*, 1974). Blantz *et al.* (1974) confirmed this using hyperoncotic albumin; these workers also came upon a group of Munich Wistar rats that did not attain filtration equilibrium under basal conditions, apparently because of low glomerular permeability. These rats had the same difference in pressure between glomerular capillaries and Bowman's capsule, but they filtered a smaller proportion of plasma than did other Munich Wistar rats, and the smaller increase in oncotic pressure left them with an effective filtration pressure of 4 to 5 mmHg at the efferent ends of their glomerular capillaries. Ordinary rats, with glomerular capillary pressures about 15 mmHg greater than those of Munich Wistar rats, and with smaller FFs, presumably have substantially larger residual filtration pressures (Ott *et al.*, 1976; Navar *et al.*, 1977; Thomas *et al.*, 1979).

The volume of fluid leaving the arteriolar end of a typical systemic capillary is less than 1% of the volume flowing onward, so that there is no appreciable increase in oncotic pressure. The hydrostatic pressure falls from, say, 35 mmHg at the arteriolar end to 15 mmHg at the venular end, so that the effective pressure for outward filtration falls to zero and then becomes negative. Ultrafiltrate therefore returns into the capillary by osmosis, and the dynamic 'Starling equilibrium' maintains the volume of plasma in the blood vessels (Robinson, 1975b). The glomerular capillaries, however, belong to a capillary bed in the course of an arteriole, and have no low-pressure, venular ends. Hydrostatic pressure is practically constant, and effective filtration pressure falls along glomerular capillaries almost entirely because oncotic pressure increases. There can be no further increase in oncotic pressure once equilibrium has been reached, and no more ultrafiltrate leaves the plasma; hence the effective filtration pressure in glomerular capillaries can never become less than zero, and ultrafiltrate does not return from Bowman's capsule by osmosis beyond the point at which equilibrium is attained. In any event, the establishment of filtration equilibrium in the course of glomerular capillaries appears to be the exception rather than the rule. In most mammalian kidneys there is a sufficient head of pressure to effect filtration over the entire length of the glomerular capillaries, and the magnitude of the mean effective filtration pressure may be a more important difference between strains or species than the presence or absence of filtration equilibrium in a portion of the glomerular capillary bed.

The balance of pressures ensures that the glomeruli could continually produce an ultrafiltrate of the plasma. To show that they do so it is also necessary to establish that the glomerular fluid has the characteristics of an ultrafiltrate, and that the glomerular membrane has the appropriate selective permeability. Other criteria depending upon the rate of formation of glomerular fluid are considered in Section 3.2.7.

3.2.4 Is the glomerular fluid an ultrafiltrate?

It is not sufficient that the glomerular fluid is practically free from protein, for most protein-free fluids are not ultrafiltrates. The cerebrospinal fluid cannot be simply an ultrafiltrate because it differs in details of ionic composition (Davson, 1956). The ocular aqueous humour was thought to be an ultrafiltrate until Davson (1954) showed that its composition was altered by dialysing it against plasma. Glomerular fluid cannot be collected in sufficient quantities to test in this way, and must be judged on its composition. Within the limits of primitive micromethods, developed for samples which were usually less than $0.5\,\mu l$, fluid from the relatively large glomeruli of frogs and *Necturi* agreed with their plasma in total concentration, pH, the concentrations of total electrolytes, phosphate, glucose, urea, uric acid, creatinine, and, when they were present, phenol red and inulin (Richards, 1938). The concentration of chloride was a few per cent greater than in the plasma, as would be expected for a Gibbs−Donnan distribution. The first analyses of glomerular fluid from guinea pigs and of proximal tubular fluid from guinea pigs and rats showed that fluid near the glomeruli closely resembled an ultrafiltrate of plasma (Walker *et al.*, 1941). In tabulated data for amphibia, guinea pigs, rats, snakes and dogs the concentrations of small molecular species were not significantly different from those predicted for an ultrafiltrate (Renkin & Gilmore, 1973). Fluid from superficial glomeruli of Munich Wistar rats also had largely the same composition as an ultrafiltrate of the plasma (Grimellec *et al.*, 1975).

These tests on tiny samples from a few accessible glomeruli or tubules gave no information directly about many thousands of undamaged glomeruli, even in the same kidneys. Attempts have been made to find the composition of pooled glomerular fluid from whole kidneys by suppressing the modifying activity of the tubules. When cyanide was added to the blood perfusing an isolated kidney in a heart-lung-kidney preparation (Bayliss & Lundsgaard, 1932), or was infused into one renal artery leaving the other kidney as a control (Nicholson, 1949), the urine increased greatly in volume and became more like an ultrafiltrate of the plasma. Chilling the perfused kidney in a pump-lung-kidney preparation to between 3 and 13°C halved the flow of blood, as expected from the increase in its viscosity, while the urine became like an ultrafiltrate of the plasma, and its output increased five-fold (Bickford & Winton, 1937). These results provide circumstantial evidence which suggests that if tubular activity could be competely suppressed so that the urine became the unmodified product of the glomeruli, this would have the character of an ultrafiltrate.

3.2.5 Selective permeability of the glomerular membrane

The 'permeability' of the barrier between plasma in glomerular capillaries and fluid in Bowman's space includes the selectivity that determines which molecules reach the glomerular fluid as well as the hydraulic conductivity that determines how fast water and permeant solutes move across under existing driving forces (Section 3.2.7).

Analyses of glomerular and proximal tubular fluids showing that albumin and larger molecules were retained in the plasma while small molecules passed through with undiminished concentrations provided the first and the most direct evidence of the selectivity of the glomerular capillary wall. The almost complete absence of plasma proteins from normal urine provides less conclusive evidence, because the epithelial cells can remove proteins from the tubular fluid (Renkin & Gilmore, 1973; Section 4.2.5). Foreign macromolecules are less likely to be removed by the tubules, and those which do not appear in the urine are more likely to have been held back by the glomerular membrane. Concentrations in glomerular fluid of substances that are neither removed nor added to the urine by the tubules can be calculated by dividing their concentrations in the urine by the proportion in which the glomerular filtrate has been concentrated by losing water; i.e. by the ratio of the concentration of inulin in the urine to its concentration in the plasma (Section 3.3.2). If the filterability, F_X, of a substance X, which is neither added to the urine nor removed by the tubules, is defined as the ratio of the concentration of X in the glomerular fluid to its concentration in the plasma, then

$$F_X = \frac{[X]_{GF}}{[X]_P} = \frac{[X]_U}{[X]_P} \div \frac{[I]_U}{[I]_P} \tag{3.5}$$

Alternatively, since $[X]_U \cdot V/[X]_P = C_X$, and $[I]_U \cdot V/[I]_P = C_I$, where C_I is the clearance of inulin, F_X is equal to the fractional clearance, or the clearance ratio C_X/C_I. This is the clearance of X expressed as a fraction of the clearance of inulin (which measures GFR; Section 3.3.2).

Wallenius (1954) developed the use of dextrans to test the selectivity of the glomerular membrane in dogs. Dextrans are flexible, linear polymers composed of D-glucopyranose units; they are elaborated by some species of bacteria and can be partially degraded to yield preparations with a range of molecular weights from 100 000 to less than 10 000. Wallenius infused polydisperse preparations into dogs and then laboriously fractionated corresponding samples of urine and blood in order to determine clearance ratios for dextrans of different molecular weights. His results are in Table 3.2, together with two results from a series using separate preparations, each with a narrower range of larger molecular weights. A discontinuity where the two series overlap may be partly due to uncertainty about molecular weights arrived at in different ways (Renkin & Gilmore, 1973).

Table 3.2 Filterability and molecular weight of dextrans in dogs

Mol. wt	8500	12500	16500	20500	24500	28500	51700	91300
F_D	0.91[a]	0.72[a]	0.49[a]	0.29[a]	0.16[a]	0.11[a]	0.04[b]	0.01[b]

References: a Wallenius, 1954
              b Giebisch et al., 1954.

The results in Table 3.2, indicating a reduction in filterability with increasing molecular size, agree with preliminary tests in rabbits (Brewer, 1951) and with measurements made in normal human subjects by using gel filtration to fractionate dextrans in urine and blood after a single injection of a preparation with molecular weights ranging from 10000 to 80000 (Mogensen, 1968).

The development of more precise and convenient micromethods for fractionating dextran by gel chromatography (Granath & Kvist, 1967) made extensive studies feasible in rats. Brenner and his colleagues chose Munich Wistar rats, so that they could obtain glomerular fluid and confirm that tubular reabsorption did not occur. They infused preparations of dextran with a wide range of molecular size, and fractionated corresponding samples of plasma and urine before calculating clearances for each fraction. The fractions were separated by size, and the results presented in terms of effective molecular radii from 1.8 nm (18 Å) to 4.2 or 4.4 nm, in steps of 0.2 nm, instead of in terms of molecular weights. The effective molecular radius (Stokes−Einstein radius), a_e, was originally obtained from a measured diffusion coefficient, D, by the formula

$$a_e = \frac{RT}{6\pi \cdot \eta DN} \tag{3.6}$$

where R and T are the gas constant and absolute temperature, N is Avogadro's number, and η is the viscosity of the solvent.

Table 3.3 shows average fractional clearances for neutral dextrans of different effective molecular radii from two sets of experiments.

Table 3.3 Filterability and effective molecular radius for dextrans in rats

a_e/nm	2.0	2.4	2.8	3.2	3.6	4.0
F_D	0.98	0.84	0.58	0.32	0.15	0.04

References: Chang et al., 1975c
              Bohrer et al., 1977.

There appears to be a filter which allows molecules smaller than inulin (a_e about 1.5 nm; Pitts, 1974) to pass freely from plasma to urine, but which

increasingly restricts the passage of larger molecules. Wallenius (1954) suggested that this selectivity could be explained by a population of circular
pores ranging from 1.8 to 5.0 nm in radius, very few of them being wide
enough for plasma albumin and large dextran molecules to pass through. A
remarkably similar estimate was made independently by measuring the distribution of solutes ranging from urea (mol. wt 60) to serum albumin (mol. wt
69 000) between particles of isolated glomerular basement membrane from
rats and the isotonic solution in which they were suspended (Gekle *et al.*,
1966). The widest pores seemed to have radii of 4.2 to 4.5 nm, and the
distribution of all the solutes could be explained by a normal population of
cylindrical pores of mean radius 2.9 nm and standard deviation ± 1 nm.

Molecular size, however, cannot be the only factor that determines whether
different substances can cross the glomerular membrane. Proteins like haemoglobin (Mol. wt 68 000, a_e 3.6 nm) and albumin (mol. wt 69 000, a_e 3.6 nm)
are almost totally excluded from glomerular fluid and urine while larger
dextrans get through. Dextrans of molecular radius 3.2 nm and 3.6 nm had
fractional clearances of 0.32 and 0.15 in rats (Table 3.3), while the fractional
clearance of albumin is less than 0.01. Dextrans of the same effective radius
have smaller molecular weights than albumin, and neither molecule is spherical. But the molecule of albumin, about 14.5 nm long and 4 nm in diameter,
has a smaller cross-sectional area than that of dextran (9 nm long and 5 nm in
diameter; Renkin, 1970), and should be able to pass through smaller pores.
Albumin, however, carries a negative electrical charge in the physiological
range of pH, while dextran molecules are uncharged. Brenner and his colleagues used modified dextrans with negative and positive charges to investigate
the effect of charge upon filterability.

Negatively charged, polyanionic, dextran sulphates were less filterable than
corresponding neutral dextrans, suggesting that negative charge restricted
movement across the glomerular capillary wall (Table 3.4).

Table 3.4 Glomerular filterability of dextran sulphate in rats (averages)

a_e/nm	2.0	2.4	2.8	3.2	3.6	4.0
F_{DS}	0.47	0.20	0.08	0.03	0.01	0.0002

References: Chang *et al.* (1975a)
           Bohrer *et al.* (1977).

Dextran sulphate of similar molecular size to albumin (a_e 3.6 nm) was restricted as much as albumin itself. Moreover, the fractional clearances in Table 3.4
agree with those for proteins of similar molecular radius excreted by dogs
(Renkin & Gilmore, 1973) and humans (Hall & Hardwicke, 1979). If penetration
of negatively charged macromolecules was restricted because the barrier itself
is negatively charged, positively charged macromolecules should pass through
more readily than neutral ones of the same size. Bohrer *et al.* (1978) tested

this in Munich Wistar rats by infusing a polydisperse preparation of positively charged diethylaminoethyl (DEAE) dextran and separating fractions with radius 1.8 to 4.4 nm in steps of 0.2 nm from corresponding samples of urine and plasma. Some of their results are quoted in Table 3.5, along with results for neutral and polyanionic dextrans from Tables 3.3 and 3.4 for comparison.

Table 3.5 Filterabilities of cationic, neutral and anionic dextrans in rats

a_e/nm	2.0	2.4	2.8	3.2	3.6	4.0
F_{DEAE-D}	0.99	0.93	0.80	0.66	0.44	0.20
F_D	0.98	0.84	0.58	0.32	0.15	0.04
F_{DS}	0.47	0.20	0.08	0.03	0.01	0.0002

Averages for cationic species from Bohrer et al., 1978.

Whatever the sign of the charge, fractional clearance decreased with increasing effective radius. For any effective radius, the positively charged forms had larger, and the negatively charged forms smaller fractional clearances than had the neutral molecules. Comparable effects of electrical charge were demonstrated in rats with derivatives of horseradish peroxidase (HRP), which were also shown not to be removed by the tubules, so that their rates of excretion in the urine reflected glomerular filterability (Rennke et al., 1978). Fractional clearances of anionic (succinyl), neutral and cationic (hexanediamino) horseradish peroxidases are compared with those of similarly sized dextrans in Table 3.6, which also shows the order of magnitude of the ratio of the fractional clearances of the dextrans to those of the horseradish peroxidases.

Table 3.6 Fractional clearances of horseradish peroxidases and dextrans of similar effective radius

	Anionic a_e 3.2 nm	Neutral a_e 3.0 nm	Cationic a_e 3.0 nm
F_{HRP}	0.007	0.061	0.338
F_{DEXT}	0.03	0.44	0.74
F_D/F_{HRP}	4	7	2

References: Rennke et al. 1978
      For dextrans, averages from Brenner's group.

Although charge affected the excretion of both kinds of macromolecule in the same direction, the dextrans crossed the glomerular membrane more readily than did horseradish peroxidases of the same size, suggesting that other factors, such as molecular shape and deformability as well as size and charge, affected penetration (Rennke et al., 1978).

The relatively loose, random coils of dextran polymers should be more deformable and hence pass through narrower spaces than more rigid globular proteins judged to have the same effective radius by gel filtration in the absence of convective or shearing forces. The mutual repulsion of like charges would, however, make the charged dextrans more rigid and more nearly spherical than the neutral dextrans, so that they should be more hindered by negative, and less helped by positive net charge. It might also be significant that the neutral dextrans have no ionic charges at all, whereas neutral protein molecules are zwitterions with positive and negative charges in equal numbers, and should interact at short range with charged surfaces. The most important difference, however, was probably the smaller cross-section of the elongated dextran molecules compared with the more spherical horseradish peroxidases.

Apart from the size, charge, shape and deformability of the molecules in the plasma, the selectivity of the glomerular membrane is affected by hae-modynamic factors. As predicted from a theoretical model (Chang et al., 1975b,c), restriction of filterability is shifted to smaller effective molecular radii as glomerular blood flow becomes more rapid (Brenner et al., 1976c); and as flow approaches zero the glomerular barrier becomes appreciably permeable to albumin which appears in the urinary space (Section 3.2.6).

Under normal haemodynamic conditions, molecular size and charge are the two most important determinants of filterability. For molecules of any size, net positive charge facilitates, and net negative charge hinders move-ment across the glomerular capillary wall. Charge also affects the size at which penetration into the glomerular fluid becomes negligible. This is about 3.6 nm for negatively charged macromolecules compared with 4.2 nm for neutral, and at least 4.5 nm for positively charged dextrans. Alternatively, dextran sulphate of effective radius 2.4 nm, neutral dextran of 3.6 nm and DEAE-dextran of 4.2 nm all had the same fractional clearance, 0.10, in Munich Wistar rats (Brenner et al., 1978).

These effects of electrical charge would be expected if the filtration barrier between plasma and glomerular fluid was itself negatively charged, repelling polyanions but attracting positively charged macromolecules into its pores. The observations that fractional clearances of dextran sulphates (Bennett et al., 1976) and DEAE-dextrans (Bohrer et al., 1978) became almost identical with those of neutral dextrans (Chang et al., 1976), so that charge became unimportant and size alone determined filterability when the glomeruli were damaged by a nephrotoxic antiserum, provided circumstantial evidence that the glomerular barrier does normally carry a negative charge.

Finally, although the importance of charge for the passage of macromole-cules through the glomerular membrane has seemed to be one of the greatest discoveries of the 1970s, it was anticipated two decades earlier. Wallenius (1954) suggested that albumin, with a radius of about 3.5 nm, and haemoglobin, with a radius about 3.1 nm, might cross the glomerular membrane less easily than dextrans of 3.5 nm radius because the proteins are electrically charged; and hence that dextrans, being neutral, would make better probes for testing the size of pores in the membrane. Further discussion requires some consi-deration of the structure of the glomerular capillary wall and of sites within it where movement of macromolecules might be restricted.

3.2.6 The glomerular capillary wall

The glomerular capillary wall has three principal layers: the capillary endothelium; the glomerular basement membrane; and a peculiar, specialized epithelium. Many of the details which are summarized diagrammatically in Fig. 3.1 were first revealed by electron microscopy (Latta, 1973).

The endothelium is attenuated, about 40 nm thick, and perforated by a large number of circular fenestrae of about 40 to 100 nm diameter. These round windows are 'glazed' in mice by diaphragms 4 to 6 nm thick (Rhodin, 1962); but in most species the plasma comes directly into contact with the proximal surface of the glomerular basement membrane. This basement membrane is the only continuous barrier between capillary blood and glomerular fluid. Its total thickness ranges from about 150 nm in rats to 300 nm in man. It can be subdivided into three equally thick layers: a lamina rara interna, immediately beyond the fenestrated endothelium; a central lamina densa; and a lamina rara externa facing the urinary space across the epithelium. The lamina densa appears as a close felt-work of fine fibrils, 3 to 5 nm thick. The two less dense laminae rarae have fewer fibrils, embedded in an amorphous matrix, and also some thicker filaments which run across from the lamina densa to the endothelial and the epithelial layers (Karnovsky & Ainsworth, 1972; Venkatachalam & Rennke, 1978).

The epithelium forms a complete visceral layer covering the glomerular tuft. It is continuous with the parietal layer lining the inside of Bowman's capsule, but consists of specialized cells (podocytes) having primary trabeculae

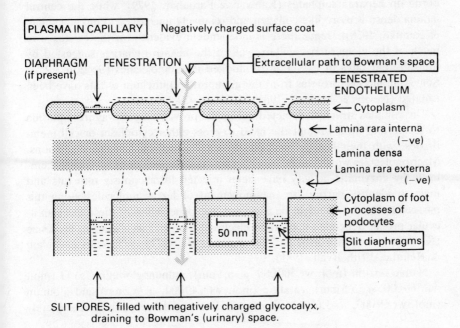

Fig. 3.1 The principal features of the glomerular basement membrane.

or arms which are wrapped around the capillaries (like the tentacles of an octopus in a dramatic reconstruction by Hans Elias, 1956). The primary trabeculae give off foot processes which interdigitate with foot processes of adjacent trabeculae like the fingers of a pair of hands clasping the lamina rara externa, and embedded in it to a depth of 40 to 50 nm. The gaps between the interdigitating foot processes form 'slit pores' 20 to 30 nm wide; these are bridged by slit diaphragms 4 to 6 nm thick, with central thickenings linked to the adjacent foot processes by cross-bridges. In rats and mice these divide the epithelial slits into rectangular pores about 4 nm by 14 nm, whose aggregate area amounts to 2 or 3% of the total area of the capillary wall (Rodewald & Karnovsky, 1974; Venkatachalam & Rennke, 1978; Ryan, 1981). Many early diagrams showed the slit pores widening rapidly beyond the slit diaphragms, but if the cytoplasm of the podocytes does not shrink during fixation the pores appear narrower, almost parallel-sided as shown in Fig. 3.1, and several hundreds of nm long (Latta, 1973).

The endothelial cells and the edges of the fenestrae have a surface coat of glycoprotein about 12 nm thick. This does not obstruct movement through the endothelial fenestrae, but a similar glycocalyx up to 80 nm thick, covering the epithelial cell surfaces and the slit diaphragms, fills the epithelial slit pores with a loose, highly hydrated, anionic mucopolysaccharide gel. The negative charges which cationic stains pick out on these surface coats are removed by neuraminidase, and hence likely to be mostly on carboxyl groups of sialic (N-acetylneuraminic) acid. The laminae rarae of the glomerular basement membrane contain other polyanionic glycoproteins, with negative charges borne on heparan sulphates (Kanwar & Farquhar, 1979), while the central lamina densa is more like collagen and relatively uncharged (Venkatachalam & Rennke, 1978). Hence there is independent evidence for the existence in much of the glomerular capillary wall of the negative charges suggested by the different rates of excretion of charged macromolecules (Section 3.2.5). Some anionic sialoproteins from the glomerular epithelium of rats have been isolated (Nevins & Michael, 1981; cf. Timpl, 1986).

The complex structure depicted in Fig. 3.1 provides a pathway from plasma to glomerular fluid without the need to cross either cytoplasm or cell membranes, with their low permeability to small dissolved molecules and ions. Macromolecules which can be localized by their electron density or histochemically by enzymatic activity have been injected intravenously into rats and mice to identify barriers to the movement of larger molecules along this paracellular path. As might be expected, the penetration of these macromolecular probes depended upon their electrical charge as well as upon their size (Karnovsky & Ainsworth, 1972; Brenner et al., 1977, 1978; Venkatachalam & Rennke, 1978; Ryan, 1981).

Native ferritin (mol. wt 500 000, a_e 6.1 nm), immunoglobulin (Ig) G (mol. wt 160 000, a_e 5.5 mm), catalase (mol. wt 240 000, a_e 5.2 nm) and albumin (mol. wt 69 000, a_e 3.6 nm), all negatively charged, were almost completely stopped at the lamina rara interna, though small quantities of albumin reached the urinary space. Neutral dextrans of mol. wt 62000 and a_e about 5.5 nm penetrated the lamina rara interna but were retained by the lamina densa of the glomerular basement membrane (Farquhar, 1975). Lactoperoxidase (mol. wt 82000, a_e 3.8 nm), myeloperoxidase (mol. wt 180000, a_e 4.4 nm) and cationized forms of ferritin (mol. wt 500000, a_e 6.1 nm; Rennke *et al.*, 1975), all larger than albumin but positively charged, crossed the glomerular basement membrane and accumulated at the slit diaphragms. Neutral horseradish peroxidase (mol. wt 40000, a_e 3 nm) passed quickly through the endothelial fenestrae and fanned out into the lamina rara interna. Later it passed on into the urinary space, unhindered by the slit diaphragms, and left the glomerular basement membrane uniformly stained. Cytochrome (mol. wt 12000, a_e 1.5 nm) passed into the urinary space without restriction (Fig. 3.2). Farquhar (1975) concluded that the glomerular basement membrane is the primary filter, and

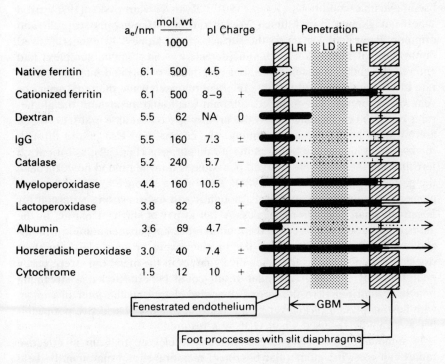

Fig. 3.2 Effect of size and charge upon the penetration of macromolecules through glomerular capillary wall, during normal flow and during capillary stasis (......).
LRI = lamina rara interna
LRE = lamina rara externa
pI   = isoelectric point
LD   = lamina densa
GBM = glomerular basement membrane.

that since positively charged macromolecules which cross it are attracted to
the negatively charged surface coats beyond, their accumulation around the
slit pores need not imply that these act as a second filter with a finer mesh.
Indeed, a much smaller positively charged polycation (hexadimethrine; mol.
wt 6000 to 8000) accumulated on the epithelial glycocalyx and laminae rarae
in rats (Hunsicker *et al.*, 1981) and, incidentally, produced a reversible
proteinuria, presumably by neutralizing the fixed negative charges, because
the chief urinary protein was albumin (though some larger but neutral IgG
also escaped into the urine). Placing the principal filter at the slit diaphragms
would have the obvious disadvantage that albumin accumulating there would
build up an oncotic pressure within the membrane and oppose filtration.
Fortunately albumin is stopped at the endothelial surface coats and the
lamina rara interna because of its negative charge, and gets carried away by
the flowing plasma without clogging the filter.

The selectivity of the glomerular membrane is critically dependent upon
haemodynamic conditions (Ryan, 1981). Ryan & Karnovsky (1976) fixed
superficial glomeruli in Munich Wistar rats by stripping the capsule and
dripping glutaraldehyde on to the surface of the kidney. In glomeruli fixed
during normal blood flow, albumin (detected as an immune complex) had
entered the endothelial fenestrae, but only traces penetrated into the lamina
rara interna and none got further. In glomeruli fixed while the renal artery or
vein, or the ureter, was occluded, albumin was found throughout the glomerular basement membrane and in the urinary space. Catalase and IgG, which
are normally held back at the lamina rara interna, had also passed through
the basement membrane as far as the slit diaphragms (Fig. 3.2), as cationized
ferritins and the positively charged peroxidases do when blood flows through
the glomeruli normally (Ryan, 1981). Thus in the absence of blood flow the
glomerular membrane behaved as though it had lost its strong repulsion for
negatively charged macromolecules. A fall in pH of stagnant plasma in the
glomerular vessels could reduce the mutual repulsion between anionic proteins
and the lamina rara interna as the proteins were brought closer to their
isoelectric points, and as fixed negative charges in the membrane were partly
neutralized by protons. A similar result could be expected if a streaming
potential contributed to the normal negative charge on the filter in contact
with flowing plasma. Whatever its mechanism, the loss of selective permeability was rapidly reversed when GBF was restored.

In summary: positively charged macromolecules up to 6 nm in effective
radius can cross the glomerular basement membrane, and may then be held
up at the slit diaphragms pending removal by phagocytosis. Neutral dextrans
are held up predominantly by the glomerular basement membrane, and are
not further hindered by the slit diaphragms. Negatively charged macromolecules are held back by the proximal, negatively charged layer of the glomerular
basement membrane (lamina rara interna). Although positively as well as
negatively charged and neutral macromolecules have been used to test the

permeability of the glomerular capillary wall, it is important that the major macromolecular species of the plasma are negatively charged like albumin. With anionic plasma colloids and a negatively charged filter it is possible to have larger pores than would be required to achieve the same selectivity by size alone. The glomerular capillary wall can therefore have a greater hydraulic conductivity and allow faster transfer of water and solutes of low molecular weight without losing the important large molecules from the plasma. Only a little albumin and traces of plasma globulin reach the urine under normal conditions, but albumin can cross the full thickness of the glomerular capillary wall during vascular stasis.

3.2.7 The rate of formation of glomerular fluid

Although there is a sufficient excess of hydrostatic over oncotic pressure to transfer fluid from plasma in the glomerular capillaries into Bowman's space by ultrafiltration, and although the membrane is suitably selective, and samples of glomerular fluid have the chemical characters of an ultrafiltrate, it still needs to be established that ultrafiltration can account for the actual rate at which glomerular fluid is produced. Measurements by methods to be discussed in Section 3.3.2 indicate that the two human kidneys together form about 2 ml of glomerular fluid every second. This amounts to a rate of about 1 nl/s for each glomerulus; and rates for other mammals are comparable (Renkin & Gilmore, 1973).

On the assumption that the glomerular fluid is indeed an ultrafiltrate, it is possible to define an ultrafiltration coefficient, K_f. This is the rate of formation of fluid by a single glomerulus per mmHg of effective filtration pressure, $\triangle P_F$, defined by equation 3.1 (Section 3.2.3); i.e. the rate of filtration by a single nephron

$$\text{SNGFR} = K_f \triangle P_F \qquad (3.7)$$

K_f can be regarded as the product of the hydraulic conductivity, k, and the area, S, of the glomerular capillary wall across which ultrafiltration is presumed to occur; i.e. $K_f = k.S$ (Brenner et al., 1976a). Hence if S can be estimated, measurements of K_f can be used to derive values of k to compare with the hydraulic conductivities of artificial membranes for which the sizes and aggregate cross-section of the pores are better known.

Taking the effective filtration pressure as 20 mmHg, and the area of a human glomerulus as 0.0047 cm^2 (Renkin & Gilmore, 1973), k for the human glomerular wall is of the order of $1/(20 \times 0.0047) = 10.6 \text{ nl/s cm}^2$ mmHg; and values quoted by Renkin and Gilmore give a similar value for dogs. Their figures for rats yield $k = 0.05/(40 \times 0.0022)$, which comes to 5.7 nl/s cm^2 mmHg; about half the conductivity of the human and canine capillary walls. These are all average values based on the assumption that the effective filtration pressure and the hydraulic conductivity are both uniform over the area across which fluid is transferred. The low value of k for rats is based on the old estimate of 40 mmHg for ΔP_F and the acceptance of any lower estimate will increase K_f and k proportionally. Thus if the average filtration pressure were closer to 5 mmHg, as suggested by the direct measurements of Brenner and others (Section 3.2.2), k would become about $8 \times 5.7 = 45$ nl/s cm^2 mmHg for Munich Wistar rats. Furthermore, if equilibrium occurs anywhere along the glomerular capillaries, S will be less than their total surface area, and dividing a measured K_f by the total glomerular area will underestimate k. Brenner *et al.* (1976a) avoided ambiguity from this source by measuring K_f under conditions which increased glomerular blood flow (plasma expansion or reduction of PCV), so that equilibrium was precluded. The ultrafiltration coefficient was 4.8 nl/min per mmHg, and taking the area S to be $0.0019 \, cm^2$ gave $k = 2.5 \, \mu l/min \, cm^2$ mmHg, $= 42$ nl/s cm^2 mmHg, for Munich Wistar rats. A similar value for K_f, 6 nl/min per mmHg, was obtained independently from the rate at which isolated glomeruli from Buffalo rats took up fluid under a gradient of oncotic pressure (Savin *et al.*, 1982). In view of residual uncertainties about the magnitude of effective filtration pressures in different species (Osgood *et al.*, 1982), it is perhaps fair to state that hydraulic conductivities of mammalian glomerular capillary walls are likely to be between 10 and 40 nl/s cm^2 mmHg.

Pappenheimer (1953) compared nonfenestrated capillaries in mammalian skeletal muscles with glomerular capillaries and with artifical membranes on the basis of Darcy coefficients of hydraulic conductivity; these include the thickness of the membrane, which was taken to be 0.3 μm for capillary walls. The most permeable collodion membrane had pores of effective radius 5 nm, but retained serum albumin, presumably because it resembled glomerular capillaries in having fixed negative charges on its surface. The Darcy coefficients, in $cm^2 \times 10^{-18}$, were 6 for capillaries in the muscle, 600 to 1200 for glomerular capillaries, and 19000 for the collodion membrane with 5 nm pores. Hence Pappenheimer concluded that 'collodion membranes which withold proteins to about the same degree as capillary membranes offer far less resistance to flow than capillary membranes'. It is also apparent that the conductivities of glomerular capillaries were two orders of magnitude greater than those of the capillaries in skeletal muscles. Pappenheimer based this comparison on old values of k, of 300 to 600×10^{-8} ml/s cm^2 cmH_2O, or 4 to 8 nl/s cm^2 mmHg for glomerular capillaries. More recent measurements showing lower capillary pressures would make these underestimates; they therefore suggest that mammalian glomerular capillaries have up to 500 times the hydraulic conductivity of capillaries in skeletal muscle, and about one sixth that of collodion membranes of comparable molecular selectivity.

Water-filled pores occupied about two thirds of the cross-sectional area of the collodion membranes, so that if glomerular capillary walls have pores of the same size, these should occupy about 10% of the total filtering area; but pores of the same size occupying less than 0.05% of their total area could account for the permeability of capillaries in skeletal muscle. These rough comparisons, indicating that the walls of glomerular capillaries are comparable in permeability with artificial membranes of similar molecular selectivity, suggest that ultrafiltration could account for the actual rate at which the glomerular fluid is formed, without the help of any cellular process of secretion.

3.2.8 The nature of the glomerular process

The process which delivers fluid into Bowman's capsule is usually called 'glomerular filtration', although filtration ordinarily implies separating a clear fluid from a mixture of liquid and solid phases without altering the composition of the liquid phase. Because the glomerular membrane retains dissolved proteins as well as the solid constituents of the blood, the glomerular process separates one homogeneous liquid (plasma) into two homgeneous liquids which differ in composition. One contains only traces of protein, and shows the small differences in concentrations of diffusible ions required for a Gibbs—Donnan membrane equilibrium. The formation of the glomerular fluid therefore conforms to the accepted definition of ultraflration as the transfer of liquid out of a solution through a selectively permeable membrane under the influence of a pressure greater than the difference in effective osmotic pressure.

Chinard (1952) suggested that each substance, including water, should be regarded as diffusing from the blood into Bowman's capsule at a rate determined by its own gradient of chemical potential and its own coefficient of (restricted) diffusion in the membrane. All the components of the plasma would have their chemical potentials increased by pressure and should tend to diffuse from the capillaries into the capsular space. The larger solute molecules, particularly the plasma proteins, which have much smaller coefficients of diffusion in the membrane, should be retarded much more than the smaller molecules, so that the final result would not be very different from that expected to arise from ultrafiltration.

Pappenheimer's (1953) analysis of the contributions of flow and of diffusion to the passage of molecules across porous membranes showed that when pores are large compared with the molecules (greater than 2 nm in radius), bulk flow is predominant. Diffusion is predominant in pores smaller than 1 nm which are too small to permit laminar flow. Between 1 nm and 2 nm there is a 'region of uncertainty' in which Poiseuille's law cannot be applied with confidence, because it was derived for hypothetical continuous liquids in which infinitesimally thin layers can be supposed to slide over each other. A more recent examination using the approach of statistical mechanics placed the changeover between hydrodynamic flow and diffusion at a smaller pore radius around 0.5 nm (Longuet-Higgins & Austin, 1966).

If the molecular selectivity of the glomerular membrane depends upon a porous structure with pores as large as 4 to 5 nm in effective radius, well outside Pappenheimer's region of uncertainty, flow across the membrane should be far more important than diffusion. Manegold (quoted by Pappen-heimer, 1953) found that even wider (but much longer) pores, up to 15 nm, restricted the diffusion of solutes as small as sucrose and inulin. These reach the glomerular fluid in the same concentrations as in the plasma water, as would be exected to result from bulk flow of water and small molecular solutes through the membrane. Moreover, Renkin & Gilmore (1973) pointed out that calculations of the hydraulic conductivities of glomerular membranes on the basis of flow through short cylindrical pores agreed remarkably well with measured values in a number of animals.

The process by which the glomerular fluid is produced is better described as ultrafiltration than as diffusion. But is it necessary to be pedantic and reject the common term 'glomerular filtration'? Garby (1955) seized upon the motion of the centre of mass to distinguish flow from diffusion. He proposed that the term 'diffusion' should be used to describe transport of molecules across a plane which does not move relative to the centre of mass. When the centre of mass moves he would speak of flow. In diffusion, individual solvent and solute molecules move independently, at different rates, and not always in the same direction; whereas in flowing solutions solvent and solute molecules move together in the same direction at the same average rate. The glomerular process is predominantly a bulk movement of water and small solute molecules together across the glomerular capillary membrane. In the light of Garby's definition, this can quite properly be described as glomerular filtration.

3.2.9 A model of the glomerular filter

Several models have been proposed to account for the selective permeability of the glomerular capillary wall. It could be explained by circular pores 3.6 nm in radius, by slits 7.2 nm wide or by fibres separated by interstices 5.2 nm wide (Renkin & Gilmore, 1973). The fibre model is probably nearest to reality. Pores have not been seen (Farquhar, 1975), and Scatchard (1956) suggested the biological membranes should not be visualized as plates punched with neat, round holes, but rather as like 'piles of sand, or brush, or tangled fishnets'. But although fibres may provide more realistic models (Michel, 1980), cylindrical pores lead to easier calculations (Deen et $al.$, 1979). It is useful to form an idea of the actual magnitudes involved by comparing the 'grain' of the filter with the sizes of molecules in the plasma and the distances between them.

A molar solution contains 6.023×10^{23} molecules (Avogadro's number) in 10^{24} nm^3 (1 litre), and may be said to have a specific volume of $10^{24}/6.023 \times 10^{23} = 1.66$ nm^3 per molecule. If this solution were made up of tiny cubes, each with a molecule at its centre, then the molecules would be $\sqrt[3]{1.66} = 1.184$ nm apart. Hence molecules in molar solutions should on average be about 1.2 nm apart. Table 3.7, which shows the approximate average distances between some solute molecules in the plasma, together with their approximate dimensions or diameters, indicates the 'grain' of the plasma. Figure 3.3

Table 3.7 Average distances between centres of some molecules in mammalian plasma

Species	Concentration mol/l	Specific volume		Average separation nm	Molecular diameter nm
		l/mol	nm³/molecule		
Water	52.5	0.019	0.032	0.32	0.38[a]
Na$^+$	0.14	7.14	11.857	2.3	0.72[b]
Cl$^-$	0.105	9.52	15.81	2.5	0.66[b]
Glucose	0.005	200	332	6.9	0.88[a]
Urea	0.005	200	332	6.9	0.51[a]
K$^+$	0.004	250	415	7.5	0.66[b]
Albumin	0.0005	2000	3 320	14.9	7.2[c]
Inulin, 50 mg/dl	0.0001	10000	16 600	25.5	2.4[a]

	Average distance between dissolved particles at 0.30 osm				
Particles	0.30	3.30	5.48	1.76	Diverse

References: a Durbin, 1960
　　　　　b Conway, 1981
　　　　　c 7.2 nm is twice the effective molecular radius; albumin in solution is regarded as a flattened, cigar-shaped particle $14.4 \times 3.2 \times 4.4$ nm (Renkin, 1970).

compares these dimensions with a diagram of the glomerular capillary wall on the same scale. The filter is represented as a set of cylindrical pores 7.2 nm in diameter in the substance of the glomerular basement membrane.

It is also of interest to compare the speed at which the filtrate moves through the capillary wall with the speed of plasma flowing along the lumen.
1　Movement across the wall. About 1 nl/s passes across the capillary wall of a human glomerulus, and the area of the glomerular surface is about 0.005 cm². Since 1 nl/s $= 10^{-6}$ ml/s, the average velocity through the membrane is $10^{-6}/5 \times 10^{-3} = 2 \times 10^{-4}$ cm/s, $= 2$ μm/s. The whole thickness of the membrane, about 0.3 μm, would be crossed in 0.15 second. If the filtrate passed through pores occupying 8% of the total area of the filtering membrane, the average velocity in the pores would be 25 μm/s. This is 250 000 nm/s, and the arrow in Fig. 3.3 shows how far the fluid should move along a pore in 0.0004 second.
2　Movement along the capillary lumen. Glomerular plasma flows of around 1.5×10^{-6} ml/s in rats and 5×10^{-6} ml/s in man imply blood flows of the order of 10^{-5} ml/s. A flow of 10^{-5} ml/s distributed through 40 capillary loops of radius 5 μm (5×10^{-4} cm) with an aggregate cross-section of $40 \times \pi \times 25 \times 10^{-8} = 3.14 \times 10^{-5}$ cm² would require an average velocity of the order of $10^{-5}/3 \times 10^{-5} = 0.3$ cm/s $= 3000$ μm/s. This is about four times the actual velocity measured by Steinhausen *et al.*, (1981) in individual glomerular capillary loops in rats, and both are much larger than the velocity of movement across the capillary wall. The albumin retained from each element of plasma converted to glomerular filtrate would be swept at least 100 μm along a glomerular capillary during the 0.15 second taken by the filtrate to reach Bowman's space, and so would not be left behind to hinder filtration.

(a)

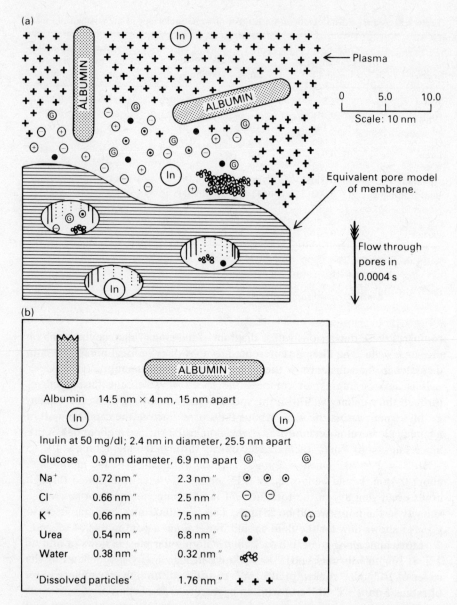

Scale: 10 nm

← Plasma

Equivalent pore model of membrane.

Flow through pores in 0.0004 s

(b)

ALBUMIN

Albumin   14.5 nm × 4 nm, 15 nm apart

Inulin at 50 mg/dl; 2.4 nm in diameter, 25.5 nm apart

Glucose   0.9 nm diameter, 6.9 nm apart

Na⁺   0.72 nm "   2.3 nm "

Cl⁻   0.66 nm "   2.5 nm "

K⁺   0.66 nm "   7.5 nm "

Urea   0.54 nm "   6.8 nm "

Water   0.38 nm "   0.32 nm "

'Dissolved particles'   1.76 nm "

Fig. 3.3 (a) An impression of the 'grain' of plasma and glomerular capillary membrane. (b) Average sizes and separations between solute particles in plasma.

3.3 THE RATE OF GLOMERULAR FILTRATION

3.3.1 Introduction

Measurements of GFR are required not only to calculate the permeability of the glomerular membrane, but also to evaluate the respective contributions of the glomeruli and the tubular cells to the elaboration of the urine. They are also helpful for assessing the severity and progress of diseases affecting the kidneys. Indeed, the clearance tests originally introduced by clinicians were essentially rough measures of GFRs.

Rates of glomerular filtration cannot be determined directly by draining fluid from undisturbed glomeruli and measuring its volume. Micropuncture techniques are limited to superficial nephrons and they require the animal to be anaesthetized, the kidney to be exposed surgically, and the overlying capsule to be penetrated or removed. Single isolated glomeruli have been perfused and rates of filtration deduced from differences between afferent arteriolar inflow and efferent arteriolar outflow, but this reveals little about how much fluid the same glomeruli would have delivered to their tubules *in vivo* (Osgood *et al.*, 1982).

Aggregated rates of filtration by all the glomeruli in intact kidneys can be measured indirectly in unanaesthetized animals and human subjects. The methods can only be used when the kidneys are producing urine, because they depend upon the rates of urinary excretion of substances which pass freely through the glomerular membrane with the filtrate and are then neither added nor removed by the tubules, which merely conduct them to the renal pelvis without gain or loss. In principle it is not actually necessary to collect the urine, if the rate at which a test substance which is removed only by glomerular filtration disappears from the blood can be measured, but it is usually more satisfactory to measure the rate of urinary excretion than to calculate it indirectly. The same methods can be extended to single superficial nephrons in the exposed kidneys of anaesthetized animals by collecting tubular fluid from punctured tubules instead of urine from the bladder or ureter, but there is some uncertainty whether removing fluid before it reaches the end of the nephron affects the rate of filtration (cf. Section 3.3.5.3).

3.3.2 The measurement of glomerular filtration rates

The rate of glomerular filtration can easily be calculated from the rate of excretion in the urine of a 'glomerular substance', G, which is excreted in the glomerular filtrate and conducted through the tubular system without gain or loss. If such a substance G crosses the glomerular membrane in the filtrate without change in concentration, its rate of delivery into the tubules (its 'filtered load') is $F \cdot [G]_P$, where F is the total rate at which plasma is filtered by all contributing glomeruli, and $[G]_P$ is the concentration of G in the plasma from which the filtrate is formed. Since all that is filtered is excreted in the urine, $F \cdot [G]_P = V \cdot [G]_U$, where $[G]_U$ is the concentration of G in the urine. Hence $F = V \cdot [G]_U / [G]_P, = C_G$, where C_G is the renal plasma clearance of G, as defined in Section 2.2.3.1. Thus the clearance of a glomerular substance (which may be called a glomerular clearance) is a precise measure of the GFR.

The glomerular filtration rate defined in this customary manner is not actually the rate at which filtrate is formed. The clearance formula gives the least volume of whole plasma from which the amount of G excreted in unit time could be derived. Proteins, which make up about 6% of the volume of the plasma, do not pass into the filtrate. Consequently the actual rate of formation of glomerular fluid is about 94% of the conventional GFR. It could be determined by calculating $V \cdot [G]_U / [G]_{plasma\ water}$, but this is rarely necessary because the filtered load of a freely filterable solute is correctly obtained by multiplying its concentration in whole plasma by the conventional GFR — which is the rate at which whole plasma is filtered (Robinson, 1954).

When timed collections of urine are made from the urinary bladder the result is the combined rate of filtration by all glomeruli of both kidneys. Results for either kidney separately can be obtained by collecting its urine through a ureteric catheter. In either case the best that can be achieved is an average rate of filtration over an appreciable period of time after a steady state has been established in which the concentrations of the test substance in plasma and urine, and the rate of flow of urine, have become constant during a continuous intravenous infusion of the substance as fast as it is being excreted. It takes 20 to 30 minutes to establish such a steady state because of delays in transit and equilibration in the urinary tract (Section 2.2.3.2). Somewhat less reliable results can be obtained during the exponential decline in concentration in the plasma following a single injection, but delay in the dead space of the urinary tract causes points on the curve of urinary concentration to fall some minutes after corresponding points on the curve of concentration in the plasma. If it can be assumed that the substance is removed from the blood by glomerular filtration and in no other way, this problem can be avoided, provided that the volume of distribution of the test substance in the body (usually about equal to the total ECFV) has become constant and is known. The rate of excretion can then be calculated from the decline in concentration in the plasma, and it is not necessary to collect the urine, which can sometimes be an advantage. This approach has even been used to measure the rate of filtration in kidneys with occluded ureters which were not delivering any urine (Harris & Gill, 1981). But such single-injection techniques are inferior in precision (Levinsky & Levy, 1973). $V \cdot [G]_U$ is usually calculated by multiplying the concentration of G determined by chemical analysis by the volume of urine collected per unit time. It has, however, become commoner to use radioactively labelled test substances, especially in clinical work; this may make it unnecessary to measure the volume of urine and calculate V, because the total amount excreted can be determined by counting the whole volume of urine collected. Measurements over short periods of time can be made while urine is still in the bladder if labels are used whose radiation can be counted from outside the body.

The use of radio-isotopes to facilitate the analysis of very small volumes has also made it feasible to measure SNGFR, using counters to measure the concentrations of labelled glomerular substances in the plasma and their rates of appearance in fluid collected by micropipettes from tubules on the surface of the kidney, or with ferrocyanide in microdissected proximal tubules after the renal pedicle has been clamped a few seconds following a bolus injection. The results are of the same order as averages obtained by dividing whole-kidney GFR by the number of contributing glomeruli, though they show much wider variations. Deeper, especially juxtamedullary glomeruli, are larger than superficial ones and seem to have substantially larger filtration rates. There are also good correlations between SNGFR, size of glomerulus and length of proximal tubule both in single kidneys and between different species of rodents (Wright & Giebisch, 1972; Renkin & Gilmore, 1973; de Rouffignac & Bonvalet, 1974).

Underlying all these methods is the important practical question of whether glomerular substances actually exist. Candidates for use as glomerular substances should not be metabolized, for that would indicate that they could enter and probably pass through cells. They must not be synthesized, destroyed or stored in the kidney, and they must not be toxic. Their concentrations in plasma and urine must be readily and accurately measurable. Other criteria, mostly laid down by Homer Smith (1937, 1951, 1956), include:

1 They should not be bound by plasma proteins and must pass freely through artificial membranes comparable in permeability with the glomerular capillary wall.

2 They should not be excreted by animals whose kidneys do not have glomeruli. Although this property makes their tubular secretion improbable, it offers no guarantee against reabsorption; glucose, which is not excreted by aglomerular kidneys, is freely filtered, and then almost totally reabsorbed by mammalian renal tubules.

3 Their clearances should not be affected by their concentrations in the plasma over a range that goes high enough to saturate specific mechanisms of transport.

An independent measurement of GFR would be necessary to establish that a substance was excreted solely by glomerular filtration. The nearest possible approach to an independent measurement is provided by using two or more test substances at the same time. The following two additional criteria are therefore of greater importance than the previous three which are essentially negative and cautionary.

4 If several glomerular substances are being excreted simultaneously, their clearances must remain equal under all conditions — even conditions which alter GFR.

5 Clearances of other substances, which are either greater or less than those of glomerular substances because of tubular secretion or reabsorption, must approach glomerular clearances when transporting mechanisms in tubular cells are saturated by high concentrations or inhibited by poisoning. This criterion makes it possible to arrive at the filtration rate without assuming that the clearance of any one substance measures it precisely. If a large number of substances are being excreted simultaneously, the rate which all

their clearances approach when tubular transport is saturated or inhibited should be the GFR.

When creatinine, inulin, mannitol, thiosulphate and ferrocyanide were found to have identical simultaneous clearances in dogs, Homer Smith (1951) argued that because they are so different chemically, the process by which they were all excreted at the same rate per unit of concentration in the plasma could not involve metabolic handling. It must be some physical process, such as filtration through the glomerular membrane followed by conduction along the tubules without gain or loss. Moreover, xylose, sucrose and glucose, whose clearances were ordinarily 75%, 70% and 0% that of inulin, all had the same clearance as inulin after the tubular cells had been poisoned with phlorizin. Hence any one of a number of substances could be used to measure glomerular filtration in dogs. Inulin, which Smith introduced and established, has generally become regarded as the most reliable, and contemporary understanding of renal function rests firmly on the foundation of GFRs measured with inulin. This is a polymer of fructose, with molecular weight about 5000 and asymmetric particles, obtained from dahlia tubers. When it is introduced parenterally into the mammalian body, it is rapidly distributed through most of the extracellular fluids, it penetrates more slowly into the extracellular phase of the denser connective tissues, and hardly enters cells. Although it may be broken down very slowly (Nichols et al., 1953), it should be safe to assume negligible penetration into cells during short experiments such as measurements of its renal clearance.

Before much was known about the specificity of mechanisms transporting carbohydrates, Ekehorn (1931; and subsequent polemics attacking Smith, in Acta Medica Scandinavica) argued that, being a carbohydrate, inulin must be reabsorbed; hence its clearance must underestimate GFR, and this could be measured better with creatinine, proposed by Rehberg in 1926. The so-called 'endogenous creatinine clearance', calculated from the rate of excretion of creatinine and its normal concentration in human plasma, happens to be approximately equal to the clearance of inulin. This agreement was first seen when the nonspecific colorimetric methods then in use overestimated the concentration in the plasma, but not in the urine, by reacting with chromogenic materials in the plasma which are not creatinine and are not excreted. If the concentration in the plasma is increased by administering exogenous creatinine, the noncreatinine chromogens are diluted and their contribution become less important; an 'exogenous creatinine clearance' is then obtained which is up to 30% greater than the clearance of inulin. When, however, sufficient creatinine is administered to raise its concentration in the plasma towards 100 mg/dl (9 mM instead of a normal concentration of about 1 mg/dl or 0.1 mM), the exogenous clearance falls to that of inulin. With low concentrations in the plasma, far larger C_{creat}/C_{inulin} ratios are normally found in chickens (1.7) and dogfish (6.0) than in man (up to 1.3); but these higher ratios also approach 1.0 as the concentration of creatinine in the plasma is increased, and phlorizin brings the exogenous clearance of creatinine down to the clearance of inulin. Indeed, the clearance to which all larger or smaller clearances converge when tubular activities are overloaded or poisoned is not that of creatinine but that of inulin, and so, by criterion (5) above, the clearance of inulin should be the best measure of glomerular filtration.

It happens that the measurements which first showed identical clearances of inulin and creatinine in dogs were made for mechanical convenience on females. Stop-flow experiments allowing the epithelial cells more time to enrich the tubular fluid showed that in male dogs the tubules secrete creatinine by a mechanism which can be inhibited by 2, 3-dinitrophenol and which exhibits competition with other transport processes (O'Connell et al., 1962; Swanson & Hakim, 1962). The clearance of creatinine also exceeds that of inulin in male, but not in female rats, and secretion by the proximal tubular epithelium can be induced in female rats by treatment with androgenic hormones (Harvey & Malvin, 1966). Most observations support the preference for inulin as a primary glomerular substance, but there are exceptions. Eggleton & Habib (1951) found that the clearance of creatinine was less dependent on concentration in the plasma than that of inulin in cats, and inulin appeared to be less freely filtered and to underestimate GFR in transplanted human kidneys (Rosenbaum et al., 1979).

The endogenous creatinine clearance has been popular for clinical use because it avoids the need to administer a test substance and minimizes discomfort for the patient. Though it is accurate enough for most clinical purposes, it suffers from the disadvantage that it is not quite certain what is being measured, especially when renal function is affected by disease (Doolan et al., 1962). Other substances, mainly radioactively labelled and offering greater convenience and ease in determination, do not involve any new principles, and their use need not need be discussed. They include such things as ^{125}I-iothalamate, ^{51}Cr-EDTA, ^{60}Co-cyanocobalamin, and their use is largely confined to clinical work where absolute accuracy is not of critical importance (Israelit et al., 1973; Levinsky & Levy, 1973; Britton, 1979; Kassirer & Gennari, 1979; Morrison, 1979).

Finally, although GFR cannot be precisely determined with absolute certainty, the clearances of a number of substances give good approximations, and of these inulin is probably the best in most animals. Even under good working conditions, however, the measurements show a variability of the order of $\pm10\%$, and this is comparable with the differences between inulin and its rivals, as well as with the variability expected for such 'physiological constants' (Smith, 1943). There seems to be no reason to change the opinion (Robinson, 1954) that taking inulin to be a glomerular substance is still acceptable as a working hypothesis.

3.3.3 The magnitudes of glomerular filtration rates

Normal GFRs depend upon species, size and age. In adult man the renal plasma clearance of inulin is usually between 100 and 150 ml/min. This seems large compared with rates of output of urine, which do not normally exceed 20 ml/min. Indeed, the need for such large rates of glomerular filtration was one basis of early criticisms of Ludwig's filtration–reabsorption theory of renal function. Heidenhain (1883) objected that it would take 70 litres of filtrate to carry the amount of urea that was excreted each day, and then at least 68 litres of water would have to be reabsorbed. The human filtration rate is now accepted as about 180 l/day, 10 times the maximal rate of sweating from an area of skin comparable with the glomerular surface. The glomerular filtration rate is about one tenth of the total flow of blood through both kidneys. The fraction of renal arterial plasma that is filtered, C_{IN}/C_{PAH}, is the filtration fraction (FF) and is about 0.2 in man.

Comparisons with other animals are usually based on the weight of the body or of the kidneys. Renkin & Gilmore (1973) published an extensive table of glomerular numbers, dimensions and filtration rates in 37 species from cyclostomes to man. The rates of glomerular filtration in man, rabbit, dog and rat are roughly 2, 3, 4 and 6 ml/min per kg of body weight respectively, and 0.46, 0.66, 0.62 and 0.75 ml/min per g of kidney weight (Smith, 1951). Rates per glomerulus in man, dog and rat are about 70, 50 and 20 to 40 nl/min respectively (Hierholzer & Ullrich, 1969). As with basal metabolic rates, there is a better correlation with the surface area than with the weight of the body. Most published results for human subjects are expressed arbitrarily per $1.73\,m^2$ of body surface. The average is then a little larger for men (130 ml/min) than for women (120 ml/min; Smith, 1951), and 125 ml/min per $1.73\,m^2$ is a convenient norm to use for people from 2 years of age upwards. The rates for adult people, rabbits, dogs and rats (about 125, 90, 50 and 70 ml/min respectively) per $1.73\,m^2$ differ less amongst themselves than the rates per unit of body weight.

The relative constancy of GFRs per unit of surface area matches the increasing size of the kidneys as the body grows. The ratio of kidney mass to body mass is larger for small animals than for large animals, ranging from 6 g/kg for mice to 0.8 g/kg for elephants, with man falling between at about 2 g/kg (Smith, 1951). What determines the ratio for each species is not known. The kidneys may grow in some proportion to the work they are called upon to do. Thus both kidneys grow bigger if adult rats are placed on a high protein diet or fed urea (McManus, 1966). A remaining kidney grows rapidly after the other one is removed, and both kidneys grow similarly if the urine of one is diverted into the vena cava (Morris, 1976). But the links between an increased work load and renal growth have not been established (Fine, 1986).

Babies and children under 2 years old have smaller filtration rates per $1.73\,m^2$ than adults, yet their kidneys excrete urea fast enough to keep its concentration in their blood no higher. Young animals are, however, more occupied in synthesizing than in breaking down proteins, and the infant's low filtration rate is matched by a relatively low rate of formation of urea, which helps to keep its concentration low in the blood. The question arises as to whether the kidneys of infants are inferior to adult kidneys in glomerular function, or whether they merely appear inferior because of an inappropriate standard of comparison. Babies at birth have lower filtration rates than adults per unit of total body water, but reach adult rates in 2 weeks instead of 2 years, and thereafter actually exceed adult rates for a year or so (McCance & Widdowson, 1952). At the other end of the span of human life, GFR gradually declines after about 45 years of age, chiefly because the number of functioning glomeruli diminishes (Davies & Shock, 1950).

3.3.4 Variations in rates of glomerular filtration

3.3.4.1 INTRODUCTION

Considerable emphasis was placed on the constancy of GFRs by Smith (1951), who remarked that the filtration rate measured 15 times over a year in one man varied only between 113 and 137 ml/min. Glomerular filtration rates of adult men, apes, dogs, cats, sheep, guinea pigs and rats do indeed often remain unchanged during large alterations in urinary output (Dicker, 1956), though filtration rates parallel urinary output in most nonmammalian species (Renkin & Gilmore, 1973). Unfortunately, GFRs can be measured most accurately when they are least likely to change. The most reliable measurements with inulin, during constant intravenous infusions after the concentrations in urine and blood have become steady, have been made upon recumbent human subjects in hospitals or clinics, and upon placid, trained dogs under resting conditions. It is less easy to measure GFR during strenuous work, athletic contests and many ordinary activities, but if mean values determined even under basal conditions have standard errors as large as ± 20% (Dicker, 1956), the apparently 'constant' values allow for considerable variations. It is now accepted that GFRs, like those of RBF, are not fixed. Moreover, changes which are not statistically significant, and therefore hard to demonstrate, may be important physiologically. Alterations of GFR less than 1% could, if nothing else altered, change the rate of excretion of sodium by more than 100%; and small changes with fluctuations in the volumes of blood and extracellular fluid could help to keep these volumes constant from day to day (Section 7.4).

Rapid fluctuations in filtration rates lasting only a few minutes are not detectable by clearance methods which give only averages over periods approaching half an hour. Early workers noticed that not all the glomeruli in amphibian kidneys might be perfused at one time. Some might become inactive as others opened up, or diuretics like caffeine might increase the total number of active glomeruli (Richards, 1922). Intermittent glomerular function was considered unlikely in mammalian kidneys because the tubules have no alternative blood supply from renal portal vessels, but it became less unlikely on anatomical grounds with the realization that few tubules in dog and man are perfused exclusively by efferent arteriolar blood from their own glomeruli (Beeuwkes, 1971; Beeuwkes & Bonaventre, 1975; Moffat, 1979). Smith's (1956) physiological argument, that there cannot be any nonfiltering glomeruli because the maximal rate of reabsorption of glucose does not increase when RPF is almost doubled during pyrexial reactions, still holds. The capacity to reabsorb glucose cannot be saturated if many glomeruli do not deliver filtrate, and should increase if inactive glomeruli open up (see a more detailed discussion by Renkin & Gilmore, 1973).

Although Smith (1951) did not discuss the variations and control of glomerular filtration explicitly, he reviewed renal function in a wide variety of circumstances and diseases and documented several dozen alterations in GFR discovered within a decade or so after he established the clearance of inulin as its best measure in human subjects and experimental animals. Some diseases subject normal kidneys to unusual demands and the conditions then may be no less 'physiological' than they are in experiments that involve extreme diuresis, large doses of drugs, drastic alterations in the pressure, volume or composition of blood, anaesthesia or surgical procedures. Pathological changes may therefore illuminate physiological mechanisms and need not be too rigidly separated for discussion.

Alterations in GFR that occur rapidly and are not sustained may be characterized as acute; slower and sustained changes as chronic, but, as with many physiological and pathological changes, the categories may overlap. Chronic changes reflect the size and state of the kidneys and adjustments to long term needs of the body to growth, climate, diet, habitual patterns of activity and chronic illness. Acute changes reflect homeostatic adjustments affecting functions of the kidney in response to postural changes, exercise and countless other activities, transient stresses and medical emergencies. Many of these affect RBF even more than glomerular filtration, but it is the alterations in glomerular filtration that are most relevant to the production of urine.

3.3.4.2 INCREASED RATES OF GLOMERULAR FILTRATION

A. Causes of acute and subacute increases

1 Reduction of renal vasoconstrictor tone. Activation of the kidney's rich sympathetic nerve supply can reduce GFR as well as RBF; and Homer Smith's (1956) 'normal' state of ideal rest is so rarely attained in waking life that increases in GFR from reductions in constrictor tone might be anticipated. Increases in filtration rate when enhanced sympathetic tone abates during recovery after stresses like cold, pain, loss of blood and surgery, are perhaps better regarded as returns to normal than as increases. Such recoveries from earlier depression can be demonstrated by denervating a kidney while sympathetic tone is enhanced by anaesthesia and surgery; but a denervated kidney in a conscious, resting animal does not have a larger filtration rate than its innervated companion (Smith, 1951; O'Connor, 1962). Earlier suggestions that immersing the body in water increased GFR in man were not confirmed (Epstein, 1978).

2 Pyrexial reactions. Substantial increases in GFR occurred when human subjects received infusions of inulin contaminated with pyrogens, but they were not so great as the simultaneous increases in RBF, and they failed to occur if the pyrexial symptoms (pains, headache, nausea and chills) and the elevation of body temperature were prevented by prophylactic treatment with aminopyrine (Smith, 1956). Similar responses occur in both innervated and denervated kidneys in dogs (Hiatt, 1942), which suggests that they depend upon some widespread action on vascular smooth muscle which lasts for several hours.

3 Increased intake of water. Parallel increases in glomerular filtration and output of urine follow ingestion of water in many nonmammalian species (Renkin & Gilmore, 1973). Uncertaintities as to whether rabbits responded in the same way were largely resolved when Forster (1952) kept the rabbits warm and contentedly nibbling during experiments which caused large alterations in urinary output. Glomerular filtration rate did not then change and averaged 5.3 ml/min per kg of body weight; in excellent agreement with maximal rates reported by 11 other authors. Rabbits are notoriously labile in vascular and renal responses, and may react to insults like the passage of stomach tubes and restraint in unnatural postures with large reductions RPF and GFR (Brod & Sirota, 1949). During recovery, the capacity of the tubules to reabsorb glucose can increase along with GFR and RPF, suggesting that a substantial number of glomeruli had been shut down (Forster, 1947).

Water diuresis in man does not require increasing GFR (Chasis *et al.*, 1938), and moderate loads of water, up to a few per cent of body weight, increase the output of urine without increasing GFR in adult rats, cats, guinea pigs, dogs and sheep. Larger loads of water, up to 10% of body weight in rats and 5% in dogs, may however increase GFR and RPF (without altering the FF) some minutes before the output of urine increases (Sellwood & Verney, 1955; Dicker, 1956).

4 Increased extracellular sodium. Isotonic infusions of sodium chloride tend to remain extracellular and affect the volume and oncotic pressure of the plasma more than similar volumes of water which are shared with the cells. Dramatic increases in GFR, rivalling pyrexial increases in RPF, can follow expansion of the ECF compartment with saline solutions. In a classical experiment Wesson *et al.* (1950) gave dogs priming injections followed by continuous infusions to replace losses in the urine over the next 6 to 8 hours. Glomerular filtration rate increased between 30 and 60%, and the FF increased somewhat after an early fall. Ladd & Raisz (1949) reported larger increases in GFR and RPF after adding solid sodium chloride to a dog's food and allowing free access to drinking water. Saline infusions seem to increase GFR

in rats as in dogs (Dicker, 1956; Landwehr *et al.*, 1967). But there are difficulties in measuring filtration rates in rats; Smith (1951) tabulated 'normal' values between 0.27 and 1.49 ml/min per 100 g of body weight from 13 publications. Brenner *et al.* (1972a), however, reported that SNGFR in Munich Wistar rats was doubled by large infusions of Ringer's solution.

Such increases have been described as totally absent in man (Smith, 1951, 1956, 1957). When Crawford & Ludemann (1951) gave 35 human subjects between 1 and 3 litres of isotonic saline intravenously, GFR increased a little in four, decreased a little in six and the average for the group showed no change. O'Connor (1962), however, objected that no greater increase than 10 to 15% should have been expected, and that the measurements showed too much scatter to demonstrate such a change. Ladd (1951) was more successful with larger doses, as were Markley *et al.* (1957), who gave young subjects 10% of their body weight of isotonic saline (about half the normal volume of their ECF) by stomach tube over 21 hours. The average GFR increased 32%, with no change in RPF and more than half of the extra sodium had been excreted by the kidneys before the end of the infusions.

Human subjects have not been challenged with the massive doses of salt that dogs can handle. Wesson *et al.* (1950) kept the ECFV 25 to 50% greater than normal for up to 8 hours. Ladd & Raisz (1949) gave 60 g of salt (enough to make 6660 ml of isotonic saline; this would correspond to 280 g of salt for a 70 kg man) daily for a week to a dog weighing 15 kg. The rate of excretion sometimes exceeded 1 mmol per minute (1440 mmol per day, which is about the salt content of 10 litres of ECF), and the dog did not develop oedema or even gain weight! Humans cannot excrete enormous loads of salt as quickly as dogs, and Pitts (1959) remarked that this leaves them 'only a salt shaker away from incipient oedema'. Dogs excrete saline as briskly as humans excrete water. Their rapid and large increases in glomerular filtration may help them to do this but it cannot be the sole mechanism because saline infusions are followed by rapid excretion of sodium even when an increase in GFR is prevented by arterial clamps (Section 7.4.4). Smith (1957) accepted the poorer human response as an unexplained difference between the species, and referred to a familiar class experiment in which some students imbibe a litre of water, and eliminate most of it in 3 hours, while others take a litre of isotonic sodium chloride and are still waiting for it to appear at the end of the day. But failures to detect a statistically significant increase in GFR with salt loading in man may be partly due to the use of smaller doses than dogs have often been given, and small increases in filtration rate paralleling expansion of the ECFV have not been excluded.

5 Osmotic diuretics. Osmotic diuretics are unreabsorbed solutes which increase the output of urine by the amount of water that has to accompany them at the prevailing urinary osmolarity. When the loads are large, this is not much less than the amount required to contain them in isotonic solution (because of limitations of the concentrating mechanism, discussed in Section

5.5.3). Though no increase in GFR is necessary for their action, osmotic diuretics might produce such an increase by withdrawing water from the cells and expanding the ECFV. Kruhøffer (1960) stated that sulphate, urea and mannitol may carry half the filtered water into the urine, and also increase glomerular filtration so much that the output of urine approaches normal (nondiuretic) filtration rates. Large doses of glucose and sodium sulphate used as diuretics to study the effect of urinary output on the excretion of urea by dogs increased the clearance of creatinine only modestly (Shannon, 1938a). Mannitol was a popular diuretic with physiologists, and it has been used to increase glomerular filtration and urinary output in patients with severe circulatory failure (Lauson et al., 1944). But when Wesson & Anslow (1948) infused dogs with 25% (1.34 osm) mannitol and produced a massive diuresis during which sodium was demonstrably reabsorbed against a sizeable gradient, there was no consistent effect on GFR. Hypertonic mannitol (3.8 osm) also failed to increase GFR in dogs on a restricted intake of water, though it provoked an impressive diuresis (West & Rapoport, 1950). The dehydration produced by losing large volumes of nearly isotonic urine may prevent expected increases in glomerular filtration in experiments such as this.

6 Infusion of plasma, plasma proteins and other colloids. Infusions of plasma, plasma proteins and plasma expanders help to restore glomerular filtration depressed by failure of the circulation, and rapid infusions of 1 to 2 litres of reconstituted human plasma increased GFR greatly in six out of 10 convalescent men (Wilson & Harrison, 1950), with RPF increasing more than GFR, so that the FF decreased. Large infusions (up to 5% of body weight) of plasma also doubled SNGFR and single nephron filtration fraction (SNFF) in Munich Wistar rats (Brenner et al., 1974). Infusions of salt-poor human albumin and of other colloids used as substitutes (because albumin is expensive and soon lost in the urine) may initiate diuresis in hypoproteinaemic patients with nephrotic syndromes by temporarily increasing plasma volume and GFR (Pitts, 1959); but current therapy relies more upon diuretics which block tubular reabsorption of sodium and upon corticosteroids and immunosuppressive drugs which influence the course of the disease (Robson, 1972). Infusions of albumin may actually depress GFR in normal subjects who are not depleted of plasma proteins (Goodyer et al., 1949). Hyperoncotic (10% and 25%) infusions of human albumin did not affect GFR in normal subjects and patients with diabetes insipidus, possibly because the increased volume and the increased oncotic pressure of the plasma had opposing effects (Welt & Orloff, 1951; Petersdorf & Welt, 1953).

7 Consumption of meat. In one dog studied intensively by Shannon et al. (1932) the clearance of sucrose or xylose increased from 40 to 135 ml/min per m^2 after feeding on meat instead of cracker meal, and GFR could be doubled in a few hours after a single meal of raw beefsteak (Smith, 1951). The rate of glomerular filtration may have been artificially increased by excessive hydration in some published studies with urinary outputs up to about 10 ml/min

(Ramsay & Coxon, 1967); but Shannon *et al.* (1932) had kept the output of urine below 0.8 ml/min. O'Connor & Summerill (1976a) re-examined the effect of meat, using a subcutaneous depot of creatinine to avoid infusions which could themselves increase GFR and urine volume. Their resting values for GFR were about 40% below many in the literature, and a meal of 10 g of meat per kg of body weight (an amount dogs ordinarily eat) increased GFR 40% without raising the flow of urine above 0.3 ml/min. Increases in GFR after larger amounts of meat (30 and 50 g/kg) were little greater (about 50% after 3 hours) but lasted longer (Summerill, 1982). Meat increased the production and the urinary excretion of urea, and enough urea given by stomach tube to yield the same increase in its concentration in the plasma (60%) increased the output of urine by 50% but did not increase GFR (O'Connor & Summerill, 1976b).

Seals, with their dramatic diving reflex, show renovascular lability like rabbits, and their glomerular filtration varies with urinary output during water diuresis (Ladd *et al.*, 1951). Seals normally depend upon preformed and metabolic water, and so do not drink (Smith, 1951), but they enjoy an impressive postprandial diuresis; a seal's GFR and RPF may increase three-fold after eating 1 kg of herring (Hiatt & Hiatt, 1942). Dicker (1956) remarked that, compared with their effects in dogs, seals and rats, meat meals produce only minimal acute effects on human GFRs; he regarded this as a species difference, like the smaller response to loading with saline. O'Connor's (1962) suggestion that it might merely be related to the larger amounts of meat that dogs ordinarily eat was supported by the more recent observations of Hostetter (1986), who gave 10 human volunteers 3.5 g/kg of cooked meat and compared the effects with those of ingesting on control days as much sodium chloride and water as the meat contained. In eight of the subjects the meat meal was responsible for an average increase of 28% (range 5 to 46%) in GFR over 3 hours, with parallel increases in renal blood and plasma flows, and a greater increase in excretion of sodium than followed similar intakes of salt and water without the meat.

8 Some diuretics and vasodilators. Old-fashioned xanthine diuretics like caffeine and theophylline increase GFR and FFs in men, dogs and rats (Chasis *et al.*, 1938; Smith, 1951; Pitts, 1959). More modern diuretics which block reabsorption of sodium from proximal tubules or chloride from thick ascending limbs of Henle's loops may depress GFR, possibly by presenting more sodium and chloride to the macula densa (Seely & Dirks, 1977). Vasodilators are equally disappointing. Acetylcholine, PGE_1 and bradykinin increased plasma flow but not filtration in whole kidneys of humans, dogs and rats (Brenner *et al.*, 1976a), and in single superficial nephrons of Munich Wistar rats (Baylis *et al.*, 1976), though PGs synthesized within the kidneys may help to preserve glomerular filtration when renal perfusion is threatened (Schnermann & Briggs, 1981). The atrial natriuretic factors (ANF, Section 7.4.4.4) are natural agents which increase GFR.

9 Diurnal changes. If GFR is taken as basal during sleep, the change to daytime values is a subacute increase. When Sirota *et al.* (1950) followed 18 normal human subjects for 24 hours using a slow, continuous intravenous infusion, the ratio of GFR by night to GFR by day was 0.96 ± 0.07, but there was a significant slight fall during deep sleep between midnight and 4 a.m. Wesson's (1964) 12 normal subjects had larger diurnal swings, with average GFR least at 4 a.m. and 23% greater at 2.30 p.m. Renal plasma flow swung 25%, not quite in phase with GFR; the largest FF, at 10 a.m., was 15% greater than the smallest at 11.30 p.m. The causes of these changes are not understood. Sympathetic nervous activity probably fluctuates during sleep (Mountcastle, 1974), and diversion of blood from the kidneys may accompany diminished cardiac output and cutaneous vasodilatation. Some patients with congestive cardiac failure show an inverted rhythm; their usually low GFR increases substantially at night (Baldwin *et al.*, 1950b: Smith, 1951; Brod & Fejfar, 1955). For a general review of human circadian rhythms see Mills (1966).

B. Causes of chronically increased GFR

1 Growth. The most important sustained increase in glomerular filration accompanies the natural growth of the body. All the nephrons in the human kidney are present at birth, but they have less than 20% of the adult number of cells, which is reached 6 months after birth. The kidney grows thereafter by increasing size of the cells then present and takes several years to reach maturity (McDonald & Emery, 1959; Widdowson *et al.*, 1972). The last nephrons to be formed are on the cortical surface and have small glomeruli at birth, with cuboidal epithelium and a relatively low permeability, restricting filtration at molecular weights above 15 000. In guinea pigs a rapid increase in GFR after birth has been explained by increasing arterial and filtration pressures combined with decreasing renal vascular resistance as the area and permeability of the glomerular filtering surface increase (Spitzer & Edelman, 1971). Developmental renal physiology was reviewed by Kleinman (1982).

Chantler (1979) published a table showing how the 50-fold increase in human glomerular filtration from 2.4 ml/min at birth to adult rates around 125 ml/min keeps pace with the growth of the body and of the kidneys. Six months after birth GFR has increased six-fold to 15.5 ml/min and is already equal to the adult rate per kg of body weight, two thirds of the adult rate per g of kidney and more than half the adult rate per 1.73 m^2 of body surface. Glomerular filtration rates per 1.73 m^2 and per g of kidney reach adult values by 2 and 4 years of age. Glomerular filtration rate per kg of body weight exceeds adult values from 9 months to 12 years, being 50% greater between 2 and 4 years of age. Moreover, GFRs per kg of body weight, per g of kidney, per 1.73 m^2 of body surface and per 1000 kJ of basal metabolic rate 1 week after birth are all approximately one third of their adult values. Hence glomerular filtration increases fairly regularly with kidney size, body size and metabolic demands throughout the growing period.

2 Trophic hormones. Bodily growth depends upon hormonal support of anabolic processes which allow cells to grow to the size and number prescribed by the individual's genetic heritage. Growth of the kidney is supported principally by the adenohypophysial growth hormone (GH), adrencorticotrophic hormone (ACTH), thyroid stimulating hormone (TSH) and the trophic hormones these control (Smith, 1951). Testosterone, mobilized by adenohypophysial gonadotrophic hormones, increases the mass of the renal tubular epithelium but has no direct effect on GFR. Apart from its main effect on the growth of the kidney, GH increased GFR by 17% in 10 out of 11 men between 26 and 53 years of age who received injections of human GH for 4 days (Corvilain & Abramow, 1962). Increased GFRs with no change in FF, presumably due to excessive secretion of GH, occur in acromegaly (lkkos *et al.*, 1956; Falkheden & Sjøgren, 1964). Thyroid hormones, which are essential for normal growth, can increase GFR in rats and dogs (Smith, 1951); and GFR and RPF are often, but not invariably, increased in hyperthyroid patients (Bradley *et al.*, 1974). Early work with adrenal corticosteroids showed that synthetic deoxycortone could expand the ECFV and increase GFR and RPF, though cortical extracts did not do this (Smith, 1951). Later work showed that cortisol can increase GFR, but aldosterone does not do so unless it expands the ECFV (Bartter *et al.*, 1974).

3 Diet. Chronic effects of dietary regimes corresponding to the acute effects of protein meals have been known since Shannon *et al.* (1932) recognized that the maintenance diet affected renal function in dogs. With more than one protein meal daily, GFR does not have time to return to basal values between meals, and it takes 4 or 5 days to return to initial values after protein meals are stopped (Smith, 1951). High protein diets may also maintain increased GFRs in rats (Dicker, 1956). The effects in man are usually small or absent unless large amounts of protein (more than 2 g per kg of body weight) are eaten each day (Pullman *et al.*, 1949), though GFR was possibly a few per cent greater in adult men on a diet containing 25% protein than on a rice diet containing 4% (Murdaugh *et al.*, 1958).

4 Pregnancy. Smith (1951) found no effects of pregnancy on renal function established by 1951, but a dozen more recent studies analysed by Davison & Dunlop (1980), including more than 300 pregnant women and 100 nonpregnant controls, showed consistently that GFR increased about 50% throughout pregnancy, while RPF was increase 65% during the first two trimesters and 45% during the third; the FF was therefore reduced at first but returned to normal or a little above normal towards term. The volumes of plasma and ECF increase, and dilution of plasma proteins reduces the oncotic pressure of the plasma by about 20% during human pregnancy (Chesley, 1972). In rats, GFR increased about 30% with no change in RPF, so that the FF was increased throughout pregnancy (Alexander *et al.*, 1980). There may be similar changes in GFR and in ECFV in pseudopregnancy (Atherton *et al.*, 1982).

5 Diabetes mellitus. Insulin-dependent diabetics, especially those with a low plasma threshold for glucose (Robertson & Gray, 1953), have their GFRs per $1.73\,m^2$ of body surface increased 20 to 40% during the early course of their illness (up to 12 years; Mogensen, 1971) before the kidneys are damaged. Renal plasma flow is also increased, but less than GFR, and the FF is therefore increased (Parsons & Watkins, 1979). The high filtration rate is accompanied by a comparable increase in the size of the kidneys, and has been said to represent a real hyperfunction because it is accompanied by an increase in the ECFV such as occurs in pregnancy (Brøchner-Mortensen & Ditzel, 1982). Treatment of newly diagnosed patients with insulin can halve the increase in GFR in a week, without reducing the size of the kidney (Christensen *et al.*, 1982). The increase in GFR cannot be attributed to the osmotic diuretic action of glucose, and it bears no relation to the concentration of glucose in the plasma (Mogensen, 1973). It might be a consequence of increased concentrations of GH in the plasma (these may be four times normal), for GH is known to increase the size of the kidneys and also GFR (Hansen & Mogensen, 1972). Both the increased GFR and the high concentrations of GH return towards normal when the disease is treated with insulin. Comparable increases in whole kidney GFR and in SNGFR (40%) occurred in Munich Wistar rats made diabetic with streptozotocin and partially treated with insulin; but GFR was less than normal in more severely hyperglycaemic rats not treated with insulin (Hostetter *et al.*, 1981b).

6 Obesity. The rate of glomerular filtration averaged 40% above normal in a dozen extremely obese patients who were 86 to 159% overweight, and returned to normal after they had lost between 23 and 79 kg following gastric bypass surgery (Brøchner-Mortensen *et al.*, 1980). The surface area of the body and the ECFV were also increased so that GFR per $1.73\,m^2$ of body surface and per unit volume of ECF were not abnormal and did not alter when the patients lost weight. Their earlier filtration rates were normal for their size.

7 Renal disease. Diseases of the kidneys usually lower GFR, but some children in early stages of nephrotic syndromes, before signs of renal failure appeared, had GFR and RPF increased to an extent rarely seen in other clinical states (Emerson & Dole, 1943; Smith, 1951). The FF was usually higher than normal, not lower as in pyrexial renal hyperaemia with a comparable increase in RPF. Smith (1951) commented upon the great labilty of these patients' glomerular function, but the low concentration of urea in their plasma suggests that their urea clearances and GFRs were high even when they were not being measured. Less is heard of this unusual finding at present, and the cause of the increase is not known, though RPF and GFR should both be increased by the low viscosity and oncotic pressure of plasma depleted of albumin.

C. Increased filtration rate per nephron

Under normal conditions, when the number of functioning glomeruli does not alter, filtration rate per nephron can only increase when whole-kidney GFR increases, or when redistribution of blood flow leads to an increase in some nephrons balanced by decreases in others. Reductions in the number of functioning nephrons, however, are often accompanied by proportionately smaller reductions in GFR, and then SNGFR must be increased. It has been known for many years that atrophy or surgical removal of one kidney is soon followed by increases in size and activity of the remaining kidney. Verney (1929) remarked that after he cut off the blood supply to one half of an isolated, perfused canine kidney, 'the remaining half suddenly and without a moment's hesitation doubled its previous rate of secretion'. The slower process of compensatory hypertrophy was reviewed by Nowinski & Goss (1969) and by Hayslett (1979).

Within a few minutes of the removal of one kidney, the rate of incorporation of ^{14}C-choline into phospholipids in cortical slices from the other kidney increases nearly 40%. Synthesis of DNA preceding cell division increases within 6 hours; faster synthesis of RNA leading to hypertrophy begins within 12 hours and continues for several weeks as the remaining kidney grows about 40% in weight. Hypertrophy (increase in size of cells) is more prominent than hyperplasia (increase in number of cells). The rate of glomerular filtration increases faster than the weight of the kidney, though the number of glomeruli does not increase. In one study in rats (Provoost & Molenaar, 1980) the GFR of the remaining kidney increased 26% in 4 hours, 40% in 12 hours, and a final increase of 64% over 4 weeks was compounded of a 35% increase in weight of the kidney and a 21% increase in GFR per g of renal tissue. Measured values of SNGFR increase along with whole-kidney GFR (Hayslett et al., 1968; Deen et al., 1974). Similar compensatory growth may follow unrelieved ureteral obstruction or ischaemic damage without removing the affected kidney from the body. Large increases in SNGFR follow the total removal of one kidney and partial destruction of the other. Single nephron filtration rate in the remnant portion of kidney doubled after uninephrectomy and infarction of five sixths of the remaining kidney in Munich Wistar rats (Hostetter et al., 1981a); glomerular capillary pressure and effective filtration pressure both increased about 10 mmHg, and filtration no longer proceeded to equilibrium. Comparable increases in GFR occur in dogs (Bradley et al., 1974a), and the remaining kidneys of healthy human donors may increase their GFR by 40% within about 2 weeks of nephrectomy. Renal plasma flow also increases, and the FF remains normal or low (Krohn et al., 1966; Pabico et al., 1975).

Compensatory renal growth requires the same hormonal support as normal growth (Reiter, 1969), and does not occur in hypophysectomized rats (Dicker et al., 1977). The enhancing effect of a large intake of dietary protein was well known to the pioneers of micropuncture, who combined it with partial nephrectomy to get hypertrophied tubules which were easier to see and to puncture (Walker & Oliver, 1941). Conversely, the increase in SNGFR and the later structural changes following subtotal nephrectomy in rats were largely prevented by a diet poor in protein (Hostetter *et al.*, 1981a). But Fine (1986) had to conclude after reviewing 242 relevant publications that the causes of renal growth and augmented function are still not fully understood. Increases in GFR and in SNGFR usually appear to be essential early events. Then the proximal tubules grow more in proportion than the rest of the nephrons, and the basolateral membranes (which carry the sodium pumps required for most tubular reabsorption) hypertrophy out of proportion to the less actively involved luminal membranes. As Oliver remarked in 1939, the sizes of the tubules come to parallel the sizes of the glomeruli they drain and larger filtered loads somehow hasten the synthesis of cytoplasmic and membrane components for the growing cells.

Whereas experimenters remove or destroy nephrons in whole kidneys or in blocks of renal tissue, ageing and renal diseases remove individual nephrons throughout both kidneys, leaving a dwindling proportion of the original population to carry on an undiminished excretory and homeostatic task. The output of urine per nephron must then increase, sometimes greatly, and the SNGFR may increase also. During healthy middle age, reductions in whole-kidney GFR lag many years behind the falling numbers of filtering glomeruli (McLachlan, 1978). Early in diseases like pyelonephritis which attack tubular tissue rather than glomeruli, both GFR per remaining nephron and measured SNGFR may increase as much as they do after healthy nephrons have been removed surgically (Bricker *et al.*, 1976). Glomerulonephritis, however, attacks glomeruli specifically and gradually reduces the kidney to an extremely heterogeneous collection of variously damaged, atrophic, hypertrophied and modified nephrons (Oliver, 1950; Franklin & Merrill, 1960). The rate of glomerular filtration is then drastically reduced; but although average SNGFR may be substantially less than normal in chronic experimental (autologous immune complex) glomerulonephritis, the range may be so large (e.g. from 5 to 90 nl/min compared with a normal of about 40 nl/min) that GFR per nephron must be greater than normal in some of the hypertrophied nephrons (Allison *et al.*, 1974).

3.3.4.3 DECREASED RATES OF GLOMERULAR FILTRATION

A. *Causes of acutely diminished GFR*

1 Change of posture. The simplest change from Smith's (1956) ideal state of rest with minimal renal vasoconstrictor tone is to sit or stand up. This reduces the rate of RPF, but the effect on the GFR of standing quietly, or of being ordinarily up and about, is no more than a few per cent, except in patients with cardiac failure whose already low GFR is depressed further (Epstein *et al.*, 1951, 1956; Surtshin & White, 1956). Suggestions that the postural fall in

GFR was exaggerated in subjects of orthostatic proteinuria (Bull, 1948; Smith, 1951) were not confirmed (Robinson, 1980). More drastic effects do occur, however, in normal human subjects who are passively up-ended on a tilt-table or who lean relaxed against a wall with no muscular activity to assist the return of venous blood from their legs. Glomerular fultration rate may then fall 20 to 30% within 15 to 30 minutes, with the FF increasing to more than 0.25 and GFR falls further if the subjects faint (Smith, 1939–40; Brun *et al.*, 1945; Smith, 1956).

2 Muscular exercise. Flow through large active muscles may divert blood from the renal circulation, but GFR is well maintained unless the exercise is uncomfortably severe (Castenfors, 1967a) and it has to be severe to depress GFR in healthy supine subjects (Castenfors, 1967b; Grimby, 1965). Walking at 3 miles per hour up a gradient of 5% on a treadmill only reduced GFR in a very hot environment which had already depressed GFR at rest (Radigan & Robinson, 1949). In fact, moderate exercise depresses GFR a great deal less than relaxation in the erect posture with consequent circulatory stasis, falling plasma volume and increasing oncotic pressure from haemoconcentration. Patients with cardiac failure, however, experience greater reductions in GFR with mild exertion than do healthy subjects (Merrill & Cargill, 1948).

3 Haemorrhage, shock and trauma. Smith (1951) reviewed experiments on dogs and work on 35 human victims of major trauma studied by Lauson *et al.* (1944). Increased vasomotor activity following the loss of substantial amounts of blood reduces GFR, but usually less than it reduces RPF. The FF therefore increases at first, but it may fall to zero if systemic arterial blood pressure falls below 60 mmHg and abolishes glomerular filtration while blood still flows through the kidneys. Rates of glomerular filtration in rabbits were reduced about 20% by the loss of a quarter of their blood, and 40% by the loss of a third, in agreement with earlier results in dogs and man (Korner, 1967).

4 Hypoxia. Moderate hypoxia corresponding to altitudes up to 7313 m had minor and inconsistent effects on GFR (Smith, 1951). Breathing 9.6% oxygen at atmospheric pressure reduced GFR in rabbits, but less than it reduced RPF, so that the FF increased. When blood pressure was less well maintained during hypoxia from breathing 0.1 to 0.2% carbon monoxide in air, GFR and RPF both fell 10 to 20% with no change in FF (Korner, 1963).

5 Pain and distress. Smith (1956) remarked that severe but tolerable pain can reduce GFR and RPF by 50%, and that Cannon had rated fright and anger as highly as haemorrhage in the list of effective sympathetic stimuli. In the patient mentioned in Section 2.2.5 who suddenly became alarmed during an investigation, GFR fell 20% while RPF fell 50% and FF increased from 0.16 to 0.25 within 30 minutes. Observations like these bear an important message for all who seek to acquire physiologically valid information from measurements on patients, healthy human subjects and conscious animals.

6 The diving reflex. The diving reflex which reduces blood flow to one tenth

of its resting rate in marine animals (Section 2.2.5; Zapol *et al.*, 1979), and the equally striking nasopharyngeal reflex of rabbits to noxious fumes (White & Franklin, 1970) must also grossly depress GFR.

7 Dehydration and depletion of sodium. Reduction of the GFR with diminishing water content of the body occurs regularly in submammalian species and contributes to homeostatic regulation of the body's water content (Knox, 1982). In reptiles this reduction in GFR is produced mainly by reducing the number of filtering nephrons (Dantzler, 1982). The amphibian antidiuretic hormone, arginine vasotocin, acts by reducing GFR not by promoting the tubular reabsorption of water as arginine vasopressin (AVP) does in mammals (Pang *et al.*, 1982).

Mammalian GFR is subject to autoregulation, and reductions with dehydration are smaller. They were, however, thought to explain the old observation that successive measurements of the clearance of inulin in one long session with the same subject get smaller (Smith, 1951). Shannon (1936) described falling GFR with dehydration in dogs, and Smith (1951) cited reductions of up to 30% after several days without water in man. The clinical and experimental dehydrations that threaten glomerular filtration most acutely are secondary to large losses of sodium in sweat, stools or urine. Their characteristics include increases in the concentration of urea in the blood (Marriott, 1950) which reflect lowered GFRs, though the clearance of urea may be depressed more than GFR itself (Jones, 1972). McCance (1936), whose classical accounts make fascinating reading, depleted human subjects of about a third of their ECF by several days of enforced sweating, and they experienced comparable reductions in GFR. Victims of cholera and infantile gastroenteritis may suffer greater losses in hours rather than days, and patients with Addison's disease (lacking aldosterone and unable to avoid losing sodium in their urine), besides being chronically dehydrated, are liable to suffer life-threatening acute exacerbations (Addisonian crises) with severe peripheral circulatory failure. Glomerular filtration is grossly depressed as a result of haemoconcentration and inadequate perfusion pressure in these and other such states of 'medical shock.'

8 Increased pressure in the ureter and renal vein. Acute increases of about 37 mmHg in ureteral pressure or 21 mmHg in renal venous pressure on one side reduced GFR reversibly by about 15% in dogs (Hall & Selkurt, 1951; Selkurt *et al.*, 1952). Renal blood flow was reduced only about 5% by the elevation of pressure, so that the FF fell.

9 Increased intrathoracic pressure. Breathing air at pressures 24 to 26 mmHg above atmospheric reduced GFR and RPF about 30% in a dozen normal human subjects (Murdaugh *et al.*, 1959), though GFR was not increased by breathing air at pressures less than atmospheric (Sieker *et al.*, 1954). Similar observations have been made on anaesthetized dogs. Although breathing against a positive pressure increases pressure in the renal veins, a more important effect is probably to displace blood away from the heart and the

large intrathoracic veins with renal effects analogous to those of haemorrhage (Gauer & Henry, 1963).

10 Anaesthesia. A great deal of experimental work on the kidney has been done on anaesthetized animals and interpreted in the hope that anaesthesia itself does not affect renal function. Light anaesthesia with barbiturates, ether or cyclopropane was not believed to affect GFR or RPF in dogs, though deep anaesthesia may depress both of these by 50%, and the effects of anaesthesia alone are aggravated by surgical trauma (Smith, 1951, 1956; Bálint, 1961).

Some barbiturate anaesthetics were later found to induce an angiotensin-mediated renal vasoconstriction in dogs, reducing RBF by more than 30% (Burger *et al.*, 1976). Moreover, effects of anaesthetics may last longer than was once thought. Valtin *et al.* (1982) found RBF and GFR still depressed 20 to 25% 3 hours after rats were catheterized under light anaesthesia with ether, and they suggested that many animals described as 'conscious' or 'awake' may not have been fully recovered. Moreover, many measurements of SNGFR and other work using micropuncture techniques are carried out during continued anaesthesia.

11 Vasoconstrictors and sympathetic nerves. The classical sympathomimetic agents, adrenaline and noradrenaline, reduce RBF but largely spare glomerular filtration. Smith (1943, 1956) showed typical reductions of about 40% in RBF and 10% in GFR with a large increase in FF in a human subject given adrenaline. Noradrenaline has a similar direct action on the kidney, but, unlike adrenaline, it does not double the flow of blood through the liver and skeletal muscles (Barcroft & Swan, 1953) and it may increase GFR by raising arterial pressure and reflexly reducing vasoconstrictor tone (Anderson *et al.*, 1981).

Moderate stimulation of renal sympathetic nerves also reduces GFR less than RPF, and increases the FF, but the traditional explanation in terms of preferential constriction of postglomerular vessels is hard to sustain if efferent glomerular arterioles are not innervated (Hollenberg, 1979). Strong stimulation of renal sympathetic nerves can halt glomerular filtration temporarily, presumably by constricting the well-innervated preglomerular vessels, and this may contribute to very low GFRs and FFs in severe shock (Lauson *et al.*, 1944).

Angiotensin II is the most powerful endogenous vasoconstrictor known, and human renal vessels are so sensitive that one thirtieth of the dose needed to raise arterial pressure can reduce RBF. Angiotensin II also reduces GFR, but increases FF in man, laboratory animals, and the isolated kidneys of rabbits, cats and dogs (Peart, 1978; Hollenberg, 1979). Both noradrenaline and AT II depressed glomerular plasma flow without reducing SNGFR in superficial nephrons of Munich Wistar rats (Brenner *et al.*, 1976a). Glomerular capillary pressure increased enough to offset the greater oncotic pressure arising from a 25% increase in FF. These results suggest constriction of the glomerular efferent arterioles, where Richards & Plant (1922) long ago suggested that adrenaline might act — because it caused the kidney to swell.

The suggestion that the renal action of noradrenaline is mediated by AT II, formed within the kidney and acting on efferent glomerular arterioles (Hollenberg, 1979; Anderson *et al.*, 1981), would readily explain the similar effects of noradrenaline, AT II and the renal sympathetic nerves. In intact animals the sympathetic nervous system can release both renin and noradrenaline within the kidney, and it can increase the concentrations of circulating catecholamines, renin and AT II. The action of AT II on postglomerular vessels could therefore provide a final common path enabling all these to work together to reduce the flow of blood through the kidneys with minimal disturbance of glomerular filtration.

12 Diurnal changes. Nocturnal reductions in GFR are the counterparts of the daytime increases mentioned in section 3.3.4.2A (9).

13 Acute renal failure. Renal failure, defined as a degree of renal insufficiency causing substantial alterations in plasma biochemistry, occurs when GFR falls below about 30 ml/min per 1.73 m^2 of body surface. Acute renal failure has many causes. Kerr (1979), citing over 500 references, discussed more than 40 categories; including diseases of the kidneys, effects of drugs, toxins and poisons, and conditions leading to shock and gross depletion of body fluids. Renal blood flow is often relatively well maintained, and FF low, suggesting that filtration pressure is diminished (Reubi & Vorburger, 1976). Thurau & Boylan (1976) referred to the nearly total suppression of glomerular filtration as an 'acute renal success' because it prevents the loss of an enormous volume of filtrate from the body when tubular reabsorption fails. Patients have lost as much as 45 to 70 litres in a day when tubular reabsorption failed and glomerular filtration was not suppressed! Thurau and Boylan proposed that GFR might be reduced by tubuloglomerular feedback as the macula densa was flooded with fluid which the tubules had failed to reabsorb further upstream. Proximal tubules in autopsy and biopsy specimens are however widely dilated, not collapsed from lack of filtrate (Bohle *et al.*, 1976), though there is little evidence of increased tubular pressure (Thurau *et al.*, 1979). Fortunately the survival value of the acute reduction in glomerular filtration when tubules fail to reabsorb the filtrate is not diminished by the uncertainties that still exist about its mechanism.

B. Causes of chronically low glomerular filtration rates

1 Ageing. Human kidneys cease growing in middle life. By the eighth decade most of them have lost about a fifth of their mass and up to half of their glomeruli have disappeared or become hyalinized and useless. Similar changes occur in rats, mice, hamsters and dogs (McLachlan, 1978). The decline in GFR with advancing age reported by Davies & Shock (1950) has since been found to be much more rapid after the fifth or sixth decade, suggesting that loss of glomeruli during middle age (but not later) may be partly offset by some hypertrophy of remaining nephrons.

2 Diet. Diets deficient in protein can significantly lower GFR in rats and dogs, but do not seem to do so in man (Dicker, 1956). Even victims of prolonged malnutrition in Europe at the end of World War II showed no reduction in GFR or RPF.

3 Chronic dehydration. Chronically low GFRs occur with depletion of ECF in Addison's disease and when sodium is lost from other causes such as pyloric stenosis. Therapeutic diets low in sodium content may also reduce glomerular filtration (Smith, 1951).

4 Lack of trophic hormones. Hypophysectomy leads to a chronic reduction in GFR in dogs, due mostly to lack of GH. According to Smith (1951), thyroidectomy produced a far smaller reduction, but Bradley et al. (1974b) described substantial reductions in GFR in hypothyroid patients and of SNGFR in hypothyroid rats compared with normal litter mates. The well established reductions in GFR in Addison's disease and after adrenalectomy are probably secondary to depletion of sodium and the reduced ECFV. McCance's (1936) subjects, depleted to about the same extent as patients with Addison's disease, had similarly depressed GFRs, though their adrenal cortical secretion should have been maximally stimulated by their severe sodium depletion and dehydration.

5 Cardiovascular diseases.

(a) Cardiac failure. The GFR is usually low and the FF increased when the kidneys receive a diminished share of the reduced cardiac output in uncompensated cardiac failure with oedema (Merrill & Cargill, 1948).

(b) Hypertension. Studies of 60 patients by Goldring et al. (1941), quoted in detail by Smith (1951), showed some reduction in GFR with increased FFs and wide variations between individuals. In a more recent study of nearly 60 patients with essential hypertension matched by paired controls, the increased FF was due solely to a reduction in RPF. The GFR was normal, and there was little variation between individuals in either group (London et al., 1981).

(c) Anaemia. Patients with severe chronic anaemia had low normal values of RPF, but RBF was depressed 30 to 40% because fewer red cells accompanied the plasma. Glomerular filtration rate was depressed about 20% and the FF was low, possibly because the lower viscosity of the cell-poor blood led to lower effective filtration pressures. Glomerular filtration rate recovered as the PCV increased when the anaemia was treated (Bradley & Bradley, 1947).

6 Miscellaneous conditions. Mechanisms of these are uncertain, and they are not discussed in detail because they throw little light on physiological regulation.

(a) Potassium depletion. Glomerular filtration was depressed in two women who were severely depleted of potassium from excessive use of laxatives (Schwartz & Relman, 1953). Although small reductions in GFR have been noted in other human subjects, and in rats and dogs, they are often absent (Jones, 1972; Massry, 1979). The laxative addicts might have been somewhat dehydrated, but their low GFRs were corrected by potassium. Sabatini &

Kurtzman (1984) considered the reduced GFR as a factor in maintaining the metabolic alkalosis associated with depletion of potassium.

(b) Magnesium depletion can apparently reduce glomerular filtration (Massry, 1979).

(c) Phosphate depletion. The GFR can be reversibly depressed in dogs and man by severe depletion of phosphate with hypophosphataemia from a large variety of causes (Massry, 1979).

(d) Hypercalcaemia. Hypercalcaemia can reduce GFR quickly and reversibly without evident structural damage to the kidney. Chronic hypercalcaemia due to hyperparathyroidism, excessive doses of vitamin D, myelomatosis, and metastatic tumours attacking the skeleton, leads to more severe and incompletely reversible impairments of filtration, with structural changes in the kidney (nephrocalcinosis, hypercalcaemic nephropathy; Jones, 1972; Massry, 1979).

(e) Gout. Glomerular filtration rate is considerably depressed when the kidneys are damaged by urate crystals in chronic gout (Smith, 1951).

7 Obstructive nephropathy. Although a transient vasodilatation may occur when the ureter is first obstructed, chronic partial or complete obstruction always reduces GFR, and there is only partial recovery after the obstruction is relieved (Wilson, 1980).

8 Glomerulonephritis. Diseases of the kidneys usually reduce GFR. Glomerulonephritis, from many causes, mostly immunological (Leaf & Cotran, 1976), attacks the glomeruli and characteristically reduces GFR more than RPF. The FF may fall to 0.10, but return later to normal or somewhat higher values with hypertension and impending renal failure late in the course of the disease (Earle et al., 1944; Smith, 1951). Early in the course of experimental glomerulonephritis SNGFR and whole-kidney GFR may be reduced similarly, with little difference between individual nephrons (Rocha et al., 1973). Single nephron filtration rate can be reduced by the loss of loops within capillary tufts, which lowers K_f as the area available for filtration diminishes (Brenner et al., 1976a). Late in chronic nephritis some nephrons may hypertrophy (Allison et al., 1974), but this fails to compensate for the destruction of others, and the typical gross reduction in whole-kidney GFR is mainly caused by loss of glomeruli. The heterogeneity of the population of remaining nephrons is most fully revealed by microdissection and micropuncture (Oliver, 1950; Kramp et al., 1974), though Smith (1943, 1951) devised ways of evaluating it during life by comparing the clearances of inulin, glucose and PAH as concentrations in the plasma were increased until tubular transport was saturated. Destruction of tubular epithelial cells reduces the capacity to secrete PAH and to reabsorb glucose; loss of glomeruli (leaving aglomerular tubules) reduces the capacity to reabsorb glucose disproportionately because glucose is not presented to all the cells that could reabsorb it. But these ingenious 'saturation titrations' were something of a *tour de force*, and they have been replaced for diagnostic purposes by renal biopsy (Muehrke & Pirani, 1972).

Finally, the most important cause of chronic lowering of GFR is destruction of nephrons in the course of progressive disease. Platt (1952) pointed out that the remaining nephrons have as much urea to excrete each day as the larger number in a pair of healthy kidneys and that the high concentration of urea that developes in the blood is not merely a laboratory sign of the presence and severity of glomerular insufficiency; it is an automatic compensating mechanism. While the concentration of urea, though high, is not increasing, urea must still be excreted as fast as it is formed, and the high concentration allows the daily load to be eliminated in a smaller volume of filtrate.

3.3.5 The control of glomerular filtration rate

3.3.5.I EXTRINSIC CONTROLS

Modifiers of GFR which impinge on the kidneys from outside include the renal sympathetic nerves and circulating hormones which back up the effects of transmitters released from nerve endings within the kidney. The sympathetic vasoconstrictor nerves act primarily to reduce RBF when there are greater demands elsewhere. During severe renal ischaemia, such as occurs in shock, especially when the action of the vasomotor nerves is augmented by circulating catecholamines, constriction of afferent glomerular arterioles may predominate and reduce glomerular filtration drastically (Korner, 1974). Moderate reductions of RBF under more physiological conditions are achieved by preferential constriction of glomerular efferent vessels, producing an increase in FF and little change in GFR (Smith, 1951, 1956).

Extreme alterations in the pressure of arterial blood with which the kidneys are perfused may also have drastic effects; but autoregulatory mechanisms protect glomerular filtration from smaller variations in blood pressure under physiological conditions. The oncotic pressure of the plasma is another property of the perfusing blood which exerts a controlling influence upon glomerular filtration. Variations in the concentration of protein in the plasma during dehydration and expansion of the body fluids are often associated with alterations in GFR in the same direction as homeostatically appropriate changes in urinary output. Dicker (1956) was unwilling to attribute increased GFRs after large intakes of water by rats and dogs to dilution of plasma proteins because plasmapheresis did not increase GFR. But after plasmapheresis the lowered volume of the plasma might offset its lower oncotic pressure, much as an increased volume of circulating plasma outweighs its greater oncotic pressure when infusions of plasma proteins restore GFR in protein-depleted patients with nephrotic syndromes. O'Connor (1962, 1977; O'Connor & Summerill, 1979) marshalled evidence that the oncotic pressure of the plasma is a major factor controlling glomerular filtration in conscious dogs, whose GFR increased about 2% for each reduction of 1 g/l in the concentration of protein in the plasma.

3.3.5.2 DETERMINANTS OF GLOMERULAR FILTRATION

Extrinsic controlling factors must ultimately act within the kidney, and Brenner and his colleagues (Brenner et al., 1976a,c) specified four 'determinants of glomerular filtration' which operate in each individual glomerulus. These are: (1) the ultrafiltration coefficient, K_f; (2) the mean pressure gradient, P', from capillary lumen to Bowman's space; (3) the oncotic pressure of afferent arteriolar plasma, π_A; and (4) glomerular plasma flow, Q_A. Separate effects of each of these determinants (assuming no change in the others) were evaluated from measurements on Munich Wistar rats with the aid of a mathematical model (Deen et al., 1972). The results are conveniently described in terms of the SNFF which is SNGFR per unit of glomerular plasma flow, Q_A. Single nephron filtration fraction can be measured in accessible glomeruli as $(1 - C_A/C_E)$, where C_A and C_E are the concentrations of protein in systemic arterial plasma (representing afferent glomerular arteriolar plasma) and in the plasma of blood removed from single glomerular efferent arterioles by micropipettes. Single nephron filtration fraction similarly calculated from afferent and arteriolar PCVs may be 80% greater than that derived from concentrations of protein in the plasma, suggesting that blood entering superficial glomeruli is richer in erythrocytes than femoral arterial blood (Jackson & Oken, 1982).

1 The ultrafiltration coefficient (K_f) is the product of the hydraulic conductivity and the area of the filtering surface. If it is large enough for filtration to proceed to equilibrium, increasing K_f shifts the point of equilibration back towards the arteriolar ends of the glomerular capillaries, but does not increase SNFF. In Munich Wistar rats, K_f is of the order of 5 nl/min per mmHg; and it can be reduced to 4 nl/min per mmHg before disequilibrium appears. The point of equilibration has then reached the efferent ends of the glomerular capillaries and a further 50% reduction in K_f depresses SNFF by about 20%. Vasoactive agents such as dibutyryl-cAMP, prostaglandins PGI_2 and PGE_2, parathormone (PTH) and vasopressin, which cause mesangial cells to contract in vitro, can reduce K_f by about 50%. Inhibitors of the AT converting enzyme prevent the effects of all these agents except vasopressin, which seem to be mediated within the kidney by renin and AT II (Dworkin et al., 1983). The magnitude and the rapidity of the alterations in K_f have suggested that the contractile mesangial cells might open or close individual capillary loops and change the area available for filtration, producing a sort of 'intraglomerular intermittence' (Hollenberg, 1979; Schor et al., 1981). Stimulation of the renal sympathetic nerves at low frequencies reduces K_f in Munich Wistar rats (Kon & Ichikawa, 1983). Increasing oncotic pressure of the plasma may increase K_f, possibly because hydraulic conductivity is increased by shrinkage of cells and widening of intercellular pathways for diffusion without changing the filtering area (Thomas et al., 1979).

2 The mean pressure gradient (P') is the difference between the mean hydrostatic pressures in glomerular capillaries and Bowman's space. In super-ficial glomeruli of Munich Wistar rats and squirrel monkeys, with capillary pressure about 45 mmHg and capsular pressure 10 mmHg, P' is about 35 mmHg and there is a negligible difference between the afferent and efferent ends of the capillaries (Maddox *et al.*, 1974; Brenner *et al.*, 1976a). Filtrate can be removed until the oncotic pressure of the remaining (efferent) plasma, π_E, reaches P', so that increasing P' makes it possible to extract more filtrate. However, SNGFR and SNFF do not increase in fixed proportion to P' because the oncotic pressure of the plasma increases more steeply than the concentration of protein.

3 The oncotic pressure of glomerular afferent plasma (π_A) is measured in plasma from peripheral blood. This is an important determinant of glomerular filtration because the closer it is to the oncotic pressure of efferent plasma at filtration equilibrium, the smaller is the amount of filtrate that can be expressed from the afferent plasma. Since SNGFR and SNFF both approach zero as π_A approaches P', the difference between π_A and P' sets an upper limit to SNFF. Munich Wistar rats and squirrel monkeys, with the same value (35 mmHg) for P', both have about 85 g/l of protein in their efferent arteriolar plasma at filtration equilibrium. But the rats have a smaller initial concentration of plasma protein (55 g/l compared with 69 g/l in the monkeys), so that their glomeruli can extract 75% more filtrate before the oncotic pressure rises to 35 mmHg; their SNFF is about 0.35 compared with 0.20 in squirrel monkeys (Maddox *et al.*, 1974). Human plasma contains about 70 g/l of protein, and the whole-kidney FF is about 0.20. Brenner *et al.* (1976a) therefore suggested that filtration might proceed to equilibrium in human kidneys, and that P' would be 35 mmHg. However, a greater capillary pressure would be consistent with the same small FF if blood left the efferent ends of the glomerular capillaries before equilibrium was attained.

4 The glomerular plasma flow (Q_A) can be evaluated indirectly in Munich Wistar rats from SNFF and the clearance of labelled inulin from plasma into tubular fluid withdrawn by micropipettes: $Q_A = \text{SNGFR/SNFF}$. When filtration proceeds to equilibrium, decreasing Q_A shifts the point of equilibration towards the afferent ends, and increasing Q_A shifts it towards the efferent ends of the glomerular capillaries. Meanwhile SNFF remains constant, and SNGFR is simply proportional to Q_A. In Munich Wistar rats studied by Brenner's group, Q_A was ordinarily about 80 nl/min, and could be increased about 30% before disequilibrium appeared. With further increases, SNFF began to fall, and SNGFR still increased with Q_A, but less steeply (Brenner *et al.*, 1976a).

The demonstration that glomerular filtration could proceed to equilibrium was welcomed because it made SNGFR a constant fraction of Q_A, and so did away with the need for an additional mechanism for autoregulation of glo-merular filtration separate from that for RBF. But filtration equilibrium is not always attained, even in the Munich Wistar rats in which it was first discovered. Some published series are too small (and their variances too large) to establish that ($P' - \pi_E$) actually reaches zero (Oken & Choi, 1981), and it may be equally difficult to prove that equilibration does not occur (Osgood *et al.*, 1982). Baylis (1981) tabulated published measurements on Munich Wistar rats from 10 laboratories, showing that equlibrium occurred in 11 studies in which the average capillary pressure was 49 mmHg, but not in five others where K_f was smaller and the average glomerular capillary pressure was 54 mmHg.

Tucker *et al.* (1977) explored the contributions of the different determinants to increasing the filtration rate in Munich Wistar rats. During filtration equilibrium, Q_A contributed 60%, π_A 27%, and P' 13% to increasing filtration rates. During disequilibrium following infusions which increased the volume of circulating plasma, Q_A was still the most important, but it contributed only 30%, P' 25%, and π_A 21%. The ultrafiltration coefficient, K_f, which only appeared to be important under rather extreme conditions and in pathological states, contributed 21%.

Since the plasma is the source of the glomerular filtrate, it is not surprising that the glomerular plasma flow should be such an important determinant of GFR, even under nonequilibrium conditions when GFR may depend upon the glomerular plasma flow partly because of flow-dependent changes in capillary protein concentration (Wright, 1982). The other three determinants control what fraction of the incoming plasma shall become glomerular filtrate. Filtration equilibrium, when it occurs, is important not so much because it fixes the ratio of SNGFR to Q_A, but rather because it creates a reserve of filtering area which can be brought into use when Q_A increases and the point of equilibration is displaced efferentwards (Thurau *et al.*, 1979). With further increases in Q_A, SNFF begins to fall, and the next most important determinants of filtration rate are π_A and P'. Since lower concentrations of plasma protein and larger capillary pressures both increase effective filtration pressure, it might be expected that the effects of lowering π_A and of increasing P' would be equivalent. But a parallel reduction in K_f which occurs when π_A is reduced partly offsets the expected increase in filtration rate, and this leaves P' as the more important variable. The pressure gradient from glomeruli to Bowman's capsule is especially important for preserving filtration when blood is diverted away from the kidneys. Moderate stimulation of the renal sympathetic nerves, and moderate concentrations of circulating catecholamines, which constrict glomerular efferent more than glomerular afferent arterioles, increase P'. The single nephron filtration fraction then increases almost enough to compensate for the reduction in Q_A, and the RBF can be reduced with little loss of GFR.

3.3.5.3 INTRINSIC CONTROLS

The four determinants of glomerular filtration are intrinsic in the limited sense that they act within the kidney. But they are also mediators for extrinsic controls which impinge upon them. P' and Q_A depend upon sympathetic nerve impulses, arterial blood pressure and cardiac output; π_A is a property of the arterial blood coming into the kidney; K_f can be modified by π_A as well as by vasoactive agents and may be partly controlled by extrinsic neural and humoral factors.

Vasoactive agents formed within the kidney are more strictly intrinsic, but in so far as they protect glomerular filtration and blood flow from external threats, they too must respond to extrinsic factors; and they often act as mediators in pathways of extrinsic control. Besides the renin–angiotensin system, these agents include catecholamines released from constrictor nerve endings as well as PGs, renal kinins, and probably dopamine (Lee, 1982), which are mainly vasodilator. The renal kinins are present almost exclusively in distal segments of the nephrons and probably do not affect GFR (Mills, 1982), while extrinsic kallikrein and circulating kinins pass into the glomerular filtrate and are destroyed by the proximal tubular epithelium (Clappison *et al.*, 1981). These agents are considered further as agents which may control the excretion of sodium in Section 7.4.4.6; and atrial natriuretic peptides (Section 7.4.4.4) should be added to the list.

The renal PGs are synthesized mainly in the cortex, but they are not considered major determinants of the resting tone of the kidney's resistance vessels, and do not increase RBF unless these vessels are constricted (Lote, 1982). By modulating the constrictor actions of AT and noradrenaline they help to maintain the circulation of blood and its optimal distribution within the kidney in the face of threats such as those posed by acute trauma (Lifschitz, 1981), salt depletion, haemorrhage and endotoxic shock (Schnermann & Briggs, 1981). They may also potentiate the dilator actions of kinins, and so help to maintain renal perfusion without much affecting GFR.

It is becoming apparent that these intrinsic vasoactive agents interact in extremely complex and confusing ways. For example, the converting enzyme which changes AT I into active AT II seems to be identical with the kininase which destroys vasodilator kinins. The PGs, especially PGE_1 or one of its stable metabolites, participate in the release of renin, yet oppose the constrictor action of AT II. Thus, although the PGs, along with catecholamines, are involved in activating the renin–angiotensin system, they oppose the vasoconstrictor actions of its endproducts as well as those of the catecholamines. Having so many actions covered by counteractions is a little like driving a car with feet on both the brake and accelerator pedals; but the system of checks and balances probably helps to maintain the stability of the renal circulation and glomerular filtration.

The most truly intrinsic mechanisms are perhaps those that subserve auto-regulation and can act in isolated, perfused kidneys. Autoregulation originally implied keeping RPF and GFR constant in spite of alterations in arterial blood pressure; and the myogenic theory (Section 2.2.7) was a plausible attempt to explain it mechanically by direct effects upon the tone of the resistance vessels. Thurau (1963), however, insisted that autoregulation should be understood in relation to total function of the kidney, and emphasis swung during the next two decades towards mechanisms linking glomerular blood flow and filtration to the fate of the filtrate downstream. Autoregulation of blood flow is severely impaired in nonfiltering kidneys (Davis & Freeman, 1976; Sadowski & Wocial, 1977); and the need for balance between glomerular and tubular functions under normal conditions is readily apparent. Each day an average human tubule receives about 12 μmol of sodium in its glomerular filtrate, reabsorbs 11.95 μmol, and allows 0.05 μmol to be excreted in the urine. If all the 2 million tubular systems in the two kidneys received 1% too much filtrate or reabsorbed 1% too little sodium, the body would lose 240 mmol each day — about one tenth of the amount of sodium in the ECF.

Kruhøffer (1960) proposed a simple, hydrostatic mechanism which could control glomerulotubular balance (GTB) in each individual nephron. If resistance to flow along the tubules was, perhaps, five times as great as resistance to filtration through the glomerular membrane, and was localized in distal parts of the nephrons, the rate of proximal reabsorption should determine GFR. If proximal reabsorption failed to keep pace with glomerular filtration, pressure should rise in the tubular lumen and be transmitted back to Bowman's capsule, where it should reduce the effective filtration pressure and the rate of filtration. A very small gradient of pressure should ordinarily be sufficient to maintain flow along the proximal tubules, because only a small fraction of the filtrate traverses the whole length of the tubules. Most of the fluid is reabsorbed from proximal segments by a process that does not need luminal pressure to drive it (Leyssac, 1963). Early measurements (Windhager, 1968) confirmed that hydrostatic pressures within the tubules dropped most along loops of Henle, and very little along proximal tubules. Proximal tubular pressure should, however, increase if outflow is prevented or if reabsorption stops; and glomerular filtration continued at reduced rates after occlusion of the ureter in rats (Selkurt *et al.*, 1965) and dogs (Taylor & Ullman, 1961), as well as after suppression of tubular activity by chilling (Bickford & Winton, 1937) or cyanide (Bayliss & Lundsgaard, 1932). Proximal intratubular pressures measured during these experiments had increased.

Kruhøffer's proposal received remarkably little notice after Thurau (1963; Thurau & Schnermann, 1965) demonstrated another mechanism, whereby glomerular plasma flow and filtration could be dramatically reduced without the intervention of an increased back-pressure. When solutions containing higher concentrations of sodium chloride were conveyed to the region of the macula densa of a micropunctured nephron through the loop of Henle or by retrograde perfusion of the distal tubule, the filtration rate in the corresponding glomerulus and the pressure in its proximal tubule both fell, indicating that the reduction in filtration rate was due to events proximal to the filter. Hundreds of publications describing and characterizing this phenomenon of tubuloglomerular feedback appeared in the next two decades, and its status was reviewed in a symposium on the JGA edited by Thurau & Schnermann in 1982.

Most filtered sodium is reabsorbed by the proximal tubule and the loop of

Henle. Fluid passing the macula densa to enter the distal tubule is hypotonic with a concentration of sodium less than 50 mM, probably between 20 and 25 mM (Schnermann *et al.*, 1982). A reduction in the rate of proximal reabsorption, or an increase in glomerular filtration unmatched by faster reabsorption, would supply the distal nephron with fluid richer in sodium and increase the concentration bathing the macula densa. Thurau (1963) originally suggested that the cells of the macula densa responded to increasing concentrations of sodium by releasing renin, which mediated a chain of events leading to constriction of the corresponding glomerular arterioles, and a consequent reduction in glomerular plasma flow and filtration; this would occur in nephrons which filtered too much sodium for the proximal tubules to deal with before the fluid passed on to more distal segments. A tendency for glomerular blood flow and filtration to increase as a result of increased arterial pressure should then be matched by arteriolar constriction, and this could account for the integrated autoregulation of glomerular blood flow and filtration in the whole kidney.

The phenomenon of tubuloglomerular feedback (TGFB) is now well established, but it is not certain whether the signal which activates the sensor is the concentration of sodium chloride; the concentration, or the rate of reabsorption, of either ion (Schnermann & Briggs, 1982; Wright *et al.*, 1982; cf. Section 2.2.7); or total concentration without specificity for individual ions (Bell, 1982; Bell & Navar, 1982). It is also not certain that the renin—angiotensin system provides the link between what is monitored by the macula densa and what happens at the glomerulus. Thurau favoured renin because the feedback was best seen in sodium-depleted animals with kidneys rich in renin. But, as already mentioned, AT formed within the kidney acts on glomerular efferent arterioles and would increase rather than decrease GFR (Frega *et al.*, 1980a; Section 2.2.7). Moreover, although autoregulatory behaviour was attenuated, it was not abolished by inhibiting the angiotensin converting enzyme (Thurau, 1981; Ploth & Roy, 1982); the renin—angiotensin system may cooperate with the renal PGs as a modulator rather than as a mediator of the feedback. Schnermann & Briggs (1986) stated explicitly that the renin—angiotensin system cannot be a mediator of the feedback response because increased concentrations of sodium chloride at the macula densa reduce glomerular filtration and suppress the secretion of renin at the same time.

Whatever may be the function of renin within the kidney, one of its most important extrarenal functions is the generation of AT in peripheral blood, which then stimulates the biosynthesis of aldosterone in the adrenal cortex. Aldosterone is concerned with the conservation of sodium by the kidney and also by other organs of external exchange like the salivary, intestinal and sweat glands. In this context it might be more appropriate for the macula densa to respond to lower rather than to higher concentrations of sodium. Davis & Freeman (1976) considered that the macula does respond to lower concentrations of sodium, as proposed by Vander (1967), but they were not convinced that the macula densa has a primary role in regulating the secretion of renin and did not regard the macular feedback as important under physiological conditions. There might be less confusion if more authors distinguished clearly between release of renin within the kidney and release of renin from the kidney into peripheral blood. Sodium-sensing by the macula densa is only one of a number of mechanisms controlling the release of renin into the general circulation, and nonfiltering kidneys (with the macula densa eliminated) can still secrete renin in response to reductions in the volume of blood.

If all the glomeruli in intact kidneys responded as dramatically to increased distal loads of sodium chloride as some in punctured nephrons have been shown to do, saline diuresis should be modest or nonexistent. Yet the enormous diuretic potency of strong (10%) solutions of sodium salts was well known to nineteenth century German pharmacologists like Dreser (1982), and Starling (1909). It then seemed to be forgotten until McCance rediscovered it in the 1940s and recorded spectacular increases in GFR accompanying saline diuresis in man (Robinson, 1954). Any feedback loop which suppresses glomerular filtration in rsponse to excess sodium chloride in the distal tubules must be overridden during extreme saline diuresis, and there is evidence that the feedback is turned off by loading the body with sodium. Wright & Briggs (1979) reviewed two dozen experimental studies, three in dogs, the rest in rats, designed to test for the existence of TGFB. About half of these showed, in animals with adequate blood pressure and not loaded with salt, that SNGFR was 15 to 20% greater when tubular fluid carrying the glomerular marker was collected from proximal tubules than when it was taken from distal tubules after flowing past the macula densa. The failure of some experiments to demonstrate the control of filtration rates by TGFB might have been due to some animal foods containing more salt than others, so that the responses were blunted by abundant intakes of dietary salt. The 'successful' experiments were carried out at constant blood pressures, and therefore yielded no direct information about a possible contribution of the macular feedback loop to autoregulation of glomerular filtration in face of variations in arterial pressure.

It is paradoxical that most attempts to demonstrate TGFB or to measure its sensitivity were made with the feedback loop broken, or open (Mason & Moore, 1982). Collecting proximal tubular fluid to measure SNGFR interrupts the flow past the macula densa into the distal tubule; perfusion of the loop of Henle and retrograde perfusion of the distal tubule interfere with the normal pattern of flow in the nephron. Mason & Moore avoided opening the loop by perfusing through early parts of the proximal tubules, and confirmed that SNGFR was reduced with a negligible increase in proximal tubular pressure. However, studies in which the continuity of the feedback loop was broken furnished some of the best evidence, not only that distal events can affect glomerular filtration, but that a restraining influence is operative at ordinary filtration rates, not merely in emergency when the distal nephron is flooded with sodium-rich fluids. Hence both increases and decreases in distal tubular flow should produce appropriate alterations in filtration rate (Briggs, 1982), and the feedback mechanism actually seems to be most sensitive around normal rates (Blantz & Pelayo, 1984). The actions of diuretics are also consistent with the notion of a feedback operating continuously under physiological conditions. Some of the older diuretics inhibit reabsorption of sodium in the proximal tubules and the extra sodium passing on to the distal tubules may activate the feedback loop and restrict the diuresis by reducing the rate of filtration. Diuretics like furosemide which have the further action of opening the feedback loop are more effective (Thurau & Mason, 1974).

It is interesting to inquire whether the sensitivity of the feedback is adequate for what is required of it. Increases in the rate of flow into the distal tubules of rats and dogs lead to reductions of comparable magnitude in the flow through corresponding proximal tubules (Thurau & Mason, 1974; Briggs, 1982; Schnermann & Briggs, 1982). Wright (1981) stated that increasing late proximal tubular flow in rats reduced SNGFR by about half as much, and that the sensitivity was increased by haemorrhage, sodium depletion and dehydration, but reduced by volume expansion. The sensitivity was not affected by acute denervation of the kidney (Takabatake, 1982). Increasing rates of perfusion through the loops of Henle by 30 nl/min approximately doubled the concentration of sodium chloride in distal tubular fluid; and SNGFR was reduced by 15 nl/min. Increasing macular sodium chloride concentration from 20 to 60 mM reduced early proximal tubular flow by 12 nl/min (Schnermann & Briggs, 1982). If two thirds of the glomerular filtrate is normally lost before reaching the distal tubule (Bennett et al., 1967), an increase in distal delivery would have to elicit three times as great a reduction in SNGFR for perfect compensation. So long as proximal tubular input is reduced less than distal tubular inflow increases, TGFB need not be overridden to permit saline diuresis to occur; the diuresis should be moderated but not wholly prevented, even if salt loading does not reduce the sensitivity of the feedback. Renal interstitial pressure in the vicinity of the JGA, which is increased by salt loading and reduced in dehydration, may affect the sensitivity of the feedback (Persson et al., 1982). Renal interstitial pressure is also increased during moderate hyperglycaemia, which can abolish the feedback response to increased flow through the loop of Henle (Blantz et al., 1982).

Direct demonstrations of TGFB were limited to superficial nephrons until Müller-Suur et al. (1982) reported that SNGFR, glomerular capillary pressure and flow into the decending limb of Henle, were all reduced by increased flow up the ascending limb of Henle in juxtamedullary nephrons. Tubuloglomerular feedback may therefore be a property of the whole population of nephrons, though this cannot be demonstrated in intact kidneys. It is, however, doubtful how far the 'normal' rates of distal tubular flow observed in punctured nephrons in the exposed kidneys of anaesthetized animals (and around which the feedback loop appears to operate with optimal sensitivity) correspond to physiological rates in intact kidneys. Thurau & Boylan (1976) suggested that during acute renal failure the feedback is active in the whole kidney, and causes the drastic reduction in glomerular filtration which conserves ECF when the damaged tubules cannot reabsorb the filtrate.

A mechanism essentially similar to Kruhøffer's (1960) was revived, without reference to the original, by Häberle & Davis (1982). They suggested that the feedback operating through the macula densa is supplemented by a 'hydrodynamic feedback that arises because the loop of Henle offers considerable resistance to fluid flow and may thus be a major determinant of proximal tubular pressure and hence, in turn, of GFR'. The macular TGFB appeared to be most sensitive in the range over 2 to 3 nl/min on either side of normal distal tubular flows, and to be reinforced by the hydrodynamic mechanism at greater deviations from normal rates of flow.

The contractility of mesangial cells may also supplement the responses of glomerular arterioles in the feedback control of GFR (Ichikawa, 1982). Faster perfusion of the loop of Henle in Munich Wistar rats reduced SNGFR by 35%, but reduced glomerular plasma flow by only 25%, so that the FF fell from 0.37 to 0.30. Direct measurements of glomerular capillary pressure showed that P' was unchanged, as was π_A; and since the fall in Q_A could not account for the reduction in SNGFR, it followed that K_f had been reduced (from 0.6 to 0.25 nl/s per mmHg) presumably by contraction of mesangial cells.

It therefore seems that at least four factors contribute to the intrinsic control of glomerular filtration rates:

1 A myogenic mechanism, which operates at the level of the vascular smooth muscle, regardless of the fate of the filtrate, and helps to hold GFR and RPF stable in the face of variations in arterial pressure.
2 The 'Kruhøffer' or some other hydrodynamic mechanism.
3 Distal TGFB from the macula densa to arteriolar smooth muscle.
4 Distal TGFB to mesangial cells.

These help to match glomerular filtration to subsequent reabsorption and prevent overloading of tubules with resultant loss of extracellular ions and water. They could also provide fine tuning for the myogenic mechanism controlling primarily RBF.

Experiments designed to reveal the time relations of adjustments to sudden increases in arterial pressure can separate the roles of these factors to some extent. Rats showed a rapid increase in renal vascular resistance within 1 second (myogenic response ?), followed by a further similar increase which was about 10 times slower and presumably followed increased delivery of fluid to the distal tubule (Marsh, 1982). Moore (1982) also distinguished a separate 'TGFB-independent' mechanism which was rapid and presumably myogenic. The myogenic component is relatively unimportant in dogs, where adjustments in vascular resistance occur in time with increases in outflow of urine (Navar *et al.*, 1982).

Finally, TGFB is not the only mechanism subserving autoregulation and glomerulotubular balance (GTB) (Schnermann *et al.*, 1984). But when other mechanisms prove inadequate, and too much is filtered into a tubule to be reabsorbed proximally so that excess fluid reaches the distal tubule, TGFB can help by reducing the rate of glomerular filtration. Besides protecting against the overloading of tubular capacity to reabsorb, TGFB may also help to keep a balance between different nephrons within the kidney by allocating filtrate to those nephrons which are best able to deal with it.

3.3.5.4 THE REGULATION OF GLOMERULAR FILTRATION RATE

Homer Smith (1951), in his great monograph, described a large number of ways in which the GFR could be disturbed, but said extremely little about how it is regulated; and there is little to add. The glomeruli function in parallel. Evidence of redistribution between superficial and deep nephrons is still confusing, and individual glomeruli are not subject to extrinsic control like motor units in skeletal muscles which have motor nerve fibres to dictate their activity.

Since no more than one sixth (often less then 1%) of filtered water is ordinarily excreted, the volume of urine must be determined downstream, independently of GFR. Neurally mediated temporary reductions in GFR with exercise, postural changes and other transient stresses usually have little effect on the daily volume of filtrate, and filtered loads of solutes like urea and creatinine can be maintained by small consequential increases in their concentrations in the plasma. More prolonged alterations in GFR with dehydration, loss of blood, high intakes of dietary protein and increased volumes of body fluids are in the same direction as the accompanying changes in output of urine, but are not necessary for these changes to occur.

The sympathetic vasoconstrictors are activated by reflexes affecting systemic arterial pressure, cardiac output and the distribution of circulating blood. Reflexes from atrial receptors which might be especially concerned with the volume of blood have not been proved to affect GFR (Linden & Kappagoda, 1982), and reflexes from the carotid sinus have much less effect than emotional stresses (Di Bona, 1982). Reflexes which reduce the renal circulation when other vascular beds take more blood may incidentally reduce GFR, but they do not primarily control it, and, except under severe stresses, they tend to spare filtration when RBF is reduced. Satisfactory functioning of the kidneys depends upon continuing glomerular filtration, but does not require its rate to be kept constant. The kidneys manage their own affairs without the more detailed extrinsic neural controls that act on salivary, sweat and other glands which secrete intermittently.

In summary: extrinsic controls by sympathetic nerves and circulating vaso-constrictors serve mainly to divert flow from the renal circulation when more blood flows elsewhere, and they incidentally reduce GFR, usually to a smaller extent. Since GFR is the aggregated SNGFR of all the nephrons, regulation and autoregulation of GFR ultimately depend upon intrinsic mechanisms affecting individual nephrons. Intrinsic vasoactive agents cooperating with extrinsic factors as mediators and modulators help to preserve glomerular filtration when RBF is threatened. Other intrinsic controls are more concerned with the kidneys' own operation. Sensors in each nephron, particularly in the macula densa, monitor changes in volume and composition of fluid entering the distal tubules, and in ways which are not yet fully clarified, restrict filtration rates to match tubular reabsorption. This TGFB may also assist the myogenic activity of vascular smooth muscle to make the GFR relatively independent of blood pressure as such, and it provides a functional link between the vascular and the secretory organs which make up the kidney.

3.4 GLOMERULAR FILTRATION AND THE FORMATION OF URINE

3.4.1 Implications for tubular functions

The rate of glomerular filtration is so large that in spite of its physiological variations, all the circulating plasma is submitted to filtration up to 50 times every day. Glomerular filtration is therefore an effective means of removing waste products from the blood, including foreign substances and surplus water and soluble constituents of the body. It is, however, quite indiscriminate. If the human kidneys consisted only of their glomeruli, urea could be excreted adequately, but all the body's water and essential solutes would be lost in a few hours. Since the lumina of the renal tubules are continuous with the external environment through the renal pelvis and the urinary tract, all the constituents of the glomerular filtrate are already outside the body. But they are not beyond recall. A comparison of the glomerular filtrate and the urine formed in 24 hours (Table 3.8) emphasizes that the tubules are not mere passive conduits. They normally reabsorb 99% or more of the water, all the glucose, most of the amino acids, potassium and calcium, and nearly half the urea that escaped in the glomerular filtrate along with water and the solutes destined to be excreted.

Reabsorption is not the tubules' only activity; they transfer some substances actively from plasma to urine, and they manufacture some constituents of the urine, like ammonium, as well as hormones. But most transport across the tubular epithelium is directed 'backwards' from the duct system to the blood, not from blood to duct as in many other glands. Glomerular filtration is therefore largely responsible for the excretory functions of the kidney, and the tubules for the renal conservation of essential solutes and water. The urine consists mostly of what gets left behind from the process of tubular reabsorption, while the most important secretory product of the kidneys is the ECF. The human kidneys add about 180 litres of ECF to the plasma every

Table 3.8 A comparison of one day's glomerular filtrate and urine: approximate amounts in round figures for an adult person

Substance	Amount in glomerular filtrate	Amount in urine
Sodium	25 000 mmol	100 mmol
Potassium	800 mmol	80 mmol
Calcium	250 mmol	5 mmol
Glucose	900 mmol	NIL
Amino acids	60 g	2 g
Urea	1000 mmol	600 mmol
Water	180 litres	0.5 to 2 litres

day, and are therefore well disposed to regulate its composition. Moreover, since far more of the glomerular filtrate is reabsorbed than goes on into the urine, the fluid which is reabsorbed resembles protein-free plasma so closely that the easiest way to discover its average composition is to analyse the plasma.

Other consequences of the relationship between glomerular filtration and tubular reabsorption in mammalian kidneys include:

1 Slight alterations in tubular activity can cause large changes in the urine. If (Table 3.8) GFR remained unchanged while the tubules reabsorbed 0.4% less sodium, the amount in the urine would increase by 100%; and if the tubules reabsorbed 0.4% more, there would be no sodium in the urine.

2 Conversely, large alterations in the volume and composition of the urine may imply only small alterations in tubular activity. This makes changes in tubular activity very difficult to detect and to measure, for they are often small compared with errors in analysing plasma and urine and in determining GFR.

3 Diuretic drugs which increase the flow of urine without increasing GFR may be inhibitors, not stimulants, of renal tubular activity.

4 Diseased kidneys may declare their failing function by producing a larger rather than a smaller volume of urine.

Measurements of GFRs by the clearance of substances like inulin first made quantitative investigations of the net activity of the renal tubules possible, by enabling the filtered loads of solutes to be compared with their rates of urinary excretion. The clearance ratio C_X/C_{IN} provides a useful criterion of the direction of tubular activity. For a given period, after a steady state has been attained

$$\frac{C_X}{C_{IN}} = \frac{C_X}{GFR} = \frac{[X]_U \cdot V}{[X]_P \cdot GFR} = \frac{\text{Amount of X excreted in urine}}{\text{Amount of X in glomerular filtrate}} \quad (3.8)$$

If C_X/C_{IN} is less than 1.0, less of X reaches the urine than was present in the glomerular filtrate, i.e. X is reabsorbed (unless it is destroyed in the tubules or was incompletely filtered). Conversely, if C_X/C_{IN} is greater than 1.0, more X is excreted than was present in the glomerular filtrate, which indicates tubular secretion of X. The net rate of reabsorption of a substance whose clearance ratio is less than 1.0 is equal to the difference between its filtered load, $[X]_P$. GFR, and its rate of excretion in the urine. The actual rate of reabsorption will be greater than this if early segments of the tubule secrete an additional quantity of the solute, which is later reabsorbed downstream; but this will not be revealed by clearance measurements alone.

It is not necessary to correct for the water content of the plasma when calculating filtered loads to compare with rates of urinary excretion. The conventional GFR overestimates the actual rate of formation of glomerular filtrate because the plasma proteins are retained and do not contribute to the volume of filtrate (Section 3.3.2). At the same time, the concentration in whole plasma underestimates the concentration in the filtrate in the same proportion as the volume of filtrate is overestimated; hence the product of the conventional GFR and a solute's concentration in whole plasma gives its filtered load correctly, at least for a nonelectrolyte.

3.4.2 Donnan ratios and filtered loads

Corrections are required for diffusible electrolytes because the negative charges on protein anions retained in the plasma affect the concentrations of diffusible ions. The Gibbs–Donnan membrane equilibrium distribution requires that

$$\frac{[Na^+]_1}{[Na^+]_2} = \frac{[K^+]_1}{[K^+]_2} = \frac{\sqrt{[Ca^{2+}]_1}}{\sqrt{[Ca^{2+}]_2}} = \frac{[Cl^-]_2}{[Cl^-]_1} = \frac{[HCO_3^-]_2}{[HCO_3^-]_1} = r \qquad (3.9)$$

where r is the Donnan ratio and the subscripts delineate concentrations in the two phases at equilibrium (Robinson, 1975b). Note the symmetry: the concentration ratio should be the same for all monovalent cations and equal to the reciprocal of the concentration ratio for monovalent anions. Davson (1956) determined concentration ratios for dialysate water/plasma water: Na^+, 0.945; K^+, 0.96; Cl^-, 1.04; Mg^{2+}, 0.80; Ca^{2+}, 0.65. The divalent cations were probably not wholly diffusible, because if the Donnan ratio is 0.95 (as it was approximately for the monovalent cations) the concentration ratio for all freely diffusible divalent cations should be $(0.95)^2 = 0.90$, and the ratio for diffusible monovalent anions should be 1.05. Some electrolytes (e.g. calcium, magnesium, thiocyanate, organic anions like phenol red) are partly bound to plasma proteins and appear in lower concentrations in the filtrate; the Donnan equilibrium distribution governs only the smaller freely diffusible fractions of the ions present. Homer Smith (1951) gave empirical factors of 1.02 for concentrations of chloride and bicarbonate, 0.95 for sodium and 0.90 for potassium; these are unsymmetrical, partly because Smith included a correction for the water content of the plasma. It is probably most satisfactory to calculate filtered loads of diffusible, monovalent ions by multiplying their concentrations in whole plasma by the appropriate (symmetrical) Donnan factors and by the conventional rate of glomerular filtration of whole plasma.

In summary: filtered load = $[X]_P \cdot r \cdot GFR$; and the net rate of tubular reabsorption is $[X]_P \cdot r \cdot GFR - [X]_U \cdot V$. If this is negative, tubular secretion must be occurring.

Note: (1) Use r^n for n-valent cations and $1/r^n$ for n-valent anions; (2) for non-electrolytes, $r = 1.0$.

Some limited information can be obtained by comparing the measured clearances of nonglomerular substances. Assuming that the (unmeasured) GFR is the same for all, their filtered loads should be proportional to their concentrations in the plasma, multiplied by appropriate Donnan factors. But glomerular clearances are required to establish absolute GFRs and rates of tubular transport in whole kidneys.

3.4.3 Flow and diffusion in the renal tubule

The linear velocity with which the glomerular filtrate travels along the renal tubule is greatest at the outset. Apart from a temporary speeding up when the channel narrows at the entrance to the loop of Henle, it becomes progressively slower as water and solutes are reabsorbed. The slower onward movement as the residual volume diminishes permits the filtrate to spend longer in late segments which complete the elaboration of the urine.

It is important that the tubular fluid shall not pass through and leave important segments of the nephron before equilibrium can be reached between the centre of the lumen and layers in contact with the wall. If the radius of the tubule is $10\,\mu m$ ($10^{-3}\,cm$), diffusion in solution between the centre and the periphery should come close to equilibrium in 0.05 second (Jacobs, 1935). Each human renal tubule receives about $10^{-6}\,ml$ of filtrate per second. Hence if the radius is $10^{-3}\,cm$, the initial average linear velocity will $10^{-6}/\pi \cdot (10^{-3})^2$ = about $0.3\,cm/s$. A radius of $15\,\mu m$ would give an initial velocity of $10^{-6}/\pi \cdot (1.5 \times 10^{-3})^2$ = about $0.14\,cm/s$. A reasonable intermediate estimate of $2\,mm/s$ is larger than, but comparable with rates of about $0.3\,mm/s$, averaged over the whole length of the proximal convoluted tubules, which Steinhausen et al. (1965) deduced from times taken by the dye lissamine green to traverse superficial proximal tubules in cats and rats.

A starting speed of $2\,mm/s$ does not seem rapid but in a tubule with a radius of $10\,\mu m$ it is 100 times the diameter per second. This corresponds to $1\,km/s$ along a river or a road $10\,m$ wide; and $1\,km/s$ is $3600\,km$ per hour! Within the renal tubule, diffusion is so rapid that the fluid would move onwards by only $0.1\,mm$ in the time taken for diffusion across the lumen to equalize concentrations between the centre and the periphery, and diffusion would be increasingly favoured by the slower flows further downstream. These simple considerations support the conclusion reached more circuitously (Robinson, 1954, p. 84 to 86) that diffusion proceeds practically to equilibrium within the lumina of normal nephrons.

CHAPTER 4
Tubular function

4.1 INTRODUCTION

Each minute about 60 nl of glomerular filtrate commences its journey along each human nephron, and between 10 nl and 0.25 nl, usually a little less than 1 nl, finally emerges, greatly modified, as urine. Von Möllendorff (1930) estimated the superficial area of a single human proximal tubule as $2.5 \, mm^2$, which would be an underestimate if the microvilli forming the prominent brush border greatly increase the surface area, but the microvilli appear to be embedded in a glycocalyx rather than free in the lumen. An estimate of $5 \, mm^2$ for each entire nephron would allow $10 \, m^2$ for the total area of tubular epithelium in two kidneys, much more than the total area of the glomerular capillaries. Hence a relatively large area of epithelium is available for the task of modifying the filtrate by selective reabsorption and secretion; and according to Winton (1956b) the superficial area of the peritubular capillaries which receive the reabsorbed fluid into the blood is greater still, between 15 and 60 times that of the glomerular filtering surface.

The epithelial tube itself differs from point to point of its length and from nephron to nephron. The great heterogeneity of the nephron population precludes a treatment of tubular function in terms of transport across a single epithelial sheet, and anatomically different segments may handle different constituents of the urine (Jacobson, 1981; Knepper & Burg, 1983). The suggestion (Robinson, 1954, p. 154) that the kidney can provide the general physiologist with 'a battery of cells specialized for transferring substances across their cytoplasm, and arranged in parallel to produce macroscopic effects which are similar to the activities of the individual cells' has lost some of its validity. But attempts to grow cultured cells in sheets are beginning to succeed (Handler, 1986); and meanwhile ingenious physiologists have managed to study the activities of cells of a kind by sophisticated micromethods applied to short segments of individual tubules *in situ* or isolated *in vitro* (Windhager, 1968, 1981).

It will be convenient to list methods of investigation, and then to begin an account of tubular function somewhat traditionally with outlines of the tubular reabsorption of some important organic substances; to deal briefly with some electrolytes and water, leaving more detailed consideration of the handling of water for Chapter 5; to follow this with an outline of tubular secretion; and finally to mention some metabolic functions. The relevant literature is so extensive that some excellent reviews have been cited rather than many of

the individual publications to which they give access. Since this book is
concerned largely with the kidneys as organs of the body, no attempt has
been made to present the membrane and cellular physiology underlying its
functions in detail. Robinson (1975b) gave an introductory outline of major
concepts, and reference is made to some more rigorous and specialized
treatments.

4.1.1 Methods for investigating tubular function

A brief outline of available methods may be useful, though it is little more
than an annotated list. For further details and references see Windhager
(1981).

1 Tubular function in intact kidneys.

(a) Clearance techniques. Simultaneous measurements on glomerular
markers and other substances by classical clearance methods reveal tubular
activity by differences between corresponding glomerular filtrate and urine.
The results are averages over all tubules from which urine is collected.

(b) Stop-flow analysis. Cushny (1926) noted that with flow stopped, 'the
epithelium of the tubules, no longer overwhelmed by the flood of filtrate, can
elaborate it more completely'. Three decades later Malvin *et al.* (1958) introduced the method of stop-flow analysis, in which small samples of urine are
collected in quick succession after release of a ureter which has been obstructed
for a few minutes during osmotic diuresis with mannitol. The first samples
presumably come from the most distal segments. Inulin and *p*-aminohippurate
injected before the obstruction is released herald the arrival of fresh filtrate
and of proximal tubular fluid. The column of tubular fluid is not quite
arrested, though the mannitol used as diuretic slows the reabsorption of
sodium and water which permits filtration to continue (Taylor & Ullman,
1961). Segments represented by later samples overlap because nephrons
differ in length, but the method has yielded useful information, particularly
about distal events in the nephron.

2 Micropuncture of individual nephrons *in situ*. Fine-tipped micropipettes
can be used to withdraw samples of freely flowing tubular fluid from accessible
parts of nephrons, or fluid from columns injected into oil drops placed in the
lumen beforehand; in the latter case reabsorption of fluid may be followed by
time-lapse photography. The use of ^{14}C-inulin has made it possible to determine SNGFR and to measure the reabsorption of water along individual
tubules. By using more than one pipette, tubular segments, peritubular capillaries, or both, can be perfused with artificial solutions and changes in the
volume and composition of tubular fluid can be measured. Electrodes can be
inserted to measure transepithelial potential differences (pd), and measurements of short-circuit current permit movements of ions to be assessed in
relation to gradients of electrochemical potential (Frömter, 1984).

These methods can only be applied to parts of the proximal and distal convoluted tubules of superficial nephrons. Loops of Henle and the collecting system are usually inaccessible except in some desert-dwelling rodents whose kidneys have a single elongated papilla that projects into the upper end of the ureter. Withdrawing or introducing fluid may affect the functions of punctured tubules, and the few superficial nephrons from which it is possible to sample may not be typical of the far greater number that cannot be entered. It is also uncertain how far a surgically exposed kidney in an anaesthetized animal can be regarded as physiologically normal, and the superficial nephrons which can be punctured seem most likely to be disturbed by exposure of the kidney and the removal of the capsule to gain access. These sophisticated and ingenious techniques have yielded a great deal of information about what some accessible tubular segments can do under rather unphysiological conditions, but it cannot be proved that all nephrons always behave in exactly the same way during life.

3 Perfusion of segments of isolated nephrons. Burg and a number of colleagues developed methods for more precise investigations of transport properties in short segments of tubules dissected from the kidneys of rabbits and other animals (Burg, 1982a). Segments a few mm long are cannulated at both ends and perfused with fluids of known composition while immersed in oxygenated bathing solutions of identical or different composition. Electrodes introduced through more complicated pipettes can be used to measure transepithelial and cellular potentials, and electrical resistances. Although the experimental conditions are somewhat unphysiological because the tubular cells are not in their natural environment, this technique can be applied to segments inaccessible to puncture *in situ*. Its substantial achievements over a dozen years were surveyed in special issues of *Kidney International* (Jacobson & Kokko, 1982; Ullrich & Couser, 1986).

4 Biochemical studies of function in subcellular fractions. Factors responsible for transport across individual cell membranes have been investigated with preparations of vesicles made from brush border and other membranes of isolated tubular cells (Kinne & Schwartz, 1978).

4.2 REABSORPTION OF SOME ORGANIC SUBSTANCES

4.2.1 Urea

In mammals urea is the metabolic endproduct excreted most abundantly in the urine, and its handling has not been proved to involve active transport, though frogs excrete it actively and marine elasmobranch fishes may reabsorb it actively (Roch-Ramel & Peters, 1981). The clearance of urea in human subjects varies between one third and two thirds that of inulin, indicating that from one to two thirds of the filtered urea is excreted (Fig. 4.1). When the kidneys produce large volumes of dilute urine, one third of the filtered urea is reabsorbed and two thirds is excreted. Conversely, when the urine is most

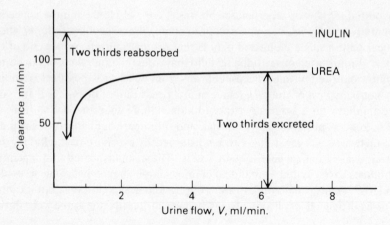

Fig. 4.1 Effect of urine flow on clearance of urea.

scanty and concentrated, about two thirds is reabsorbed and one third excreted. Thus most urea returns to the blood when the gradient from tubular fluid to plasma is steepest and most time is available for passive back-diffusion. During abnormally brisk diuresis induced in dogs by intravenous infusion of sodium sulphate, Shannon (1938b) observed that as the volume of urine approached that of the glomerular filtrate, and the gradient from tubular fluid to plasma became very small, the clearance ratio C_U/C_{IN} approached 1.0, suggesting that with no gradient and little time for back-diffusion there would have been no reabsorption.

In rats, about half the filtered urea and two thirds of the filtered water are always reabsorbed from the proximal tubules, and when the urine is dilute little more urea is reabsorbed downstream. In rats producing urine with 6.4 times the osmolality of the plasma, urea was secreted into the loops of Henle and added to the 50% remaining from the proximal tubules, so that 10% more urea than had been filtered entered the distal tubules (Lassiter, 1970). These reabsorbed 40%, and left 70% of the amount filtered to go on into the collecting system. The very low permeability of the cortical collecting tubules prevented further loss of urea in the cortex (Berry, 1982); but 57% was reabsorbed from the papillary collecting ducts, and only 13% of the filtered urea was finally excreted in the urine. Recirculation between the loops of Henle and the papillary collecting ducts maintains a high concentration of urea in the medullary interstitial fluid which can balance a similarly high concentration in the urine and this does away with the need for the terminal collecting ducts to be uniquely 'urea-proof' as Robinson (1954) had suggested. (For permeabilities of different segments of the nephron see Jacobson, 1981.) When the urine is suddenly diluted at the onset of diuresis, urea which has been stored in the renal medulla in high concentration escapes and transiently augments the rate of excretion, leading to the well-known 'exaltation of the clearance' during the first few minutes while V is increasing (Shannon, 1936; Haas *et al.*, 1965). All the transtubular shifts of urea within the kidney which underlie reabsorption and medullary recycling are believed to take place by passive diffusion. Schmidt-Nielsen (1958) considered the possibility of active reabsorption in ruminant animals that can use urea as a source of nitrogen for protein synthesis, and may excrete remarkably little; but Rock-Ramel & Peters (1981) found no compelling evidence for active transport of urea in mammalian kidneys.

Tubular reabsorption of urea is never complete enough to prevent the excretion of this important metabolic endproduct. The body of a person with 5 mM urea in the plasma and 40 kg of body water would contain 200 mmol of urea. This is substantially less than the amount filtered by the glomeruli ($5 \times 180 = 900$ mmol) and the amounts produced and excreted (around 300 to 600 mmol) each day. Moreover, the rate of excretion is automatically adjusted to meet alterations in production of urea or in glomerular filtration. Increased consumption of dietary protein increases GFR (Section 3.3.4.2) as well as production of urea. If production increases more than GFR, and excretion lags behind, the rising concentration of urea in the plasma helps to increase its filtered load. If glomeruli are destroyed and the production of urea is unchanged, the original filtered load can still be delivered in a smaller volume of filtrate by increasing its concentration. Hence an increasing concentration urea in the plasma during progressive disease of the kidneys is not merely a laboratory index of renal failure; it is at the same time a compensating factor which maintains the rate of excretion (Platt, 1951). Moreover, damaged kidneys soon fail to make the urine more concentrated than the plasma. The minimal urinary volume then increases towards 2 ml/min, beyond which the clearance of urea is nearly maximal (Fig. 4.1). Two thirds of the filtered load of urea is then excreted, and 1.5 times the clearance of urea gives a fair indication of GFR.

4.2.2 Glucose

Glucose is typical of many solutes which are reabsorbed actively and far more completely than urea. About 900 mmol (160 g, equivalent to a third of the human body's store of carbohydrates) is temporarily lost every day in the glomerular filtrate, but none normally appears in the urine. The clearance ratio C_G/C_{IN} of zero indicates that reabsorption is complete, but does not reveal the mechanism or which portion of the tubule is responsible. The earliest analyses of fluid removed with micropipettes showed that glucose had almost disappeared half way along the proximal tubules of amphibia (Walker & Hudson, 1937) and of rats and guinea pigs (Walker *et al.*, 1941). Increasing the filtered load by increasing the concentration of glucose in the plasma displaced the point of disappearance distally, and glucose which passed the end of the proximal tubule went on into the urine. The reabsorption of glucose therefore appeared to be a function exclusively of the proximal tubule, and to be of limited capacity.

Saturation of this transporting mechanism is well illustrated by the human kidney's handling of glucose. When the filtered load exceeds about 1.2 mmol/ min, the tubules of least capacity begin to be saturated, and glucose appears in the urine. With a normal GFR of 120 ml/min this happens when the concentration of glucose in the plasma reaches 10 mmol/l (mM), and the 'renal threshold', at about twice the normal concentration in the plasma, provides a margin of protection against losing glucose in the urine after meals or with other physiological fluctuations. Since the limiting factor is the capacity of the tubules to deal with the filtered load of glucose, the threshold is inversely proportional to GFR, and would be 20 mM if GFR were 60 ml/min. Severely dehydrated diabetic patients with greatly depressed GFR may therefore have no tell-tale glucosuria despite high concentrations of glucose in their plasma.

Although a few tubules show saturation when the filtered load of glucose reaches 1.2 mmol/min, it takes about 2 mmol/min to saturate the transporting mechanism in all tubules. With a normal GFR of 120 ml/min, this load is reached at a plasma concentration of 17 mM, which has been called the 'saturation limit'. Figure 4.2 shows the relations between the filtration, reabsorption (= filtration − excretion) and excretion of glucose as its concentration in the plasma is varied while GFR remains constant at 120 ml/min. According to traditional accounts, the rate of reabsorption reached at the saturation limit is maximal, about 2 mmol/min, and all additional glucose filtered as the concentration in the plasma is elevated further is excreted in the urine. The maximal rate of reabsorption reached at the saturation limit has been called the tubular maximum reabsorption rate for glucose, Tm_g. This was proposed by Homer Smith (1951) as a measure of the mass of healthy tubular tissue supplied by functioning glomeruli with glucose to reabsorb.

It has, however, been pointed out that many of the measurements which seemed to establish Tm as a fixed upper limit to the rate of reabsorption were made with nonspecific methods, sometimes employed beyond the range of concentrations in which they were reliable (Davison & Cheyne, 1974; Davison & Dunlop, 1980). It now seems that the rate of reabsorption continues to increase (though more slowly) at high concentrations, so that there may be no true saturation limit. This does not necessarily rule out a sharp upper limit to the rate of the principal active reabsorptive mechanism in the proximal tubule. Above 30 mM the concentration of glucose may increase with distance along the tubule as water is reabsorbed (Baeyer, 1981), and this should promote a component of reabsorption by passive diffusion (Barfuss & Schafer, 1981). However, if the filtered load is increased by increasing GFR rather than the concentration of glucose in the plasma, the resulting increased reabsorption of sodium enhances the reabsorption of glucose. This should increase the traditional Tm; but the rate of reabsorption *per unit of GFR* appears to become constant and maximal at high loads (Van Lieuw *et al.*,

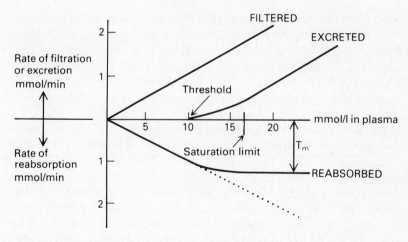

Fig. 4.2 Filtration, reabsorption and excretion of glucose.

1967; Schultze & Berger, 1973). It has also been realized that glucose may be reabsorbed beyond the proximal tubule. Concentrations up to about a quarter of those in the plasma may remain at the end of dogs' proximal tubules (Baeyer, 1981), and similar concentrations in the final urine despite the reabsorption of a great deal of water indicate that glucose must have been removed beyond the end of the proximal tubules (Deetjen, 1970). Studies of single nephrons have confirmed reabsorption from the loop of Henle and the collecting ducts in rats (Bishop & Green, 1983). Although the proximal tubules remain the major site for reabsorption of glucose under normal conditions, more distal sites may become more important when the proximal system is overloaded or damaged (Kramp & Lorenz, 1982).

The principal mechanism which reabsorbs glucose actively from the proximal nephron shows specificity for D- as opposed to L- isomers, and a substantial preference for glucose over galactose; mannose and fructose are reabsorbed only passively (Ullrich, 1976). There is also a specific inhibitor. The glucoside phlorizin, found in the bark and roots of fruit trees, has been known since 1885 to cause excretion of glucose in the urine even with a normal concentration in the plasma. Large doses increase the clearance of glucose to match that of inulin in a variety of animals including man (Smith, 1951). There is good evidence that glucose is recovered from the lumen of the renal tubules by the mechanism proposed by Crane (1965) for absorption from the small intestine. One glucose molecule and one sodium ion combine simultaneously with a mobile carrier in the luminal cell membrane; the positively charged complex then crosses the membrane, releases glucose and sodium to the sodium-poor cell interior, and returns for more. Glucose is accumulated in the cell at the expense of energy provided by the electrochemical gradient causing sodium to enter passively from the lumen with the positively charged glucose—sodium—carrier complex. The electrochemical gradient is maintained by the 'sodium pump' which extrudes sodium actively across the basolateral cell membrane and keeps its concentration low in the interior of the cell. See Frömter (1979, 1981) for a more detailed account of the electrical aspects of this process.

Glucose which is accumulated in the cells leaves across the basolateral border to the peritubular fluid by means of another carrier which is less specific, does not require sodium and is inhibited by the aglycone phloretin rather than by its glucoside phlorizin (Ullrich, 1976; Giebisch, 1978; Ullrich & Papavassiliou, 1985). The common carrier acting as a shuttle across the luminal membrane links the reabsorption of glucose to that of sodium and water. Sodium is needed to support the reabsorption of glucose, and glucose promotes the reabsorption of sodium and water. Like the small intestine which absorbs glucose in a similar manner, the proximal tubule has a brush border. Vesicles prepared from the brush border membrane take up glucose and sodium, and possess receptors with a high affinity for phlorizin in competition with glucose. Vesicles prepared from basolateral cell membranes also take up glucose, but independently of sodium, and their uptake of glucose is inhibited by phloretin rather than by phlorizin. It is expected that receptors in these membranes will turn out to be parts of the carrier systems which mediate the co-transport of glucose into the proximal tubular cells with sodium and its independent transport out. Genetically determined abnormalities of the carrier systems occur in the rare familial renal glucosurias in which glucose is excreted in the urine although the concentration of glucose in the plasma is not elevated. There are two forms of these, in one of which the threshold and the Tm are both low, presumably because of a deficiency in the number of transport sites; in the other form Tm is not reduced and the low threshold is presumed to result from a low affinity of the carrier for glucose (Scriver *et al.*, 1976).

Note on some other sugars: Smith (1951, 1956) and Pitts (1974) stated that D-xylose and D-fructose as well as D-galactose were reabsorbed actively, though incompletely, and shared the same transport system with D-glucose (but with smaller affinities for the carrier), because saturation with glucose blocked reabsorption of the others, and phlorizin blocked the reabsorption of all four. The position of fructose is, however, complicated, because it can be converted to glucose within the kidney (Cohen & Barac-Nieto, 1973).

4.2.3 Amino acids

Like glucose, the amino acids are essential metabolites which are easily filterable, but almost absent from the urine. Detailed knowledge about their reabsorption is relatively recent, because there are a score of amino acids and there were no specific methods for assaying them individually until the 1940s (Young & Freedman, 1971). They were thought to be reabsorbed from the proximal convoluted tubules because glucose, which was known to be reabsorbed there, is also excreted in some hereditary diseases characterized by abnormal losses of amino acids in the urine. Stop-flow methods (introduced by Malvin *et al.*, 1958) first established in the 1960s that amino acids are reabsorbed from the same tubular segments which reabsorb glucose and secrete PAH. More precise localization by micropuncture techniques showed that they are normally removed completely in the first third or half of the proximal convoluted tubule. With increasing filtered loads reabsorption extends along the convoluted tubule and into the pars recta, but not to the distal tubule.

Silbernagl (1981) tabulated clearances, usually less than 1% of the filtered loads, for 22 amino acids in rat, man, dog and rabbit; and their reabsorption shows striking resemblances to that of glucose. The naturally occurring (in this case L-) isomers are preferred. The reabsorption of amino acids across the luminal membrane depends upon the presence of sodium, and they promote the reabsorption of sodium and water. Their co-transport with sodium is rheogenic. The amino acid—sodium—carrier complex must cross the luminal cell membrane bearing a positive charge, for the luminal membrane is depolarized when an amino acid is added to the solution bathing it. The acidic amino acids, aspartate and glutamate, probably bind another cation, potassium or hydrogen, as well as sodium in order to carry the observed positive ionic current from lumen to cell (Frömter, 1981). Reabsorption may be inhibited (though not as completely as that of glucose) by phlorizin, and thresholds and saturation kinetics can be demonstrated. There may even be competition between glucose and amino acids, for infusions of glucose impair the reabsorption of some amino acids, and amino acids such as lysine, glycine and alanine depress the reabsorption of glucose.

The reabsorption of amino acids is more complicated than that of glucose, for one common carrier cannot serve them all and they fall into groups competing with each other for transport. The reabsorption of one amino acid at its maximal rate is inhibited by infusing another amino acid of the same, but not of a different group. In experiments on individual tubules, the further depolarization observed when a second amino acid is superposed is less when this is a member of the same group as the first, whereas depolarizations by members of different groups are additive (Ullrich, 1976). The existence of separate transport systems or carriers for groups of amino acids is also suggested by the occurrence of familial aminoacidurias characterized by low renal thresholds leading to abnormal losses of one or more amino acids in the urine.

Silbernagl (1981) indicated transport systems for seven groups of amino acids alongside the corresponding aminoacidurias (Table 4.1). These include systems of high capacity and low specificity transporting many amino acids and also highly specific systems of low capacity transporting a single amino acid or a small group. Overlapping between groups suggests that some amino acids are transported by more than one system.

Table 4.1 Transporting systems and corresponding aminoacidurias

Amino acids transported	Aminoacidurias
1 ACIDIC: aspartate, glutamate	Acidic
2 BASIC: arginine, lysine, ornithine, and cystine	'Classical' cystinuria
NEUTRAL AMINO ACIDS IN FIVE SUBGROUPS	
3 Cystine/cysteine	Isolated cystinuria
4 IMINO ACIDS: proline, hydroxyproline and glycine	Iminoaciduria
5 Glycine	Isolated glycinuria
6 Alanine, glycine, histidine, isoleucine, leucine, methionine phenylalanine, serine, threonine, tryptophan, tyrosine, valine, and perhaps asparagine, glutamine and citrulline	Hartnup disease
7 Beta-alanine, taurine (and gamma-aminobutyric acid)	Taurinuria (in mice)

In classical cystinuria the basic amino acids are lost as well as cystine; the recognition of group 3 depends on the existence of a condition in which cystine is the only amino acid lost in excess. Glycine may be lost alone, or with other amino acids in Hartnup disease, suggesting that it is reabsorbed both by its own specific system and also by the one that handles most neutral amino acids. The genetic defects and their implications were reviewed in detail by Scriver *et al.* (1976). Often they are not confined to the kidney; the corresponding carrier system may also be deficient in the intestinal mucosa and other tissues.

It seems reasonable to conclude that the amino acids are reabsorbed in the same way as glucose, entering the tubular cells by co-transport with sodium across the luminal membrane, driven by the electrochemical gradient maintained by active extrusion of sodium across the basolateral cell borders. Vesicles prepared from brush border membranes take up amino acids with sodium as they do glucose. Much less is known about the exit step across the peritubular border.

Thus the important metabolites, glucose and amino acids, which need to be circulated to all cells and which inevitably escape into the glomerular filtrate, are almost completely reabsorbed from the proximal tubules by processes which have enough capacity in reserve to make them independent of ordinary fluctuations in concentrations in the plasma. Although different carriers are needed for different substances, energy for the whole recovery operation is supplied through the sodium pumps in the basolateral cell membranes facing the blood. Deetjen (1981) suggested that about 80% of this task is completed in the first 10% of the length of the nephrons.

4.2.4 Proteins and peptides

Proteins and peptides are treated separately because they are not metabolites, and are not handled like amino acids. It is convenient to consider three more or less distinct groups: proteins of molecular weight greater than about 50000; smaller 'low-molecular-weight proteins' (LMWPs); and much smaller oligopeptides. The members of these three groups are treated differently by the tubular epithelium. Maack et al. (1979) gave an excellent review of renal handling of proteins, with detailed references; see also Carone et al. (1979) for small linear peptides.

The old doctrine that neither the glomerular filtrate nor the urine normally contain protein was an oversimplification which rested on the relative insensitivity of early methods for detecting proteins in solution. Even now there are no satisfactory methods for small proteins in the volumes that are obtained by puncturing nephrons (Maack et al., 1979). Boylan (1979) pointed out that the glomerular filtrate and the urine contain a multitude of plasma proteins and that excessive permeability of the glomerular membranes, inadequate tubular reabsorption and increased production causing the filtered load to exceed normal reabsorptive capacity, may lead respectively to glomerular, tubular and overflow proteinurias. The urine may also contain proteins secreted by the kidney (Tamm–Horsfall urinary mucoprotein; IgA) or derived from other tissues, including myoglobin and enzymes such as phosphatases, esterases and lactic dehydrogenase (LDH).

A. Proteins

The concentration of plasma albumin in rats' glomerular fluids is not zero, but of the order of 10 mg/l (contrasting with about 40000 mg/l in the plasma). Reported glomerular sieving coefficients of the order of 0.0003 would give a concentration of $40000 \times 0.0003 = 12$ mg/l in the filtrate. A similar concentration in human glomerular fluid would imply the filtration of nearly 2 g of albumin daily, and the normal excretion of about 30 mg/day (Robinson, 1980) would require 98% of filtered albumin to be reabsorbed. The proportion depends upon species, for 2 to 13% of the filtered load of albumin may remain in the urine of rats contrasted with 0.1 to 1.0% in men and dogs (Baumann, 1981). The capacity to reabsorb albumin is limited, and in rats the urinary excretion is substantially increased by modest increases in the concentration of albumin in the plasma. With Tm close to the normal filtered load, the threshold for excretion is close to the normal plasma concentration.

The principal site of reabsorption is the proximal tubule, but, unlike glucose and amino acids, the reabsorbed proteins are not returned to the plasma. There does not appear to be anything corresponding to the uptake of whole protein molecules which enables new-born animals to acquire immunoproteins by intestinal absorption from colostrum. Filtered protein is taken into the cells of the proximal tubule by a process of endocytosis that is almost entirely confined to the apical or luminal cell membranes. The process requires energy and is inhibited by cytochalasin-B which interferes with endocytosis in other tissues. Endocytic vesicles containing the protein are formed between microvilli in the depths of the brush border and move into the cells where they fuse with lysosomes whose enzymes digest the proteins and release the constituent amino acids. These may then cross the basolateral membranes along with amino acids reabsorbed by the transport systems described in the previous section, 4.2.3. Endocytosis seems to start with adsorption onto the cell membrane, and the specificity and limited capacity of this process may account for the threshold behaviour of albumin.

B. Low-molecular-weight-proteins

The so-called low-molecular-weight-proteins include insulin (6000), bovine PTH (9000), lysozyme (14600), myoglobin (16900) and rats' GH (20000). These have molecular sieving coefficients between 0.6 and 0.9. Indeed proteins with molecular weights less than 25000 and effective radius 2.3 nm generally attain concentrations in the glomerular filtrate greater than half their concentrations in the plasma, so that their daily filtered load is far greater than the corresponding plasma pool (Maack *et al.*, 1979). Their clearances are however less than 1% of GFR, so that they are almost entirely removed between the glomeruli and the renal pelvis; but they are unlike albumin in that their Tm values are far greater than the normal filtered load. Maack *et al.* (1979) commented that, although an estimate of 3 mg/min for the Tm of myoglobin in the dog might appear small, 'it is at least two orders of magnitude above the normal filtered load of any particular circulating endogenous protein smaller than 20000 daltons'. They also commented that although the capacity to reabsorb small proteins is high in relation to their own normal filtered loads, the absolute amount of albumin filtered is much larger than that of all the small proteins combined.

The mechanism for reabsorption of LWMPs is essentially the same as has just been described for larger proteins. They are removed from the proximal tubule by endocytosis and hydrolysed by lysosomal enzymes inside the cells. Uptake across the peritubular cell membrane appears to be negligible because the necessary endocytic apparatus is absent. Some hormones like insulin and PTH which have receptors in the peritubular membranes may be taken up to a small extent from the plasma as well as from the glomerular filtrate. The proximal tubule takes up LMWPs avidly from the tubular fluid, and the process appears to have a great capacity in relation to normal filtered loads, but not to be highly specific. The proteins are temporarily accumulated in the cells and then broken down at different rates. The half-life in renal tissue has been quoted as less than 10 minutes for PTH, several hours for lysozyme, and a few days for the foreign protein, horseradish peroxidase (Baumann, 1981).

C. Oligopeptides

Small peptides with 10 or less amino acid residues, like AT, bradykinin, oxytocin and vasopressin, are more filterable than the LMWPs. They have similar concentrations in the glomerular filtrate and the plasma but they disappear from the filtrate in the proximal tubules and are not excreted in appreciable amounts in the urine. These small peptides are not taken up into the tubular cells but undergo contact digestion; being hydrolysed by peptidases in the brush border membrane (Carone et al., 1979), to release amino acids which are then free to be reabsorbed by the mechanisms outlined in Section 4.2.3. When, for example, labelled AT II is infused into a dog's renal artery, about 75% is metabolized in one passage through the kidney, hardly any labelled material is excreted in the urine, and nearly 99% of the label is recoverable in the renal venous blood.

D. General significance of tubular handling of proteins and peptides

No matter whether the filtered proteins and peptides are broken down within tubular cells or by contact digestion in the lumen, they are not returned to the plasma in their original form. But the amino acid building blocks from which they were formed are taken in and made available for future use. In the alimentary digestion of proteins initial hydrolysis takes place in the lumen; small peptides may undergo contact digestion at the brush border and the amino acids released are subsequently absorbed, as in the renal tubule. In both cases proteins from the external environment (in gut or renal tubule) are not allowed to enter the body whole.

The entire filtered load of proteins and peptides is removed from the plasma, though hardly any of it is excreted in the urine. The kidney effectively eliminates these substances without actually excreting them. But they are not cleared from the blood by nonfiltering kidneys (Hierholzer et al., 1981) and their concentrations in the plasma may increase in renal failure. The initial process which makes the kidney an effective sink is glomerular filtration. The removal of LMWPs by the kidney serves to avoid large increases in their concentration in the blood. The faster removal of the more freely filterable oligopeptides, many of which are hormones, shortens their half-life in the circulation. The destruction of the whole filtered load means that they are removed at rates proportional to their concentrations in the plasma. This prepares the way for their active concentrations to be controlled by the rates at which they are released into the bloodstream. The kidneys are therefore able to perform an important homeostatic function for these biologically active molecules, not by excreting them in the urine, but by extracting them from the plasma and destroying them.

4.3 REABSORPTION OF SOME IONIC SPECIES

4.3.1 Sodium

All cells actively extrude sodium, keeping its intracellular concentration low. Like many other epithelial cells, the cells lining the renal tubules are polarized.

They extrude sodium actively across their basolateral membranes, facing the peritubular fluid, and allow it to enter from the luminal fluid across the apical membranes. All except the cells lining the thin limbs of the loops of Henle show high activities of the Na-K-ATPase, which is an essential component of the sodium pump in cell membranes. Greatest activities are in the mito-chondria-rich proximal and distal convoluted tubules and the thick ascending limbs of the loops of Henle, especially its medullary portion, but the collecting system also shows substantial activity (Jacobson, 1981). The sodium pump is rheogenic, since it takes two potassium ions into the cell for each three sodium ions extruded. The exchange carries net positive charge out of the cell, and this, together with the diffusion potential arising from potassium diffusing out down its concentration gradient, leaves the interior of the cell about 60 mV negative to the surrounding fluids. Passive movements of ions through the apical and basolateral cell membranes, with their different per-meabilities, tend to reduce the potential difference (pd) across the cell membrane, and also lead to transepithelial (or tubular) pds which are generally smaller than the cell membrane potentials, and which play a part in the reabsorption of ions through their influence upon movements between the luminal and peritubular fluids through the paracellular pathways between the cells.

Since Tamman (1896) pointed out that organic compounds account for only a few per cent of the osmolality of the glomerular filtrate, it has been apparent that the tubules mainly reabsorb a solution of sodium salts. The fact that the kidneys' suprabasal expenditure of energy (measured by oxygen consumed) is proportional to the rate at which filtered sodium is reabsorbed (Lassen *et al.*, 1961) pointed to the active transport of sodium as a major driving force for tubular reabsorption. Wesson & Anslow (1948) obtained circumstantial evidence of active transport of sodium during extreme diuresis in dogs infused with hypertonic (20 to 25%) mannitol. The flow of urine reached two thirds of GFR; the urine was approximately isosmolal with plasma and had a lower concentration of sodium because of the contribution of the mannitol. Since only 30% of the filtered sodium was excreted, two thirds had been reabsorbed against a difference in concentration of up to 60 mmol/l. The tubules must have reabsorbed sodium actively under the conditions of these experiments and it seemed reasonable to expect active tubular reabsorption under normal conditions.

Proof of active transport of an ion requires measurements of electrical potential as well as concentration in order to establish a gradient of electro-chemical potential (Robinson, 1975b). The first measurements of transepithe-lial potential in rats (Solomon, 1957) indicated a difference of about 20 mV between the proximal tubular and peritubular fluids, lumen-negative, so that even with no difference in concentration, sodium would have to be reabsorbed against a sizeable gradient of electrochemical potential. Later measurements established much smaller pds of around 2 mV, lumen-negative near the glo-merulus, becoming positive a few mm along the proximal convoluted tubule.

The small magnitude of the pd reflects the permeability of the leaky epithelium and does not negate active transport of sodium. Giebisch *et al.* (1964) measured short-circuit currents indicating reabsorption of sodium at a rate (7.5 × 10^{-9} mmol cm^{-2} sec^{-1}) comparable to its filtered load. Under the conditions required for measuring short-circuit currents the gradients of concentration and of electrical potential must both be set to zero (Ussing & Zerahn, 1951) so that electrochemical gradients contribute no driving force and any transport of sodium must be active. The classical micropuncture experiments of Walker *et al.* (1941), showing that bicarbonate was reabsorbed before chloride, offered an explanation for the change of sign. As bicarbonate disappeared from the early part of the rat's proximal convoluted tubule, the concentration of chloride in the tubular fluid increased to 20 to 40% above that in the plasma, while the concentration of sodium remained unaltered. The small, lumen-negative potential associated with active reabsorption of sodium along with glucose, amino acids and bicarbonate, is therefore apparent in the early part of the proximal tubule, but is later masked by a lumen-positive diffusion potential set up by passive diffusion of chloride from tubular fluid to peritubular plasma (Rector, 1983).

Most, perhaps 70%, of filtered sodium is reabsorbed from the proximal tubule; about 20% from the thick ascending limb of the loop of Henle, 5% from the distal convoluted tubule and 2 to 3% from the collecting ducts. Beyond the proximal tubules the epithelia become 'tighter', with lower permeability and greater electrical resistance (Jacobson, 1981). Transtubular differences in potential (except in the thin limbs of the loops, where there is no evidence of active transport) are larger than in the proximal tubules. The concentration of sodium may approach zero and the transtubular pd exceed 50 mV, lumen-negative, in the distal and collecting tubules under conditions when reabsorption is enhanced by aldosterone (see Section 7.4.3, where regulation of the rate of reabsorption is considered). There can be little doubt that reabsorption is active in these circumstances, but the thick ascending limb of the loop of Henle has posed a problem. The fluid emerging into the distal tubule is hypotonic, with a low concentration of sodium and chloride (around 60 mM), but the pd in the thick ascending limb was found to be of the order of 5 to 10 mV, *lumen-positive*, suggesting that reabsorption was driven by a chloride pump and that sodium was reabsorbed passively! However, there is no evidence of a chloride-activated ATPase; the thick limb is rich in the Na-K-ATPase, and its inhibition by ouabain, which specifically inhibits the conventional sodium pump, inhibits the transport of sodium chloride and depresses the lumen-positive pd. Hence it seems that the manifest active transport of chloride is secondary to primary active transport of sodium, but the manner of coupling within the epithelium which reverses the expected pd is uncertain (Burg, 1982b).

There have been other suggestions that substantial fractions of reabsorbed sodium are transported passively. Ludwig (1844) proposed that the increased oncotic pressure of plasma concentrated by the loss of the protein-free filtrate could recover most of the filtrate simply by endosmosis. Bayliss (1956) revived this theory a century or so later to help to explain the reabsorption which continued in kidneys that had been chilled (Bickford & Winton, 1937) or poisoned with cyanide (Bayliss & Lundsgaard, 1932). Swann (quoted by Selkurt, 1963) suggested that the glomerular tufts correspond to the arteriolar, and the postglomerular capillaries to the venous ends of systemic capillaries, and that Starling forces (Section 7.4.4.1) should promote the reabsorption into the peritubular capillaries of fluid filtered out at the glomeruli. But addition of protein to the lumen and alterations in the protein content of peritubular plasma have negligible direct effects on proximal tubular reabsorption (Giebisch, 1978).

Surprisingly, small differences of hydrostatic pressure applied to the inner surface of frog skin profoundly affect the rate of active intake of sodium (Nutbourne, 1968), and such an effect could link the rate of reabsorption to the oncotic pressure of peritubular capillary plasma indirectly. Reduced oncotic pressure should slow the uptake of reabsorbed fluid into the capillaries and increase interstitial fluid pressure, leading to a dilation of the intercellular spaces which might facilitate passive back-diffusion of reabsorbed sodium from peritubular fluid to the lumen (Section 7.4.4.3). The net rate of reabsorption of sodium could therefore be diminished without any direct inhibition of primary active transport (Rector, 1983). The small lumen-positive potential associated with diffusion of chloride down its concentration gradient should oppose back-diffusion of sodium from peritubular fluid to lumen and so promote its net reabsorption. An investigation by the methods of irreversible thermodynamics led to the conclusion that a third or more of the proximal reabsorption of sodium might be passive (Frömter et al., 1973). But even if not all of it is active, the reabsorption of 25 000 mmol of sodium every day represents a major call upon the metabolic energy released in the kidneys.

4.3.2 Anions

A glomerular ultrafiltrate containing 140 mM of sodium will have about 115 mM chloride and 28 mM bicarbonate as its principal anions (Robinson, 1975b). As with sodium, more than 99% of these anions are usually reabsorbed, mostly from the proximal tubules. Chloride is reabsorbed across the tubular epithelium directly, without change of state; but bicarbonate is reabsorbed indirectly. Most of the filtered bicarbonate is destroyed in the tubular lumen, and an equal amount of new bicarbonate formed in the cells is added to the plasma.

A. Reabsorption of chloride

About three quarters of the filtered chloride is reabsorbed from the proximal tubules, a fifth from the thick ascending limbs of loops of Henle, and most of the remainder from the collecting system. A three-fold increase in the concentration of filtered inulin with no change in the concentration of sodium showed that about two thirds of the filtered water and sodium are reabsorbed from the proximal convoluted tubules. In the first part of the proximal tubules, where glucose, amino acids and bicarbonate all enhance fluid reabsorption and the small tubular pd is lumen-negative, bicarbonate is reabsorbed in preference to chloride. Further on, after the nutrient substances and bicarbonate have largely disappeared and the concentration of chloride in the tubular fluid has increased by 20 mM or so, the reabsorbate resembles an isosmolal solution of sodium chloride, and the diffusion potential resulting from the greater luminal concentration of chloride changes the tubular pd to lumen-positive (Rector, 1983). The driving force for reabsorption of chloride is the rheogenic active reabsorption of sodium; negatively charged chloride ions follow positively charged sodium ions. The chloride does not, however, pass through the cells but mostly through the lateral intercellular spaces, which cover a substantial fraction of the area of the proximal tubular epithelium and contribute 90% of its remarkably large transepithelial electrical conductance (Schafer, 1984). The free movement of anions through this paracellular pathway keeps the difference of potential resulting from the transport of sodium very small. Thus sodium ions extruded by the basolateral pumps into the intercellular spaces attract chloride ions electrostatically from the luminal fluid; and the sodium and chloride ions collected in the intercellular spaces attract water osmotically, both from the cells and from luminal fluid across the tight junctions (Burg, 1976a). The resulting saline solution then flows across the basement membrane, and the colloid osmotic pressure of plasma concentrated by the loss of glomerular filtrate provides a driving force for uptake into the peritubular capillaries, which are closely apposed to the basement membrane. Alterations in the concentration of protein in the peritubular plasma might be expected to affect movement through the paracellular pathways; they also have a further influence on the rate of reabsorption of chloride which remains to be clarified (Rector, 1983).

In the thick ascending limb of the loop of Henle, the pump is organized to transport chloride against an electrochemical gradient, and the tubular pd is lumen-positive by up to 10 mV (Section 4.3.1). Some efficient diuretics like mercurials, ethacrynic acid and furosemide, known as 'loop diuretics', inhibit the reabsorption of chloride and reduce the tubular pd (Burg, 1976b).

In the distal convoluted and collecting tubules the concentrations of both chloride and sodium can become extremely low. The epithelium is typically 'tight', and the transtubular pd larger, up to 60 mV, and lumen-negative, indicating a passive reabsorption of chloride secondary to active transport of sodium.

B. Reabsorption of bicarbonate

An adult person loses between 4000 and 5000 mmol of bicarbonate into the glomerular filtrate every day, and the recovery of this most important of the body's buffers is a vital task for the renal tubules. When it was thought that the acidification of the urine did not begin before the distal convoluted tubules, Pitts & Lotspeich (1946) suggested that any bicarbonate which had got so far was reabsorbed indirectly. They proposed that bicarbonate ions were decomposed in the tubular fluid by hydrogen ions secreted to make the urine acid, and that an equal number of bicarbonate ions, left in the cells as a byproduct of the generation of hydrogen ions, entered the plasma along with reabsorbed sodium ions i.e.

In the cell: $CO_2 + H_2O \rightarrow H_2CO_3 \rightarrow H^+ + $ (new) HCO_3^- (to plasma with Na^+)
In the lumen: $H^+ + $ (filtered) $HCO_3^- \rightarrow H_2CO_3 \rightarrow H_2O + CO_2$

Because equal numbers of bicarbonate ions are destroyed in the lumen and added to the plasma with the same number of sodium ions, this whole operation is electrically neutral. It is, however, uphill from a lower concentration of bicarbonate in the tubular fluid to a larger concentration in the plasma. The cells lining the tubules were known to contain the enzyme carbonic anhydrase, which catalyses the otherwise rather slow hydration of carbon dioxide to form carbonic acid. When Berliner & Orloff (1956) found in dogs that after inhibition of carbonic anhydrase the urine became alkaline and half the filtered bicarbonate was excreted, it became apparent that the proximal tubular epithelium could also secrete hydrogen ions (since amply confirmed), and that bicarbonate was probably 'reabsorbed' in this same indirect way proximally. After much further work and the use of more effective inhibitors of carbonic anhydrase it has come to be accepted that most of the filtered bicarbonate is replaced in the plasma in this manner. The process and its physiological regulation are described in more detail in Chapter 6 on the contribution of the kidney to maintaining acid−base balance; and also in a small book (Robinson, 1975c) on this topic.

Of more immediate interest here is the manner in which the hydrogen ions responsible for the proximal tubular reabsorption of most (about four fifths ordinarily) of the filtered bicarbonate are secreted. While bicarbonate is present in the lumen to take up hydrogen ions, the tubular fluid is only minimally acidified, and there are no large differences in concentration of hydrogen ions between the plasma, the interior of the cells, and the tubular fluid. Studies with membrane vesicles (Rector, 1983) have confirmed the presence in apical, but not in basolateral membranes, of a sodium/hydrogen antiporter which can exchange one intracellular hydrogen ion for one luminal sodium ion; the exchange is electrically neutral, and the luminal/intracellular gradient of sodium concentration can drive it to secrete hydrogen ions into the tubular fluid, using energy ultimately supplied by the basolateral sodium pump which keeps the intracellular concentration of sodium low. Workers in Burg's laboratory showed, using isolated, perfused tubules from rabbits' kidneys, that reabsorption of bicarbonate required the presence of sodium in the luminal fluid; and that it was inhibited by inhibition of sodium transport (Rector, 1983).

In the distal tubule, after bicarbonate has been removed, secreted hydrogen ions are taken up by other buffers, principally phosphate, and the tubular fluid becomes increasingly acid. Smaller quantities of hydrogen ions are involved at this stage, but they are secreted against an increasing gradient. Passive secretion of hydrogen ions in exchange for sodium ions could possibly account for acidification of the tubular fluid to about pH 6.4, at which no more than about 2 mM bicarbonate would be left. This is 1 pH unit more acid than the plasma, and according to the Nernst equation the corresponding concentration ratio (H^+_{urine}/H^+_{plasma}) of 10/1 could be sustained by a tubular pd of about 60 mV, lumen-negative (Robinson, 1975b). It can therefore be concluded that, although a separate mechanism for active secretion of hydrogen ions would be required to acidify the urine below pH 6.4, passive secretion secondary to active transport of sodium should suffice for the 'reabsorption' of most of the filtered bicarbonate.

C. Reabsorption of phosphate

Phosphate is a buffer base of variable valency. In the physiological range of pH, inorganic phosphate (Pi) consists of a mixture of $H_2PO_4^-$ and HPO_4^{2-} with negligible amounts of PO_4^{3-}. Since pK for the second dissociation is 6.8, the mixture at pH 7.4 contains four HPO_4^{2-} to each $H_2PO_4^-$, and the effective valency is 1.8. Unlike bicarbonate, which can be rapidly generated in unlimited amounts from metabolic carbon dioxide, the total quantity of phosphate is relatively fixed; it depends upon the balance between dietary intake and renal excretion. Binding makes a few per cent of phosphate in the plasma unfilterable, enough to offset the influence of the Donnan membrane distribution, so that Pi has the same concentration in the glomerular filtrate as in whole plasma (Bijvoet, 1980). Renal handling is well reviewed in an editorial (Knox et al., 1973), updated by a book (Massry & Fleisch, 1980). Fishes, amphibia, reptiles and birds filter less Pi than their daily intake, and supplement filtration with tubular secretion, but tubular secretion has not been convincingly demonstrated in mammals, which filter substantially more than their dietary intake and require net reabsorption to maintain balance.

Adult persons with a little over 1.0 mM Pi in their plasma lose about 200 mmol each day in the glomerular filtrate, and it is important to recover this. Fasting animals with low plasma Pi may excrete hardly any phosphate, but ordinarily about 80% of the filtered load is reclaimed; 60 to 70% from the proximal convoluted tubule, 10 to 20% from the proximal straight tubule and little or none from more distal parts of the nephron, except perhaps in thyroparathyroidectomized animals. Pitts (1933) observed a rapid increase in the clearance ratio, C_{Pi}/C_{In}, when the concentration in the plasma was raised, suggesting that reabsorption was carrier-mediated and saturable. The strongly negative cell interior and the higher intracellular concentration of Pi require some form of active transport, and vesicles prepared from brush border membranes take up Pi with sodium ions *in vitro*. Hence co-transport with sodium can convey Pi from the tubular lumen into the cells by means of energy provided indirectly by the basolateral sodium pump which maintains the gradients driving uptake of sodium. Sodium in the tubular fluid promotes, and ouabain inhibits, the reabsorption of Pi. Reabsorption of Pi therefore somewhat resembles the reabsorption of glucose and amino acids, and although phosphate undergoes many reactions with organic compounds, and the cells contain a large number of phosphorus-transferring enzymes, none of these has been specifically associated with the process of tubular reabsorption. For cellular mechanisms see Gmaj & Murer (1986) and Hammerman (1986).

The ratio; concentration of Pi in tubular fluid to concentration in ultrafiltrate or plasma, (TF/UF)Pi, is reduced from 1.0 to about 0.7 very early in the proximal convoluted tubule, and then remains unchanged in normal rats studied by micropuncture methods. Parathyroid hormone increases this ratio to 1.0, depressing tubular reabsorption and increasing the rate of excretion of phosphate in the urine. Its first action may be to increase GFR. Parathyroid hormone then acts on receptors in the basolateral membranes of tubular cells, increasing the synthesis of cyclic adenosine monophosphate (cAMP); this initiates a train of events that retards the intake of Pi through the apical cell membranes. After parathyroidectomy reabsorption is enhanced, and the ratio falls to around 0.3. Calcitonin may alter the ratio in the same direction as PTH, but its phosphaturic action is much smaller, and not always observed.

Biologically active metabolites of vitamin D depress (TF/UF)Pi, at least temporarily, towards 0.35, reducing the urinary excretion of phosphate.

Infusions of phosphate which increase the concentration of Pi in the plasma appear readily to saturate the reabsorptive process, and the ratio (TF/UF)Pi increases above 1.0 along the proximal convoluted tubule as urinary constituents which are not reabsorbed become more concentrated through the reabsorption of water.

Infusions of saline solutions which expand the ECFV increase (TF/UF)Pi and increase the rate of excretion of phosphate as well as that of sodium. So many interacting factors are involved that the mechanism of this effect has not been elucidated. One possibility is that the secretion of PTH is increased, secondarily to a reduction in the concentration of calcium, as the infusion dilutes the plasma.

Alterations in the concentration of calcium in the plasma have variable and rather unpredictable effects. Increases tend to raise the concentration of Pi (possibly by depressing secretion of PTH), but also to make it less filterable.

The rate of excretion of phosphate shows a substantial diurnal variation. In man it may increase more than two-fold between early morning and late evening, paralleling smaller oscillations in the concentration in the plasma (Mills, 1966). The variation is not simply related to intake of food, it presumably results from multiple causes and is still unexplained. It is important to keep this spontaneous variation in mind when planning or interpreting studies of the effects of other factors on the excretion of phosphate.

Finally, an important mechanism by which the renal tubules can adapt their rate of reabsorption to alterations in dietary intake and bodily requirements (as for growth) appears to be independent of cAMP, and is not yet explained. This adaptive mechanism, which is powerful enough to restrain the phosphaturic action of PTH probably plays an important part in the regulation and maintenance of phosphate homeostasis (Bonjour & Fleisch, 1980).

D. Reabsorption of sulphate

Sulphate is handled similarly to phosphate. The concentration maintained in the plasma is also a little more than 1 mM; it passes freely into the glomerular filtrate, and is normally almost completely reabsorbed, actively, by a saturable mechanism with Tm a little greater than the normal filtered load. A carrier system which can take up sulphate through the apical cell membrane by co-transport with sodium has been found in vesicles prepared from brush border membranes. The Tm for sulphate is of the same order of magnitude as that for phosphate, and there is evidence of competition between sulphate and phosphate for reabsorption, in that saturation with either reduces the transport of the other; but the inhibition is small, suggesting competition for energy rather than for a common carrier. Reabsorption of both phosphate and sulphate is depressed by saturation of the glucose-transporting system, and increased by phlorizin which stops the transport of glucose. Reabsorption of sulphate is, however, inhibited by large concentrations of more mobile ions like chloride, nitrate or thiocyanate, whereas Tm for phosphate is unaffected by these but variable in response to bodily needs and agents like PTH (Pitts, 1974).

E. Reabsorption of some organic anions

1 Lactate is a useful metabolite which is freely filtered and almost completely reabsorbed until its concentration in the plasma reaches around 7 mM in man and 10 mM in dogs (Pitts, 1974). This is far above the normal concentration in the plasma and serves to retain lactate unless its concentration rises sufficiently to threaten acid−base balance by displacing bicarbonate. Lactate is one of the anions whose presence promotes the uptake of sodium by isolated, perfused proximal tubules (Burg, 1976a), and vesicles prepared from brush border membranes take up lactate with sodium (Murer et al., 1981; Rector, 1983).

2 Metabolic substrates such as α-ketoglutarate, acetoacetate and β-hydroxybutyrate are almost completely reabsorbed at normal plasma concentrations, though saturation and coupling of uptake with sodium can be demonstrated, and they may be partly or wholly metabolized in the tubular cells and not returned to the plasma (Smith, 1956; Pitts, 1974).

3 Citrate is a normal constituent of the urine, where it helps to keep calcium in solution. Increasing its concentration in the plasma leads to increased rates of both reabsorption and excretion; no Tm can be demonstrated at tolerable concentrations in the plasma. Krebs cycle intermediates compete with citrate for reabsorption and increase its rate of excretion (Pitts, 1974). Like lactate, citrate promotes reabsorption of sodium by isolated perfused proximal tubules and is taken up with sodium by brush border membrane vesicles.

4   Ascorbate, or vitamin C, is reabsorbed rather like glucose, with a Tm of around 2.2 mg/min, which would correspond to about 1 mM in plasma or glomerular filtrate (Smith, 1951).

5   Urate appears to be handled only by the proximal tubules, but in a more complicated manner, because it is secreted as well as reabsorbed. The amount excreted is about one tenth of the filtered load, but the urate in the urine is not all residual urate that was filtered. Probably the proximal convoluted tubule reabsorbs most of the filtered load, but the proximal straight tubule then secretes urate into the tubular fluid. Lang (1981) listed 100 factors (including 11 hormones) and 27 diseases and other conditions affecting renal handling of urate in a review with 356 references.

4.3.3 Some 'lesser' cations

The term 'lesser', used here to distinguish cations other than sodium, refers to their concentrations in the plasma and glomerular filtrate, and the quantities filtered and subsequently reabsorbed. These cations are certainly not lesser in importance. Potassium is the predominating intracellular cation, and its small concentration in the ECFs is especially important for the normal functioning of excitable cells. Large (two- to three-fold) deviations in either direction can paralyse skeletal (including respiratory) muscles and stop the heart. Calcium and magnesium also have small extracellular concentrations which are important for controlling the function of excitable cells. The kidney plays an important part in conserving the body's stores of these cations and regulating their critically important extracellular concentrations.

A. Reabsorption of potassium

The human renal tubules receive a filtered load of about 700 mmol of potassium every day. With normal dietary intakes around 100 mmol, and faecal losses of the order of 10 mmol each day, at least 85 to 90% of the amount of potassium filtered must be reabsorbed. This may be increased to 99% during potassium depletion, when the amount excreted may be reduced to between 4 and 10 mmol per day (Squires & Huth, 1959). The tubules can also secrete potassium into the urine, for example after excessive loading with potassium, during osmotic diuresis, and sometimes in renal disease. The ability of the kidneys to switch their activity between net reabsorption and net secretion enables them to conserve potassium avidly when intake is deficient or extrarenal losses threaten the body's stores; at other times to maintain metabolic balance by eliminating surplus potassium from the diet; and to protect against dangerous increments in extracellular concentration by excreting potassium rapidly after excessive loading or escape from cells. Reabsorption and secretion most likely go on simultaneously in different segments of the nephrons, and it is generally agreed that most of the filtered load is normally reabsorbed proximally while most of the potassium excreted in the urine is secreted by the distal and collecting tubules (Giebisch, 1975, 1976; Wright, 1977). An outline of tubular reabsorption is sketched here. Details of the secretory phase, about which much more has been published, are deferred to Section 4.4.3 on tubular secretion.

Studies of single nephrons *in situ* by micropuncture techniques and perfusion of isolated tubular segments have provided useful information about tubular reabsorption. In rats on normal diets, on diets low in potassium and on diets high in potassium, the concentration of potassium in proximal tubular fluid became a little less than the concentration in the plasma, and was less than half of this in fluid entering the distal convoluted tubules. In animals on high or normal potassium diets, the concentration in the tubular fluid increased greatly along the distal tubules to reach 10 to 20 times the concentration in the plasma. But in animals on low-potassium diets it increased much less, despite reabsorption of water, and the concentration ratio of potassium/inulin compared with that in the plasma was lower in the final urine than at the end of the distal tubule, indicating reabsorption of potassium from the collecting ducts (Malnic *et al.*, 1964). This may be a function of specialized cells in the medullary collecting ducts of rats, which occupy a greater proportion of the luminal surface during deprivation of potassium (Stetson *et al.*, 1980).

Hence the proximal tubules, the loop of Henle and the collecting ducts can all reabsorb potassium, but it is uncertain to what extent this reabsorption is active. Most of the filtered load is recovered from the proximal tubule where reabsorption of potassium roughly keeps pace with reabsorption of water and there is little or no difference in concentration between tubular fluid and peritubular plasma (Wright & Giebisch, 1978). In the later part of the proximal convolution, where the transtubular potential is lumen-positive, the electrical gradient could move potassium ions with chloride ions along the paracellular pathways. In the early proximal convoluted and the proximal straight tubules, where the pd is lumen-negative, it would need active transport to shift potassium ions from lumen to plasma. The basolateral sodium pump, which takes in two potassium ions for each three sodium ions extruded, keeps the concentration of potassium in the cells of the order of 100mM higher than in the tubular fluid or peritubular plasma. This difference in concentration opposes uptake into tubular cells from the lumen, but uptake is favoured electrostatically because the interior of the cells is about 60mV negative to the lumen. Potassium taken into the cells either passively or actively presumably mixes with the cytoplasmic potassium and joins the diffusive efflux across the peritubular membrane between pumping sites.

Reabsorption from the thick ascending limb of the loop of Henle may be passive, driven by the transtubular pd of up to 10 mV, lumen-positive. In the distal and collecting tubules the transtubular pd is much larger, of the order of 50 mV, and lumen-negative, which makes the transepithelial pd, attracting potassium ions from the lumen into the cell, correspondingly smaller. Uptake into the cells would therefore seem to require active transport, unless increasing concentration through reabsorption of water sufficiently reduces the difference of concentration between the interior of the cell and the tubular fluid.

In summary: most of the filtered potassium seems to be reabsorbed in a routine process of conservation which normally takes place mainly from the proximal tubule and the thick ascending limb of the loop of Henle, but can be augmented in times of scarcity by special cells in the medullary collecting ducts.

B. Reabsorption of calcium

An adult person has about 1 kg of calcium in the skeleton, and the concentration of ionized calcium in the ECFs is kept around 1.3 mM, where it is important for regulating the permeability of membranes and the performance of excitable tissues. Total plasma calcium is about 2.5 mM; about 60% is filterable, four fifths of this being ionized. The renal tubules receive about 250 mmol of filtered calcium each day and reabsorb about 99% of it; half from the proximal convoluted tubules, 20 to 30% from the pars recta and loop of Henle, 10 to 15% from the distal convoluted tubules and up to 10% from the collecting system (Agus *et al.*, 1981; Sutton, 1983).

Classical studies suggesting that calcium and sodium were handled together have been confirmed, at least for the proximal convoluted tubule, where reabsorption of calcium keeps pace with that of sodium and water. The epithelium is highly permeable to calcium, and reabsorption is probably mostly passive, partly active; both the active and the passive components depend upon reabsorption of sodium. If the concentration in the tubular cells is kept small, less than 0.1 mM, as in other cells (Borle, 1967), uptake from the lumen will be down gradients of both concentration and electrical potential. The basolateral membrane has a Ca-ATPase and a system for sodium–calcium exchange, both of which extrude calcium from the cell into the peritubular fluid, the first using energy from ATP directly, the second indirectly by way of the sodium gradient. In the proximal straight tubule, which is less permeable, calcium can be reabsorbed in excess of water by an active process which, unlike transport of sodium, is not inhibited by ouabain.

The thin limbs of the loop of Henle do not transport calcium, but there is significant reabsorption from the thick ascending limb, driven by the lumen-positive transtubular pd. This passive phase occurs in the medullary portion of the thick limb in perfused rabbit tubules and is not affected by PTH. There is also an active reabsorption from the cortical portion which is stimulated by PTH.

Beyond the loop, where permeability is low and the transtubular pd relatively large and lumen-negative, reabsorption is probably active, and it is stimulated by PTH and by cAMP. The granular segment of the distal convoluted tubule and the early, granular portion of the cortical collecting duct, which between them reabsorb up to 10% of the filtered calcium, appear to be the major sites for regulating the ultimate rate of excretion.

The parathyroid hormone is probably the most important physiological factor controlling reabsorption of calcium, which it stimulates. It acts in the proximal tubules, the thick ascending limb of the loop of Henle, and in the granular portions of the distal convoluted tubules and cortical collecting ducts, all of which exhibit adenyl cyclase activity. If, as some early studies indicated, PTH inhibits reabsorption from the proximal convoluted tubules, this effect can be overridden by greater reabsorption from the granular segments downstream, which may be the major site for action of PTH. Calcitonin does not seem to have any consistent direct effect on the renal handling of calcium.

1 Disturbing factors. These also seem to affect the granular segments.

(a) Loop diuretics reduce the lumen-positive transtubular pd and inhibit reabsorption of calcium proportionally more than of sodium.

(b) Metabolic acidosis inhibits, and alkalosis promotes reabsorption of calcium.

(c) Phosphate depletion increases the excretion of calcium; perhaps partly by increasing the filtered load, by reducing PTH activity and by a direct action in the distal nephron.

(d) Expansion of the ECFV by infusing saline solutions inhibits the reabsorption of calcium as well as of sodium; presumably by some distal action, because reduction of GFR does not prevent the increased excretion of calcium.

2 Alterations in plasma calcium, and homeostasis. There does not appear to be a Tm for reabsorption of calcium; increased deliveries from the proximal tubules can be taken up downstream. Increased rates of excretion follow increases in filtered load due to increased concentrations in the plasma, but not those due to increased GFR, possibly because the reabsorption of more sodium promotes reabsorption of calcium. Hence alterations in plasma concentration are followed by homeostatic changes in excretion. A circadian rhythm with greater rates of excretion by day than by night may be due to increases in plasma calcium related to intake of food and accompanied by reduced PTH activity. Homeostasis overall appears to be mediated largely by PTH which directs the kidneys to stabilize the extracellular concentration of calcium regardless of the amount stored in the body. Nevertheless, with 99% of the filtered load regularly being reabsorbed, the tubules' activity can be summed up as a routine conservation of the body's stores so long as extrarenal

factors retain the bulk of the calcium in the skeleton. Excessive loss from bone tends to raise the concentration in the plasma, and calcium is excreted and lost from the body to limit this. Primary renal losses tend to lower the concentration in the plasma (which stimulates secretion of PTH), and calcium is withdrawn from the skeleton to sustain the extracellular concentration.

C. Reabsorption of magnesium

Magnesium is the second most abundant cellular cation. The concentration in the plasma is kept a little less than 1 mм. Four fifths is filterable, and 70 to 80% of this is ionized, giving a daily filtered load of about 120 mmol. Most of this is reabsorbed, leaving 4 mmol to be excreted in the urine and balance a similar amount absorbed from the alimentary tract. The amount excreted daily can be reduced to almost zero during deficiency of magnesium. It can also be increased to over 200 mmol to avert the threat of a dangerous increase in extracellular concentration, but there is no convincing evidence of tubular secretion.

The permeability of the proximal tubules to magnesium is low, and they reabsorb only about a third of the filtered magnesium by an undefined mechanism. Little or no more is reabsorbed from the loop of Henle until the tubular fluid enters the thick ascending limb with the concentration of magnesium increased substantially by reabsorption of water. The thick ascending limb reabsorbs 50 to 70% of the filtered load, and may lower the concentration to half that in the original ultrafiltrate. Microperfusion studies *in vitro* showed that this phase of the reabsorption is voltage-dependent, and its rate can increase indefinitely as the concentration in the lumen is increased — provided that the concentration in the peritubular capillaries is not allowed to increase. Reabsorption thus appears to be driven passively by the lumen-positive transtubular pd in the thick ascending limb, and inhibited by a higher concentration in the peritubular plasma. The distal tubules can reabsorb up to 5% of normal filtered loads, and the collecting system little or none. When the concentration of magnesium in the plasma is increased in intact animals, proximal reabsorption increases as well as the filtered load, but the effect of this is offset by slower reabsorption from the loop, giving an apparent Tm for the kidney as a whole.

Calcium seems to compete with magnesium for reabsorption; an increase in the plasma concentration of either increases the excretion of both. Loop diuretics, which reduce the lumen-positive transtubular pd in the thick ascending limb of the loop of Henle, inhibit the reabsorption of magnesium more than that of calcium and sodium. Other diuretics have relatively little effect on the final rate of excretion. Expansion of the ECFV, possibly affecting reabsorption at all three sites, increases the fractional excretion of magnesium more than that of sodium. Parathyroid hormone can enhance reabsorption from the ascending limb and distal convoluted tubules in hamsters, but the most important physiological factor regulating the excretion of magnesium is probably the inhibitory effect of rising plasma concentration upon the major phase of reabsorption from the ascending limb of the loop of Henle. This composite sketch, based upon observations in several species (see Dirks, 1983, for references), suggests that the tubular reabsorption of magnesium is an operation of routine conservation, adjusted, like the reabsorption of calcium, primarily to control the concentration of the ion in the ECF.

4.4 TUBULAR SECRETION

4.4.1 Introduction

In mammalian kidneys with daily GFRs far greater than the total volume of the extracellular fluids, a major activity of the renal tubules must be the reabsorption of most of the filtered water and solutes, which have clearances less than that of inulin. In animals with aglomerular kidneys the clearance of inulin is zero and the renal tubules secrete all the constituents of the urine. Tubular secretion also occurs in mammals where it is responsible for the elimination of some endproducts of metabolism and a few normal constituents of the body, as well as of some foreign substances which provide the most striking examples.

The first substance proved to be secreted into the urine by mammalian renal tubules was the anion of the indicator dye phenol red (phenol sulphone phthalein, PSP; Fig. 4.3), a weak organic acid (Marshall & Vickers, 1923; see Smith, 1937, 1951; and Weiner, 1973, for much historical detail). By 1936 Sheehan had demonstrated the transfer of three quarters of the dye from arterial blood into the urine in one passage through the dog's kidney, although only about one quarter was filterable, the rest being bound to plasma proteins. Since so much more was excreted than appeared in the glomerular filtrate, the dye must have been secreted by the renal tubules. Diodone (diodrast, iodo-pyracet, introduced as a radio-opaque medium for radiography of the renal tract) and PAH are largely free in the plasma, and the kidneys can remove nearly 90% in one passage. This remarkably effective tubular secretion which made PAH useful for indirect measurements of RPF has been mentioned (Section 2.2.3.2). Twenty per cent passes into the tubules in the glomerular filtrate, and the tubules remove most of the remainder from postglomerular blood on its way through the peritubular capillaries.

Traces of o-aminohippurate appear in normal human urine, as a metabolite of tryptophan (Musajo & Benassi, 1964), but PAH is not a normal urinary constituent, and substances like diodone and some penicillins which have almost identical clearances, are also wholly foreign. Although it is desirable that the kidney should be able to remove foreign substances from the body expeditiously, it is nonetheless remarkable that the tubules can act so efficiently on substances they have never encountered in the course of their evolution.

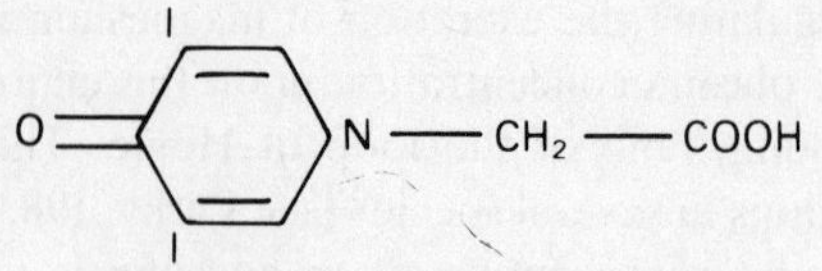
Diodone

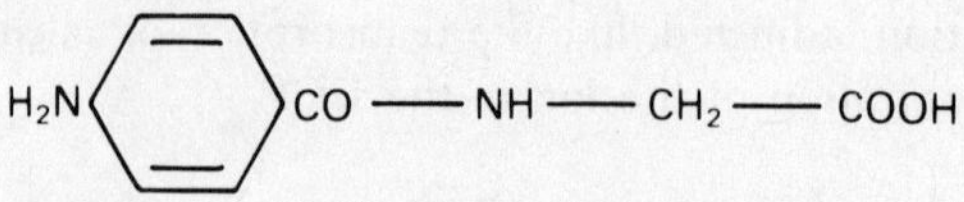
p-aminohippuric acid

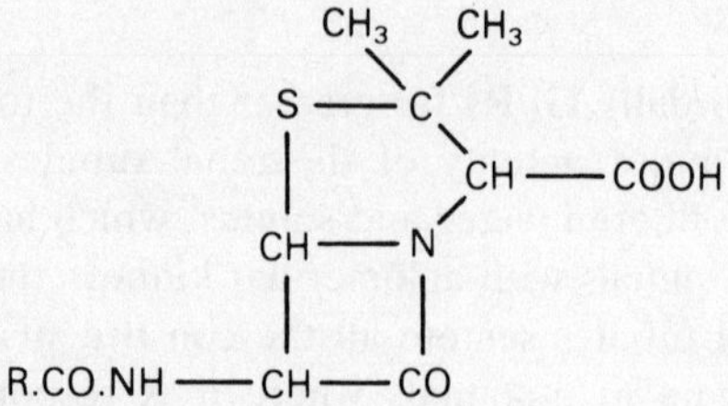
Penicillin

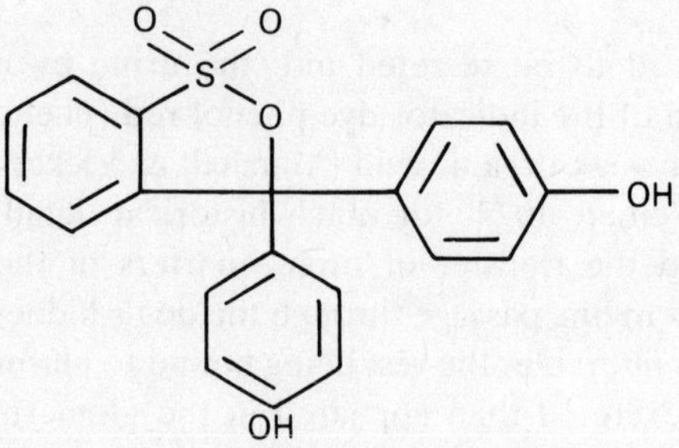
Phenol red

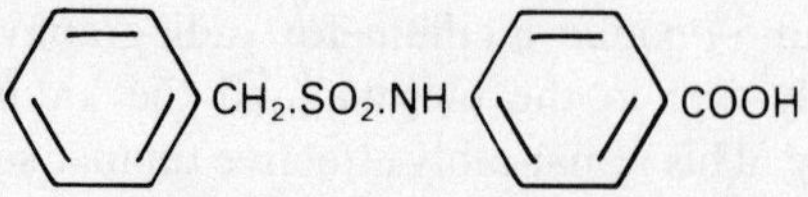
Carinamide

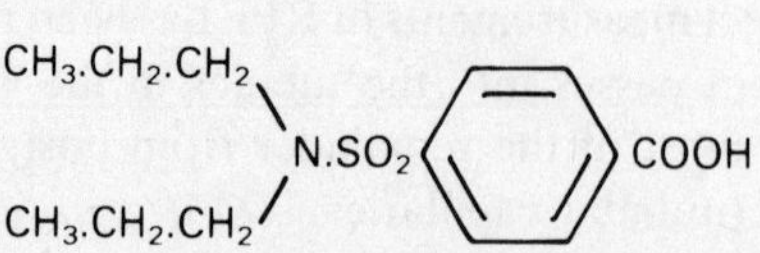
Probenecid

Fig. 4.3 Structures of some substances which are actively secreted: and of two inhibitors.

It will be convenient to deal briefly with the tubular secretion of foreign substances, and then to give an outline of tubular secretion of physiological substances.

4.4.2 Tubular secretion of foreign organic anions

Since the first demonstration of tubular secretion of phenol red, many other organic anions have been found which are excreted in a similar manner. Their tubular secretion is active, from low concentrations in the plasma to far larger concentrations in tubular fluid and final urine, and it is inhibited by cooling, by anoxia and by metabolic poisons. Since Marshall & Crane (1924) showed the rate of excretion of phenol red plateauing while that of urea continued to increase with rising plasma concentrations in the dog, it has been well established that the secretory mechanism is of limited capacity. Para-aminohippurate is typical, well studied and can serve as an example to illustrate the handling of most members of the group.

As the secretory capacity of the tubules becomes saturated, only the direct contribution of the filtered load to excretion continues to rise in proportion with the plasma concentration. Consequently the total rate of excretion fails to keep pace with a rising concentration in the plasma, and the clearance diminishes, to approach the clearance of inulin asymptotically at concentrations large enough to make tubular secretion negligible in comparison with the filtered load (cf. Smith, 1951, Fig. 45). This fall with rising concentration was called the 'self-depression of the clearance', and the concentration (sufficient to saturate the tubules of lowest transporting capacity) above which it began was called the 'self-depression limit' (Fig. 4.4). This corresponds to the threshold at which excretion begins when tubules and glomeruli act in opposition in the handling of glucose or amino acids (Fig. 4.2). There is also a saturation limit above which all tubules are saturated and the rate of excretion can only increase with rising concentration because the filtered load increases. Above the saturation limit the difference between the rates of excretion and filtration becomes constant and maximal, and defines a secretory Tm analogous with the reabsorptive Tm_g, but operating in the opposite direction. Homer Smith (1943) called this the 'tubular excretory mass', though 'maximal tubular secretory capacity' would be a better term today (cf. Robinson, 1954). Smith regarded it as a measure of the total amount of healthy tubular tissue perfused with blood to bring it PAH to secrete; whereas Tm_g excludes tubules with damaged glomeruli that fail to supply them with glucose to reabsorb.

The limited capacity of tubular secretion is also revealed by mutual competition between members of the group for maximal rates of secretion. This might be due to competition for available energy, or for a carrier-mediating active transport. When penicillin was scarce and extremely expensive, attempts were made to develope drugs which would inhibit its rapid excretion during the treatment of systemic infections. These were substances excreted by the same mechanism. One of the first, carinamide (Fig. 4.3), was excreted too rapidly and was soon displaced by probenecid (formerly benemid). All these substances possess an ionizable carboxyl group attached to some kind of ring

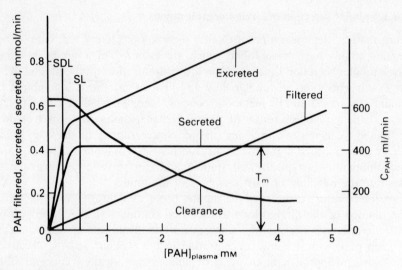

Fig. 4.4 Filtration, secretion, excretion and clearance of PAH.
SDL = self depression limit
SL   = saturation limit.

structure, and this was thought to be a requirement for transport by the system, but was shown to be unessential when PAH-hydroxamate, with the COOH group covered, was found to be excreted like PAH itself (Smith, 1956). Indeed, it hardly seems possible to go beyond Weiner's (1973) conclusion that attempts to define the structural characters necessary for secretion have not been wholly sucessful, and Häberle (1981) concluded after an extensive review that it is still not certain that these organic anions are all secreted by one common mechanism, even when they inhibit each others' secretion. There are puzzling differences between species; thus the physiological anion urate is a competitor with PAH in rat, rabbit and cebus monkey, but they seem to be secreted by different mechanisms in snake, man and chimpanzee. There are also anions which seem to be handled by other transport systems. For example, ethylenediaminetetraacetate (EDTA, Foreman *et al.*, 1953) and diphosphonates (Troehler *et al.*, 1975) are strongly secreted without competing with each other or with members of the other groups.

It is interesting that Tm values of several members of the main group are of the same order of magnitude (diodone, 0.2; PAH, 0.4; phenol red, 0.1; creatinine, 0.14 mmol/min in man), as might be expected if they were all secreted by the same mechanism. These values are not identical; but Weiner (1973) warned that the rate of actual tubular secretion would be underestimated if appreciable reabsorption occurred, because what had been secreted and then reabsorbed would not contribute to the net rate of excretion and would therefore be missed. Passive reabsorption by nonionic diffusion might be anticipated if the acids were lipid-soluble and weak enough for acidification of the urine to convert a high proportion to the unionized form; but this does not seem to be a problem for PAH or diodone, which are not especially weak acids (pKa 3.8 and 2.7) and have very low lipid-solubility. Probenecid, which has a similar pKa, 3.4, is much more soluble in lipid solvents than in water and probably owes its low renal clearance to the great lipid-solubility which enables so much of it to be reabsorbed passively by back-diffusion (Deetjen, 1970).

Earlier surmises that the secretory process is located in the proximal renal tubule have been confirmed. Evidence that the proximal straight tubule secretes organic anions more vigorously than the convoluted portion (Tune *et al.*, 1969) received interesting support from a chance observation (Grantham, 1976) that collapsed segments of proximal straight tubules isolated from rabbits rapidly became re-inflated with secreted fluid when PAH was added to the bath, whereas this did not happen in several hundred observations with proximal (or distal) convoluted tubules. Fluid secretion was maximal with 1 mM PAH in the bath, and was inhibited by ouabain. It was also abolished by cooling to 25°C, which used to be a normal American room temperature, and one which has often been used for experiments on isolated mammalian tissues. The secreted fluid was isosmolal with the bath and contained 40 mM PAH, so that the mechanism underlying the secretion of fluid was almost certainly primary active secretion of PAH into the lumen, leading to uptake of water by osmosis. The transepithelial pd was changed from + 0.3 to −1.3 mV (lumen-negative), suggesting that the anion was secreted actively. The osmotic uptake of water reduces the concentration of PAH built up in the lumen and therefore the gradient against which secretion must occur, and which tends to cause a loss of secreted solute by back-diffusion. Hippurate, benzoate and *o*-hydroxyhippurate (a metabolite of aspirin) also provoked influx of water.

Micropuncture techniques have confirmed that PAH is secreted by the proximal tubule, especially by the straight portion, with a saturation limit around 1 mM PAH. An observation that the maximal rate of secretion of PAH varied in parallel with alterations in GFR in whole kidneys was also confirmed for SNGFR in single nephrons (Häberle, 1981). The kidney's consumption of oxygen parallels GFR, and acetate, which stimulates respiration, also promotes the secretion of PAH. Another variable linked with the GFR and the rate of consumption of oxygen is the filtration and subsequent reabsorption of sodium, and there are indications that the uptake of PAH into isolated tubules or tissue slices depends on the presence of enough sodium in the medium. But the inhibition of PAH-linked fluid secretion by ouabain suggests that uptake through the peritubular membranes might depend upon the sodium gradient maintained by the pump rather than on movement of sodium through the cell in the opposite direction. Häberle (1981) concluded that if PAH/sodium co-transport is involved, it is not the only mechanism for cellular uptake of PAH. It still seems to be generally accepted that there is active uptake into the cell from the peritubular fluid and passive escape into the lumen. This passive exit across the apical membranes may also be carrier-mediated; it is inhibited by phlorizin, which actually increases the antiluminal uptake.

Despite a large amount of work during the past three decades, so much is still uncertain that Homer Smith's (1956) somewhat despairing comment about reabsorption; 'our knowledge of the enzymatic and cellular mechanisms involved in tubular reabsorption comprises almost a blank page', is still applicable to tubular secretion in either direction! Smith did add, 'but useful information is beginning to be inscribed' and indeed, a great deal of information has been inscribed, though it has not yet led to much certain knowledge.

4.4.3 Tubular secretion of foreign organic cations

Tubular secretion of organic cations was discovered two decades after that of organic anions, when Sperber (1947) and Rennick et al. (1947) demonstrated that N-methylnicotinamide (NMN, a metabolic endproduct of nicotinic acid) and the strong quaternary ammonium base tetraethylammonium (TEA) were excreted in part by tubular secretion. Since then many more examples have been found (reviewed by Rennick, 1981). They are primary, secondary, tertiary or quaternary amines, and include alkaloids, catecholamines, procaine, quinine and amiloride. Some, like isoproterenol, which have profound pharmacological actions, have been studied in chickens by injecting them into the renal portal circulation to avoid sytemic effects interfering with renal function. Almost all have pKa values above the physiological range of pH, and the resulting positive charge on the nitrogen atom appears to be the essential requirement for secretion, which can be inhibited by positively charged antimony, arsenic and sulphur compounds as well as by other organic cations (Weiner, 1973).

The organic cations may be as vigorously excreted as organic anions when concentrations in the plasma are small. Tetraethylammonium might even be better than PAH for measuring the RPF in uraemic patients; it had the same clearance in normal dogs and its secretion was not inhibited by azotaemia like that of PAH (McNay et al., 1976). Tubular maximum secretory rates have been demonstrated for some compounds, and the tubular secretion of organic cations shows mutual competition and saturation as with organic anions. Both are inhibited by chilling, poisons and anoxia, but temperature and pH optima differ. Secretion of cations is not inhibited by probenecid, but has its own specific inhibitors, a dye, cyanine 863, mepiperphenidol, and quinine, which correspond to probenecid in relation to the anion-secreting system. Krebs cycle intermediates that inhibit anion secretion do not affect cation secretion; and acetate, pyruvate and lactate do not promote it as they do the secretion of anions.

Stop-flow and micropuncture studies have confirmed that the organic cations are secreted by the proximal renal tubules, but organic cations do not compete with organic anions for secretion. Indeed, their active transport systems appear to be at opposite poles of the proximal tubular cells. Both luminal and antiluminal membrane vesicles take up NMN, but only vesicles from luminal membranes show uphill countertransport. This is driven in the first instance by a proton gradient, which may in turn be maintained by the sodium/hydrogen antiport system, and so depend indirectly on the sodium gradient. Basolateral uptake is probably passive, the cations being attracted into the negatively charged interior of the cells. So the cations seem to undergo active secretion into the lumen following passive uptake from the peritubular fluid, while organic anions are taken up actively across the basal membranes and diffuse passively out into the lumen.

4.4.4 Tubular secretion of physiological substances

Among endogenous substances whose excretion involves tubular secretion, Homer Smith listed creatinine, uric acid, hippuric acid and many derivatives, pantothenic acid, urobilin, guanidine, NMN, glucuronides, and phenolsulphuric ester. Smith (1956) remarked that tubular secretion 'as a supplement to filtration, appears to be a means of facilitating the excretion of certain types of compounds, especially aromatic nuclei, which cannot otherwise be disposed of by metabolism'. Most of these substances, and autacoids like the catecholamines, require only brief comments, for they fall into the same classes as the organic compounds already discussed. Rather more needs to be said about three important but chemically less complex cations not included in Smith's list; namely potassium, hydrogen and ammonium. The second two of these are peculiar in being manufactured in the renal tubular cells rather than transferred to the urine from the blood.

A. Organic anions

1 Ethereal sulphates. The phenolsulphuric ester of Homer Smith's list is a typical representative of what used to be known picturesquely as the ethereal sulphates, which account for around 10% of the urinary sulphur. They are formed in the liver by conjugation of sulphate with compounds that are mostly produced by bacterial fermentation of aromatic amino acids in the gut; phenylalanine, tyrosine and tryptophan yield phenol, p-cresol and indoxyl. Morphine and some of its derivatives are secreted unchanged as foreign organic cations, but they are also partly converted by the kidney into ethereal sulphates for excretion (Rennick, 1981).
2 Urate. This presents a complicated picture because it is subjected to both active secretion and active reabsorption in the proximal tubule, with important differences between species (Mudge et al., 1973). Secretion predominates; always in birds and reptiles, giving clearances many times greater than the

GFR, usually in Dalmatian coach-hounds and guinea pigs, in some rabbits but not (unpredictably) in others; and reabsorption is predominant and leads to urate clearances of the order of 10% of GFR in man, other primates and most dogs. Much of the work on the mechanism of secretion appears to have been done in snakes, where transport from blood to cells across the peritubular membrane is active (against an electrical gradient for the anion), and movement into the lumen is passive; but despite this resemblance the transport system may be separate from that for other organic anions (Dantzler, 1981).

3   Oxalate. In the urine, this amounts to 0.3 to 0.4 mmol daily in man and is mostly endogenous, derived from ascorbic acid and glycine. Although the food contains about 1 mmol per day, only about 40 µmol of this is absorbed. Since it has been realized that the concentration in the plasma is low, in the micromolar range (a satisfactory method for measuring it is still lacking), it has become clear that the urinary oxalate is secreted actively by the proximal tubules, probably by the common system for many organic anions, because secretion of oxalate is inhibited by probenecid and competitively by secretion of PAH and of urate (Greger, 1981).

5   Creatinine. This is one of the most abundant endogenous urinary organic ions. Human urine contains around 8 to 20 mmol per day, less for women than for men (Doolan et al., 1962). Rennick (1981) listed it among the organic cations, but Pitts (1974) described it as a buffer base that makes an appreciable contribution to the titratable acid of the urine (Section 6.3). With a pKa of 4.97 it should be present mostly as an anion in the plasma and in all but the most acid urines. Rehberg suggested its use for measuring GFRs in 1926, and it was widely employed, even after it was known to be actively excreted by aglomerular and other fishes, and by birds, with clearances up to six times GFR. Its secretion by some male mammals or by females treated with androgenic hormones was appreciated later (see Section 3.3.2 for references). The tubular secretion of creatinine in man has a limited capacity with a Tm value of about 0.14 mmol/min, but it can increase the creatinine/inulin clearance ratio to as much as 1.3 when the concentration in the plasma is not augmented with exogenous creatinine. The tubular secretion of creatinine suffers competitive inhibition in man and rat by diodone and PAH (Pitts, 1974), which compete in the system that transports organic anions. But Weiner (1973) noted that in some species tubular secretion was also depressed by inhibitors of the system transporting cations, and listed creatinine as an 'unclassifiable' compound.

B. Organic cations

1   N^1-methylnicotinamide. This was the first physiological substance of this group to have its tubular secretion demonstrated, in the chicken, by Sperber (1947). It is a quaternary ammonium base produced as an endproduct of the metabolism of nicotinic acid and nicotinamide, and only small amounts are normally excreted (less than 0.1 mmol daily in man). The mechanism of its

secretion has already been outlined in Section 4.4.3. Clearance ratios MNM/ inulin as high as 4 have been recorded in dogs at low plasma concentrations, and a Tm has been demonstrated in rats and dogs. Micropuncture studies have confirmed active secretion by the proximal tubules (see Rennick, 1981, for further details and references).

2 Choline. This is ordinarily present in the plasma at a concentration around 0.01 mM. This concentration should be low enough to permit very effective tubular secretion, but the amount of endogenous choline in the urine of dogs, chickens, rats and men is not more than a few per cent of the filtered load. A Tm is reached at about 10 times the normal concentration, and secretion is inhibited by quinine and cyanine 863. The renal handling of choline is, however, complicated by extensive reabsorption, probably active and also in the proximal tubule, as well as by oxidation to betaine in the kidney. Some related compounds, in very small concentrations, enhance the excretion of choline, probably by competing for reabsorption so that tubular secretion is unmasked. These include thiamine, lysine, quinine, triethylcholine and ace-tylcholine. Rennick (1981) suggested that the kidney plays a role in homeos-tasis by reabsorbing choline when its concentration in the plasma is low and excreting it when the concentration is high.

3 Catecholamines. This is a group of extremely potent vasoactive agents and neurotransmitters, including adrenaline, noradrenaline, dopamine, 5-hydroxytryptamine and histamine. They are normally present in the blood in small but physiologically effective concentrations. At larger concentrations they would exert profound pharmacological actions, and the early studies were made by Sperber's technique, which avoided systemic actions by delivering them to the tubules by way of the renal portal vein in chickens. These studies have been supplemented by infusion into the renal artery in dogs or the use of the isolated, perfused kidney in rats (see Rennick, 1981). The tubular secretion of these potent autacoids is important because they are bound to plasma proteins and would partly escape filtration. If their removal by excre-tion helps to keep their concentrations in the plasma low and more immedi-ately controllable by their rate of liberation, it may serve a similar homeostatic purpose as the removal of LMWPs by tubular destruction.

C. Potassium

Although the amount of potassium leaving the kidney in the urine is usually much less than was filtered, indicating that most is reabsorbed, the clearance of potassium sometimes exceeds that of inulin, for example after loading with potassium, during osmotic diuresis, especially with urea or unreabsorbable anions like ferrocyanide, and in renal disease when glomerular filtration is greatly depressed (Berliner, 1961; Giebisch & Windhager, 1964). In these circumstances excretion must be augmented by tubular secretion. Early ob-servations that considerable reductions in filtered load hardly affected the rate of urinary output of potassium suggested that the rate of excretion might depend mainly upon distal secretion, and it came to be supposed that all or most of the filtered load was routinely reabsorbed, so that tubular secretion determined the renal output of potassium. Moreover, samples representing distal segments in stop-flow experiments contained higher concentrations of potassium. The finding that after most of a dose of radioactive potassium given to human subjects had been taken up into cells, the specific activity of potassium in the urine was similar to that in cells and renal venous blood and far greater than in arterial plasma and glomerular filtrate, also suggested that the potassium in the urine came from tubular cells (Black *et al.*, 1956), but did not prove this because filtered potassium might have exchanged with cellular potassium on its way through the tubules.

Studies with micropuncture techniques provided more direct and conclusive confirmation that the rate of excretion was substantially independent of the filtered load. For example, Malnic *et al.* (1964) compared groups of rats on diets providing low, normal and high intakes of potassium. Some rats on high-potassium intakes also received an inhibitor of carbonic anhydrase (dichlor-phenamide) and infusions of potassium chloride and sodium sulphate, all known to promote the excretion of potassium. Average urinary outputs were about 3% of filtered potassium on the low-potassium diet, 20% on the control diet (raised to 60% by dichlorphenamide), and 150% on the high-potassium diet with measures promoting excretion. Tubular fluid/plasma ratios for potassium concentration and for potassium/inulin were remarkably similar along the accessible proximal tubules in all groups. The concentration of potassium was reduced a little below that in the plasma; even in the high-potassium group at least 70% of filtered potassium had been reabsorbed by the end of the proximal tubules, and only about a quarter of filtered potassium entered the distal tubules. From then on there were striking differences. Net reabsorption continued in the low-potassium group, but in all the others potassium was added on the way along the distal tubules, and in the high-potassium group this led to the excretion of more than had been filtered.

Such experiments established that, even under control conditions, when much less potassium was excreted than filtered; about 75% of the potassium in the urine was secreted by the distal tubules and collecting ducts. The common statements that all the filtered potassium is reabsorbed proximally, and all the potassium in the urine is secreted by distal segments of the nephron are oversimplified. Wright & Giebisch (1978) concluded in a valuable review, that 'the major fraction of excreted potassium is contributed by the potassium-secreting cells of the cortical distal nephron'. Later work identified potassium-secreting cells in the connecting tubule and the early part of the cortical collecting tubule, but not in the distal convoluted tubule itself (Stanton *et al.*, 1981).

It used to be taught that sodium was reabsorbed in exchange for hydrogen ions or potassium by an active process which was stimulated by aldosterone. The kidney's ability to excrete potassium therefore depended upon sufficient sodium reaching the exchange site, while excessive amounts of sodium passing through the distal nephron could augment the excretion of potassium and deplete the body's stores. More recently the idea of any strict coupling between movements of sodium and potassium has receded, and it seems more likely that the active process tends to set the ratio of luminal to intracellular potassium concentration, so that the rate of secretion is roughly proportional to the flow of tubular fluid past the secreting cells. Sodium is still important, because the rate of delivery of sodium ions to the distal nephron affects both the flow of tubular fluid and the pd which promotes the excretion of potassium (Khuri *et al.*, 1975). The principal factors controlling the secretion of potassium may be conveniently summarized by reference to the features of typical distal tubular cells (Fig. 4.5) The numbers correspond to numbered features in the diagram.

1 The concentration of potassium in the plasma. Increases enhance uptake by the sodium−potassium exchange pump in the basolateral cell membrane; which in turn promotes secretion by raising the concentration of potassium in the cells.

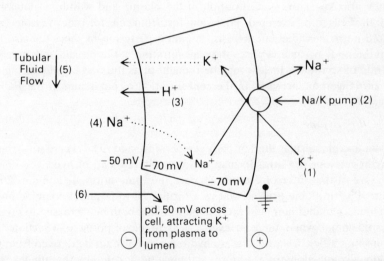

Fig. 4.5 Principal features of distal nephron cells affecting excretion of potassium.
Factors *increasing* excretion of potassium:
1 Increased potassium concentration in ECF (increases pump rate);
2 Increased aldosterone concentration;
3 disturbances of acid−base balance (except acute acidosis);
4 increased sodium concentration in tubular fluid;
5 increased rate of flow of tubular fluid;
6 increased transepithelial pd.
   Excretion of potassium is *reduced*: by decreases in 1, 2, 4, 5, 6; temporarily by acidosis; and by active reabsorption across luminal borders of cells when the need for conservation is great.

2 Aldosterone. This adrenal cortical hormone enhances the activity of the sodium—potassium pump, promoting renal retention of sodium and excretion of potassium.

3 Acid—base balance. Most disturbances promote the secretion of potassium by complex mechanisms (Section 6.4).

4 Sodium in the local tubular fluid. Higher concentrations promote exchange across the luminal membrane and flux of sodium through the pump, thus favouring peritubular uptake of potassium as well as its transport into the lumen. More unreabsorbed sodium increases the flow of tubular fluid.

5 Rate of flow of tubular fluid, which carries potassium from the secreting site.

6 The tubular pd. An increase in the lumen-negative pd (produced for example by aldosterone and the presence of anions that cannot be reabsorbed) promotes secretion by attracting potassium ions into the tubular fluid.

Other things being equal, the rate of secretion controlled by these factors is usually regulated to stabilize the concentration of potassium in the plasma in face of alterations in dietary intake. Extrarenal losses that lower the concentration in the plasma reduce the rate of secretion. Abnormal losses by the kidney also lower the concentration in the plasma and withdraw potassium from the cells to be excreted. Potassium lost from cells for other reasons (e.g. steroid hormones, diabetic ketosis, impaired perfusion in shock) is also lost from the body because it raises the concentration in the plasma and increases the rate of secretion. Its loss may be thought of as the cost of minimizing the risk of dangerous increases in the concentration of potassium in the ECFs.

D. Hydrogen ions

Plasma and glomerular fluid at body temperature and pH 7.4 contain 40 nmol of hydrogen ions per litre. In man the daily filtered load of hydrogen ions is therefore of the order of 7 μmol, whereas the urine normally contains 20 to 30 mmol as titratable acid as well as a further 30 to 50 mmol combined with ammonia as ammonium, and these quantities can both be increased to several hundred mmol when there is excess acid to be disposed of (Section 6.3; Robinson, 1975c). Clearly all these hydrogen ions cannot be derived from the blandly alkaline glomerular filtrate, and must be secreted by the tubules. The ordinary formula would yield a value for the clearance of at least $50/0.000040 = 1\,250\,000$ l/day; more than 1000 times greater than the RPF! Moreover, the reabsorption of some 4500 mmol of filtered bicarbonate requires the secretion into the tubular fluid of a further 4500 mmol of hydrogen ions which are not excreted in the urine. The clearance formula can strictly be applied only to substances which are transferred quantitatively from plasma to urine, and are not stored, created or destroyed in the kidney. The ridiculous value obtained above is the result of an illegitimate calculation, because the hydrogen ions are not transferred to the urine from the plasma but generated in the tubular cells. This process and its regulation will be dealt with in more detail in Section 6.4 on the renal control of acid–base balance.

E. Ammonium

Ammonium is another physiologically important cation which must be secreted by the tubules because far more appears in the urine than could be supplied by the glomerular filtrate. Again, a clearance cannot be calculated. Ammonium, produced in the tubular cells from glutamine and some amino acids, leaves the kidney in both the urine and the renal venous blood, which contains more than the arterial blood entering the kidney. Partition between venous blood and urine depends upon their rates of flow and pH, the urine taking an increasing share as it is made more acid by secretion of hydrogen ions (Section 6.3.3).

4.5 METABOLIC ASPECTS OF TUBULAR FUNCTION

4.5.1 Introduction

Renal tissue has an unusually large rate of consumption of oxygen per g; around half that of the heart and twice that of the brain. The human kidneys are responsible for about 0.5% of the weight of the body and 10% of the resting consumption of oxygen. In a book on metabolic aspects of renal function, Lotspeich (1959) admitted that we could not then account for the use the kidneys make of 99% of their metabolic energy. Today we would assign the bulk of it to keeping 300 g of cells filled with a potassium-rich intracellular fluid (ICF) while passing over half their volume of sodium-rich glomerular filtrate back to the plasma every minute; and to special urinary functions.

Other important renal functions that require energy include:
1 Interconversion of substrates; this helps to conserve energy as well as to regulate the composition and reaction (pH) of the plasma.
2 Synthesis of specific substances and humoral agents, for local use in the kidney or for export. Substances generated include hydrogen ions and ammonium (Section 4.4.4), glucose, active forms of vitamin D, and guanidinoacetate, which the liver converts to creatine. Humoral agents include renin, erythropoietin and PGs.
3 Synthesis of structural materials to maintain the kidneys' machinery and cell membranes. Synthesis of glycoproteins probably makes a major call on the rapid metabolism of the glomeruli, which make up 5% of the kidneys' mass and use 5% of their oxygen.

The following brief sketches of some of the kidneys' considerable contributions to the body's overall turnover of metabolic substrates are based on a handful of reviews (Cohen & Barac-Nieto, 1973; Weinstein, 1974; Cohen &

Kamm, 1976; Guder & Wirthensohn, 1981; Ross & Lowry, 1981; Simpson, 1983; Guder & Ross, 1984). These give ready access to some 500 more specific references.

4.5.2 Energy metabolism

Although the medulla appears to be fuelled principally by glucose, this is not true for the kidney as a whole. The fuels utilized vary with concentrations presented in the arterial plasma and with other factors. A suggested typical distribution might be: fatty acids e.g. palmitate, 15%; glucose, 10%; lactate, 20%; glutamine, 35%; and citrate, 10%. This allows 10% for other substrates. These include small amounts of pyruvate, 2-oxoglutarate, glycerol, 'ketone bodies', some amino acids, fructose (which the kidney can convert to glucose), and inositol which the kidney alone is able to oxidize to D-glucuronate by inositol oxidase. The metabolic mixture gives a respiratory quotient (RQ) close to 1.0; but Guder & Wirthensohn (1981) emphasized that because substrates have a variety of fates other than oxidation, their renal uptake does not precisely measure the fuels consumed. Moreover, not all of the energy-yielding substrates are completely oxidized to carbon dioxide; options include incomplete aerobic oxidation, glycolysis and anaerobic oxidative decarboxylation (e.g. of 2-oxoglutarate to succinate), according to the prevailing oxygen tension; this depends upon blood flow and activity, but even more on intrarenal location.

The kidney as a whole is so well supplied with blood (Section 2.2.1; 2.2.4) that the arteriovenous difference for oxygen is remarkably small despite a rapid rate of metabolism. But the cortex, which makes up about three quarters of the kidneys' mass, receives most of the rich blood supply, and the partial pressure of oxygen is much lower in the medulla (Section 2.3). The medulla is also more richly supplied with glycolytic enzymes (Ullrich, 1959; Guder & Ross, 1984) than the cortex. The rate of glycolysis in outer medullary tissue is greater than that in cortical tissue and increases more rapidly with falling oxygen tension; while the papilla, where oxygen tension is lowest, seems most committed to glycolysis, regardless of oxygen supply (Cohen, 1979). Slices of medullary tissue are also unique in increasing their consumption of oxygen greatly in hypertonic saline media (Ullrich, 1959). Notwithstanding Thurau's (1964) assurance that even the inner medulla, with 10% of the cortical rate of consumption of oxygen, enjoys a much greater blood supply than resting muscle, Brezis et al. (1984) suggested that their heavy demands for energy for transport cause the thick ascending limbs of the loops of Henle to operate 'on the verge of anoxia' and that the outer medulla is greatly at risk when the renal circulation is threatened. The mitochondria and their energy-mobilizing enzymes are more highly concentrated in the thick ascending limbs and distal tubules than they are in the proximal tubules which reabsorb at a greater rate but against smaller gradients.

Comparisons between the cortex and the medulla are not straightforward because neither is homogeneous. The cortex contains distal tubules and glomeruli as well as proximal tubules. The medulla contains collecting tubules and vasa recta as well as loops of Henle, though the principal cellular structures in the outer medulla are the thick ascending limbs of the loops. It is probably fair to conclude that energy metabolism in the cortex is almost wholly aerobic, while the medulla and the papilla employ both aerobic and anaerobic reactions, and that more than 90% of the kidneys' applicable energy in the form of ATP is generated by aerobic oxidations, the minor part by glycolysis, mostly in the medulla.

4.5.3 Metabolism of particular substances

A. Glucose

Each day the human glomeruli filter about 900 mmol of glucose and the proximal tubules reabsorb all of this by a process that does not involve its metabolism (Section 4.2.2). A little glucose is utilized by the kidney, but it is hard to detect any difference between the concentrations in arterial and renal venous blood because the kidney also produces about 20 mmol per day. This is ordinarily a little more than is utilized, but osmotic diuresis can cause a shift from net production to net utilization. All the kidney's structures can utilize glucose as a fuel, but the proximal tubules normally use very little. Most of the glucose consumed as fuel is oxidized to carbon dioxide and water through the Krebs cycle or by the hexose monophosphate shunt pathway. Some is oxidized incompletely along the glycolytic pathway, particularly in the medulla, where glucose is a major substrate (cf. 4.5.1 above). Utilization of glucose is directly responsible for less than a tenth of the whole kidney's consumption of oxygen and production of carbon dioxide.

Although the kidneys have about one fifth of the mass of the liver and store little glycogen, they make a substantial contribution to the body's synthesis of glucose, notably from lactate released by glycolysis in active muscles. The kidney can also convert citrate to glucose for other tissues which are unable to utilize citrate directly. The renal cortex, per unit weight, has actually a greater capacity for producing glucose than the liver, and kidney slices from animals that have been starved or kept on diets low in carbohydrate synthesize glucose twice as fast as slices from the kidneys of well-fed animals. As with the liver, renal gluconeogenesis (GNG) is increased in diabetes mellitus and by glucocorticoids, but it differs in being sensitive to the reaction (pH) of the blood, and in being increased by depletion of potassium, possibly because this lowers pH in the cells. Kidney slices from acidotic or potassium-depleted animals show accelerated GNG from glutamine, glutamate, 2-oxoglutarate and other Krebs cycle intermediates. The conversion of organic anions like lactate to neutral glucose is a nonexcretory way of disposing of unwanted acids, and the rate of conversion is enhanced by acidosis and reduced by alkalosis. Moreover, GNG from glutamate is a part of the kidney's mechanisms for generating ammonium and regenerating bicarbonate, to be dealt with in Chapter 6.

Within the kidney itself, the sites where glucose is produced and utilized are separate. Only the cortex, where proximal tubular cells possess the necessary enzymes, can produce glucose for local consumption or export; while the medulla, with its rich endowment of glycolytic enzymes, is the principal local consumer.

B. Lactate

The kidney can oxidize lactate completely to carbon dioxide and water, and this can account for a fifth or more of the renal consumption of oxygen. A small fraction of the lactate taken up by the kidney may be converted into amino acids e.g. glutamate, but up to 40% (when lactate is the only substrate) can be converted to glucose. The production of glucose from excess lactate when this is present in high concentrations in the plasma is one of the kidney's most important metabolic interconversions. It supplements the action of the liver as a supplier of glucose to other tissues, and it also helps to preserve the normal bland alkalinity of the ECFs.

C. Lipids

A fifth of the dry mass of the kidneys consists of lipids, chiefly phospholipid. The kidneys have a high rate of oxidation of free fatty acids (FFAs) compared with other organs, and are responsible for nearly a tenth of the body's turnover of FFAs. All parts of the kidney are capable of oxidizing FFAs, but this occurs mainly in the cortex in so far as the FFAs rely upon the PAH transporting system to get them into the cells. Because the rate of their uptake tends to vary in parallel with the reabsorption of sodium, FFAs have been claimed to be a major renal fuel, and the preferential substrate for the cortex. However, their oxidation probably accounts for no more than 10 to 20% of the kidneys' production of carbon dioxide, and most of the FFA's taken up by the kidneys are not burned for fuel but exported as phospholipid or triglycerate. The rate of utilization increases with the concentration of FFAs in the plasma, and it is also increased by lactate, which enhances the release of FFAs from the fat depots.

D. Citrate

The kidney is a major metabolic sink for citrate which is released into the blood from stores in the bones. The liver and kidney are the only organs that can ulilize it, but the kidney can also convert citrate into glucose for other organs to use. Oxidation of endogenous citrate accounts for less than 10% of renal consumption of oxygen, but this can be increased to as much as 40% by greatly increasing the concentration in the blood. Mammalian plasmas contain between 0.005 and 0.3 mM, all present as triply ionized citrate at physiological pH (pKa values for dissociation of the three protons of citrate are 3.09, 4.75 and 5.45). Human subjects excrete between 10 and 35% of the amount of citrate filtered, rats between 3 and 5%, and dogs even less. But more citrate disappears from the kidney than it excretes. Proximal tubular cells can take up citrate actively from postglomerular plasma across their peritubular borders as well as from the lumen, and accumulate it to several times the external concentration. Utilization of citrate by the kidney is therefore not limited to the amount that can be reabsorbed from the glomerular filtrate.

The great sensitivity of the rate of excretion of citrate to acid–base metabolism has been known for half a century, and studies on tissue slices and isolated tubular segments have confirmed that alkalosis inhibits the intracellular metabolism of citrate. In mitochondrial suspensions buffered with bicarbonate an increase of 0.3 in pH can reduce the rate of oxidation by half. The gradient of pH between the mitochondria and the cytosol is a major factor in controlling metabolism in the cells. Before it can be oxidized, citrate must cross the inner mitochondrial membrane. This is impermeable to most anions, but a tricarboxylate carrier allows citrate, isocitrate and aconitate to enter at rates depending on their concentrations and the pH gradient. In alkalosis, when cell pH and bicarbonate concentration are elevated, uptake into the mitochondria is inhibited and citrate accumulates in the cytosol; this slows both peritubular uptake and tubular reabsorption, so that the utilization of citrate is diminished and its rate of excretion is increased. Precursors like malate, succinate and fumarate, which increase the intracellular concentration, and metabolic inhibitors including fluorocitrate, fluoracetate and malonate, also increase the excretion of citrate; so do calcitonin and vitamin D. In acidosis the steeper pH gradient favours entry of citrate into the mitochondria, and falling concentrations in the cells favour both peritubular uptake and reabsorption, so that less citrate is excreted. The rate of excretion is also diminished by inhibitors of carbonic anhydrase, by potassium depletion (which may make the cells more acid), by starvation and by expansion of the ECFV.

E. Glutamine

Glutamine can be an important fuel for the kidney. It resembles citrate in being taken up both from the glomerular filtrate and from postglomerular plasma; its metabolism is also predominantly in the mitochondria and is very sensitive to acidity. In the course of catabolism, glutamine is first converted to glutamate and then to 2-oxoglutarate, yielding a molecule of ammonium at each step. The remainder of the molecule may be completely oxidized to carbon dioxide and water, or else used for the production of glucose. The rate of catabolism is several times greater during acidosis than during alkalosis, and the generation of ammonium is important for eliminating hydrogen ions in the urine. (See Section 6.3.3 on the kidneys' defence of acid—base balance.)

Filtered glutamine is all reabsorbed from the first third of the proximal tubules, but glutamine is taken up from postglomerular blood along their whole length. In dogs the kidney can extract more than half the glutamine from the renal arterial blood, three fifths of this from peritubular capillary plasma and two fifths from the glomerular filtrate (Silverman *et al.*, 1981). Catabolism begins mainly in the mitochondria because the first step is catalysed by a mitochondrial enzyme, phosphate-dependent glutaminase (PDG), which is most active in the proximal convoluted tubules during acidosis, but otherwise in the distal convoluted tubules (Guder & Ross, 1984). The main pathway continues through glutamine dehydrogenase (mitochondrial), oxoglutarate dehydrogenase and the mitochondrial enzymes of the Krebs cycle. The activity of oxoglutarate dehydrogenase is increased by falling pH, and Pitts (1974) pointed out that the increased metabolism of glutamate with the change from alkalosis to acidosis is accompanied by a roughly equivalent decrease in metabolism of lactate.

The kidney can synthesize glutamine, but the enzyme glutamine synthetase is outside the mitochondria, and mainly in cells of the proximal straight tubules, so that glutamine is produced and consumed in different tubular segments. This enzyme is absent from canine and human kidneys and is probably of little importance for production of ammonium (Tannen, 1978).

4.6 CONCLUDING REMARKS ON TUBULAR FUNCTION

The kidneys probably take so large a share of the body's resting consumption of oxygen because, like the heart, they never rest. Even when the body appears to be resting, all its cells are busy, using energy released by resting metabolism to keep their potassium inside and sodium out; for their membranes are permeable to both these cations. In addition to maintaining this steady state of dynamic equilibrium, the kidneys' cells have to reabsorb and pass on about half their own volume of sodium-rich glomerular filtrate every minute, and the suprabasal part of the renal metabolic rate parallels the reabsorption of sodium.

Shared carriers in the apical membranes of proximal tubular cells enable the sodium gradient maintained by the basolateral ion pumps to effect the reabsorption of glucose and amino acids as well as of sodium and accompanying anions. The same gradient drives the secretion of protons that destroy filtered bicarbonate, and the sodium—calcium exchange that extrudes calcium through the peritubular membranes. The ion pumps operating through the Na-K-ATPase in the basolateral cell membranes are also responsible for the strongly negative intracellular potential that attracts cations in from the lumen; and indirectly for the transepithelial potential gradients that assist reabsorption of ions. Since water follows reabsorbed solutes from the proximal tubules osmotically, a major part of the kidneys' routine conservative function is driven directly or indirectly by the active transport of sodium outwards across the peritubular cell membranes (Fig. 4.6).

Like the liver, the kidneys can synthesize glucose from shorter chain substrates and from fructose, and release it into the circulation; they also supplement the liver's metabolic functions in other ways. But whereas the liver appears relatively homogeneous, with each cell competent to carry out most metabolic functions (cf., however, Jungermann, 1985), the kidney's cells are more specialized. Investigations, mainly in rats, by microdissection and microchemical methods, have suggested that some enzyme systems are localized in distinct segments of nephrons (Guder & Ross, 1984). For example, GNG is confined to the proximal tubules, while enzymes for utilization of glucose by glycolysis are concentrated in the distal nephron. Only the proximal tubules metabolize fructose and glycerol, and produce the active metabolites of vitamin D. Glutamine synthetase is restricted to the proximal straight tubules, whereas glutaminase is normally most active in the distal nephron but becomes much more active in proximal convoluted tubules during acidosis. Such differences may reflect the fact that the liver is primarily a metabolic organ, while some metabolic activities of renal cells are more closely related to their urinary functions.

These urinary functions are carried out by selective tubular reabsorption,

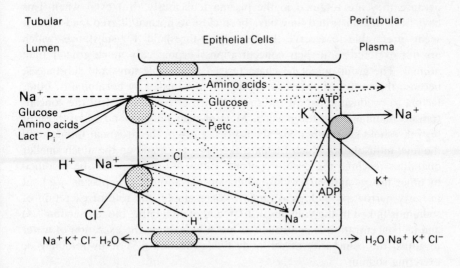

Fig. 4.6 To illustrate the dependence of proximal tubular reabsorption upon the basolateral sodium pumps. Diffusion along the paracellular pathway (. . . . . .).

supplemented by tubular secretion which may involve synthesis. The kidney's
handling of different substances can be summarized in terms of a modified
version of Cushny's (1926) classification by renal thresholds.

1   No-threshold substances are excreted no matter how small their concentrations in the plasma may be. Examples include foreign substances like inulin
and PAH, as well as endproducts like creatinine and urea, which are reabsorbed passively if at all. Parallel alterations in concentration in the plasma
enable excretion to keep pace with differing rates of production or administration and the kidney simply removes these substances from the body without
regulating their concentrations in the plasma as such. Proteins and peptides
which the tubules destroy are removed like no-threshold substances, but
without being excreted in the urine.

2   High-threshold substances include metabolic substrates like glucose, amino
acids and lactate, which disappear from the tubular fluid early in the proximal
convoluted tubules and are normally not excreted. Their maximal rates of
reabsorption are well above normal filtered loads, and the kidneys routinely
conserve them. Their concentrations in the plasma are determined by metabolic events, and meanwhile, their high renal thresholds ensure that they are
not excreted and lost during upward fluctuations within the physiological
range.

3   Medium-threshold substances. The kidneys play a major role in regulating
the concentrations in the plasma of substances like sodium, potassium, calcium,
magnesium, chloride, bicarbonate and phosphate, all of which tend to be
excreted or retained when their concentrations exceed or fall below normal
values. Cushny (1926) classed many of these as high-threshold substances
because they are retained in the plasma tenaciously. But even when Tms
have been demonstrated they have been close to normal filtered loads, and it
seems preferable to reserve the term 'high-threshold' for substances which
are not excreted until their concentrations become very much greater than
normal. The group might be characterized as variable-threshold substances,
because their rates of reabsorption are often adjusted by hormonal or other
factors to produce apparent thresholds which effectively control the concentrations maintained in the plasma. Most of their filtered loads, like those of
high-threshold substances, are reabsorbed early in the proximal tubules and
the final adjustments which regulate excretion are made on the much smaller
quantities reaching the distal nephrons. Rates of excretion may be modified
by other factors and vary widely while concentrations in the plasma are kept
in fairly narrow physiological ranges. For example, the rate of excretion of
sodium is linked to the volumes of ECF and of circulating blood (Section 7.4)
and its concentration is controlled as much by varying the excretion of water
to adjust the osmolarity of the body fluids (Section 5.5) as by retaining or
excreting sodium.

    There is an interesting and useful analogy between the mammalian distal
nephron and the amphibian urinary bladder. When the collecting ducts were

found to be performing functions like reabsorption of sodium and secretion of potassium, hydrogen ions and ammonium, they came to be regarded almost as honorary segments of the distal nephron. Not much exchange with blood takes place in the urinary bladder, which is the most distal part of the mammalian collecting system. But amphibian urinary bladders share functions of the mammalian distal tubules and collecting ducts and they have the added advantage that their secreting epithelia can be spread out in sheets and mounted between oxygenated solutions in suitably designed chambers which allow detailed studies of these functions to be carried out more conveniently (Macknight *et al.*, 1980). As Alex Leaf (1982) remarked in his Homer Smith Award Lecture; 'this tissue mimics many of the important functions of the more complex distal nephron and collecting duct of the human kidney. The basic transport mechanisms are common to both'.

Finally, the renal tubules conserve water and essential soluble constituents of the body, and help to regulate the concentrations of many of these in the plasma. At the same time they permit, or even hasten, the removal of unwanted solutes, including foreign substances or products of their degradation and normal bodily constituents in excess of requirements. They secrete daily into the blood many times its own volume of a reabsorbed fluid, which is in some respects a mirror-image of the urine, and which becomes the body's constantly renewed ECF. And besides all these 'urinary' homeostatic activities, they make significant contributions to intermediary metabolism.

CHAPTER 5
Renal handling of water

5.1 INTRODUCTION

Each minute the human kidneys extract about 120 ml of glomerular filtrate from 1250 ml of blood, and they finally produce between 0.5 ml of concentrated and 20 ml of dilute, watery urine. With a maximal rate of physiological diuresis around 20 ml/min, most of the filtered water is destined never to reach the urine. Homer Smith spoke of an obligatory reabsorption of about five sixths of the filtered water from the proximal tubules and the descending limbs of the loops of Henle, followed by a facultative reabsorption of more or less of the remainder. He located this variable process, which determines the final volume of the urine, in the distal tubules. More recent studies by micropuncture techniques in single nephrons have confirmed that the bulk of the filtered water is reabsorbed proximally, but have placed most of the final phase beyond the distal tubules in the collecting system.

The 'leaky' proximal tubular epithelium is so permeable that water can follow reabsorbed solutes, glucose, amino acids and major electrolytes, freely; changes in osmolarity of the tubular fluid were too small for early investigators to detect. Beyond the proximal tubule the permeability of the epithelium to water changes greatly. The thick ascending limbs of the loops of Henle are almost impermeable, and water left behind after solutes are reabsorbed makes the fluid entering the distal tubules hypotonic. In the absence of ADH (Section 5.3) the distal and collecting tubules are also almost impermeable to water, and continued reabsorption of sodium chloride makes the tubular fluid increasingly dilute as it advances along them; these tubules, together with the thick ascending limbs are known collectively as the 'diluting segments' of the nephron. The antidiuretic hormone greatly increases the permeability of the collecting system, and also of the late distal tubules in some animals, allowing water to return to the plasma and leave the tubular fluid more concentrated and smaller in volume. The last stage of reabsorption from the papillary collecting ducts may reduce the volume so much that the final urine is made more concentrated than the plasma. This facultative reabsorption of water allows the osmolarity of human urine to be varied between about one tenth and four times that of the plasma. Some desert rodents living on dry food can achieve concentrations up to as much as 20 or 30 times the osmolarity of their plasma, and so minimize the obligatory loss of water in their urine.

It will be convenient to describe the phenomena in more detail, and then to look at what is known or conjectured about the underlying mechanism of the concentrating process and its control.

5.2 THE PROXIMAL, OBLIGATORY PHASE OF REABSORPTION OF WATER

Ludwig (1884) proposed that water was reabsorbed with solutes of low molecular weight by the osmotic attraction of plasma proteins that had been concentrated by loss of the glomerular filtrate. This was not unreasonable before anything was known about the magnitudes of osmotic pressures, and Ludwig even proposed that concentrated urine could be produced in this way. Hoppe (1859), however, found that dogs' urine took up water from serum across a dialysing membrane, and when Tamman (1896) showed that a difference of 5000 mmHg would be needed to produce a urine one tenth as concentrated as the plasma, while Starling's (1899) first measurements of colloid osmotic pressure indicated that not more than 25 mmHg could be available from this source, Ludwig's physical theory became untenable. It could, however, still account for the reabsorption of an isotonic crystalloidal solution (see the discussion of possible passive reabsorption of sodium in Section 4.3.1).

Following the classical micropunctures of Walker *et al.* (1941) it was generally accepted that reabsorption from the proximal tubule did not alter the osmolarity of the tubular fluid, so that proximal tubular reabsorption was of water and solutes together in isosmotic proportions; the transport of water could be passive, secondary to the active reabsorption of solutes. Early experience with extreme diuresis showed that the 'obligatory' phase of reabsorption was not invariable, since large doses of solutes which were not reabsorbed greatly hindered the reabsorption of water. Shannon (1938b) found up to a third of the filtered water in the urine of dogs after large doses of urea, while up to half the filtered water was excreted during extreme diuresis with sulphate or glucose. In Wesson & Anslow's (1948) heroic experiments with mannitol, the urine contained two thirds of the filtered water and was approximately isotonic with the plasma. About half the water in this urine accompanied a third of the filtered sodium that had escaped reabsorption (the other two thirds being reabsorbed against a substantial gradient; see 4.3.1); the other half of the water in the urine accompanied mannitol.

These experiments established that the reabsorption of the bulk of the filtered water depends upon reabsorption of solutes, and pointed to sodium, with accompanying anions and co-transported organic solutes as the major solutes involved. Homer Smith came to speak of the 'obligatory' phase as an obligatory reabsorption of sodium accompanied by passive reabsorption of water, even though Wesson and Anslow had shown that the reabsorption of a third of the sodium was not obligatory under their extraordinary conditions. Moreover, the form of coupling between movements of water and movements of solutes was something of a mystery. Primary reabsorption of solutes, with water following by osmosis, should leave the tubular fluid hypotonic; it was inconceivable that so much water could be transferred without a substantial osmotic gradient. Ullrich & Rumrich (1963) estimated that a difference of about 23 mosm (corresponding to a difference in freezing point of 0.04°C) would be needed to drive proximal reabsorption in the rat, and it had to be supposed that the necessary gradient was somehow hidden within the epithelium. According to the standing gradient hypothesis of Diamond & Bossert (1967), sodium and chloride were secreted into lateral intercellular spaces, which thus came to contain a hypertonic solution. This attracted water from the cells osmotically, and became diluted to form an isotonic solution which flowed across the tubular basement membrane. Thus isotonic fluid left the lumen and was delivered to the plasma, maintaining the appearance of an isotonic transport, although it was in fact driven by a concealed osmotic gradient. This hypothesis was originally developed to account for isotonic transport out of the gall bladder, which has well defined lateral intercellular spaces and a relatively tight epithelium with a permeability smaller by one or two orders of magnitude than that of the proximal renal tubule (House, 1974). The proximal tubular epithelium has intercellular spaces which are not so well organized to maintain standing osmotic gradients, and recent measurements have shown its permeability to be so large (2000 to 3500 μm/s) that small, barely detectable, osmotic differences, of the order of a few mosm, are sufficient to account for observed rates of reabsorption of water (Schafer, 1984).

Moreover, figures taken to indicate that the reabsorbed fluid was isosmolar with the glomerular filtrate did not exclude the possibility that it was actually somewhat more concentrated. On the basis of the experiments of Walker *et al.* (1941), Homer Smith (1951) believed that the fluid in the lumen was hypotonic, as might be expected following active reabsorption of sodium. He admitted that only two of 21 samples from rats were hypotonic, but suggested that this might have been because the animals were uninephrectomized and loaded with sucrose or saline. Later (Smith, 1951, Fig. 60), he labelled proximal tubular contents as 'slightly hypotonic' and regarded the thin segment of the loop as 'a region that is highly permeable to water, wherein the variably hypotonic proximal urine is brought to osmotic equilibrium with the plasma' (Smith, 1951, p. 328). Later measurements supported Smith's prescient view. Bishop *et al.* (1979) reported that the ratio for the osmolality of tubular fluid/plasma during free flow in rats averaged 0.973 ± 0.004, so that the tubular fluid was significantly hyposmolal ($p < 0.001$). Green & Giebisch (1984) perfused proximal convoluted tubules and peritubular capillaries of Sprague–Dawley rats with identical sodium chloride solutions and found they generated luminal hypotonicity up to 5 mosm. Osmolality measured by Ramsay's method on samples of tubular fluid removed from proximal convoluted tubules of Munich Wistar rats during free flow reached 8 mosm below plasma and 5 mosm below capsular fluid (Liu *et al.*, 1984). Such results suggested that the tubules reabsorbed a slightly hypertonic solution and left the tubular fluid somewhat hypotonic.

Direct confirmation of this suggestion came from studies on isolated, perfused rabbits' tubules placed in warm (38°C) mineral oil, so that droplets of absorbed fluid that collected around them could be removed for analysis. Rates of reabsorption were of the order of 1 nl/min per mm, comparable with those from rats' tubules *in situ* (Green & Giebisch, 1984); and the absorbates were significantly hypertonic, up to 15 mosM above the luminal perfusate. Details, and an excellent discussion of their implications, will be found in Schafer's (1984) Robert F Pitts Memorial Lecture on 'Mechanisms Coupling the Absorption of Solutes and Water in the Proximal Nephron'. Schafer pointed out that the preferential reabsorption of glucose and bicarbonate, with reflection coefficients close to unity, early in the proximal tubule leads to a greater difference in effective than in total osmolality. When tubular fluid has 20 to 30 mM more chloride and less bicarbonate than plasma, the smaller reflection coefficient (? 0.8) for chloride should make the tubular fluid effectively hypotonic even when the total osmolalities are the same. Berry (1983) was less impressed with the importance of differences in reflection coefficients, but agreed that luminal hypotonicity combined with intercellular hypertonicity accounts for solute–solvent coupling. Since a difference of 1 mosM is roughly equivalent to an osmotic differential of 20 mmHg, gradients of hydrostatic pressure are unlikely to have important direct effects upon the reabsorption of water. The reabsorption of sodium is, however, surprisingly sensitive to small changes in hydrostatic pressure (Section 4.3.1). Rector (1983) in his Homer Smith Award Lecture emphasized that while a reduction in Starling forces (the balance of hydrostatic and oncotic pressures) promotes back-diffusion by increasing paracellular permeability, a low concentration of protein in peritubular capillary plasma also inhibits transcellular transport of sodium chloride by some still unknown mechanism.

The fraction of filtered water that undergoes 'obligatory' reabsorption can only be regarded as roughly constant under ordinary physiological conditions; it has been seen to be altered by the fate of the solutes dissolved in it and it is likely to differ from one species to another. Estimates based on the increase in concentration of solutes which are not reabsorbed, notably radioactively labelled ^{14}C-inulin, indicated that two thirds to three quarters of the filtered water was usually reabsorbed from the first 70% of the proximal convoluted tubules in rodents (Gottschalk, 1962–3), and at least half the filtered water by half way along the proximal convoluted tubules in dogs (Clapp *et al.*, 1963); but it is not possible to extrapolate confidently beyond those parts of the tubule which can be punctured. Moreover, saline infusions administered before and during experiments may affect the results. The reabsorption of sodium and water from punctured proximal tubules in dogs was reduced as much as 30 to 40% by saline infusions which expanded the volume of extracellular fluid (Dirks *et al.*, 1965). Proximal tubular reabsorption is no less variable in rodents. In a paper primarily on distal tubular transport of sodium and potassium in rats, Malnic *et al.* (1966) tubulated a large number of observations of tubular fluid/plasma concentration ratios for inulin based on fluid from proximal convoluted tubules under a variety of experimental conditions. The ratio 60% of the way along the proximal convoluted tubule was never greater than 3.0 and was reduced to well below 2.0 by diuresis provoked by infusing 4% sodium chloride. The lowest ratios, averaging 1.3 by half way along the proximal convoluted tubule, were in rats on low-sodium, high-potassium diets given an infusion of 10% mannitol in isotonic potassium chloride. These low ratios were not associated with increased rates of filtration, for GFRs were less than in the control animals. In many cases the tubular fluid/plasma ratios were still less than 4.0 even some way along distal convoluted tubules, so that nothing approaching the often stated five sixths of the filtered water can have been reabsorbed from the proximal tubules. Obligatory reabsorption might be expected to be greatest during antidiuretic conditions, when no additional solute is present to keep water in the lumen. Bennett *et al.* (1967) found that dogs during antidiuresis reabsorbed 45% of filtered water from the superficial proximal convoluted tubule and a further 25% from long loops of Henle. Human nephrons have not been punctured, but Bennett *et al.* (1968) found in rhesus monkeys that 70% had been reabsorbed in the first nine tenths of the proximal convoluted tubules, and that 25% was still left early in the distal tubules.

In conclusion: most, up to five sixths under ordinary physiological conditions, of the filtered water is destined to be reabsorbed from the mammalian renal tubules. The 'obligatory' phase occurs early in the nephron, recovering two thirds to three quarters of the filtered water from the proximal convoluted tubules and up to another one sixth from the proximal straight tubules and descending limbs of Henle's loops. But one of the most impressive characteristics of this so-called 'obligatory' reabsorption is its variability, which reflects the fact that it is a passive process in which the water follows by osmosis upon a reabsorption of solutes which is itself variable.

5.3 WATER DIURESIS

The most dramatic alteration in the rate of flow of urine which occurs under ordinary physiological conditions is the large increase to 10 or 20 times the 'resting' rate which follows the ingestion and absorption of large amounts of water. The increase in volume is accompanied by a roughly proportional fall in osmolarity to as little as one tenth that of the plasma, as the rate of excretion of solutes hardly changes, while the facultative reabsorption of water left over from the obligatory phase is suppressed. This copious output of a dilute, watery urine in response to loading the body with water is appropriately known as water diuresis. The kidneys quickly remove excess water and restore the normal volume and concentration of the body fluids.

If a person who is producing a small volume of concentrated urine drinks a litre of water fairly quickly on an empty stomach, there is typically a delay of 20 to 30 minutes, and only then the flow of urine begins to increase rapidly from its initial rate of 1 ml/min or less to between 10 and 20 ml/min, the peak of the diuresis occurring between 1 and 2 hours after the water is ingested. Thereafter the rate falls back to be near its initial value after 3 to 4 hours, by which time most of the extra water has been excreted. All the changes in output are accompanied by inversely proportional changes in concentration, as much the same amount of solute per minute is excreted with more or less water.

Rates of glomerular filtration of the order of 120 ml/min in man provide ample water for urinary volumes up to 20 ml/min without invoking any increase in filtration rate. Chasis et al. (1938) found no increase in clearance of inulin after human subjects took a litre of water; and Sellwood & Verney (1955) found no increase in filtration rate in dogs unless the water load exceeded 2% of their body weight. Dicker (1956) concluded that moderate loading with water did not increase GFR in rat, guinea pig, cat, dog, sheep or man, though large loads increased GFR in rats as in dogs. But since physiological water diuresis does not encroach upon the obligatory reabsorption of water, there is no need to postulate any change in activity of the proximal nephron. The increased flow of urine can be wholly attributed to a more or less complete failure to reabsorb water from the distal and collecting tubules, so that water diuresis results from a modification of the facultative phase of reabsorption.

Much of what is known about how the renal excretion of water is controlled was established by Verney, who had worked with Starling at University College, London, developing the heart-lung and heart-lung-kidney preparations, and was later Professor of Pharmacology at Cambridge. His group showed that the renal nerves played no part in water diuresis in the dog, for rates of output of urine from denervated and innervated kidneys in the same water-loaded animal were identical (Klisiecki et al., 1933). Verney was greatly impressed by the delay between the administration of water and the onset of the diuresis, which seemed too long to be accounted for by delay in absorption, and Rioch (1930) had described a delay of 15 to 20 minutes between dilution of the blood and water diuresis in human subjects. A direct action of diluted blood within the kidney was definitively excluded by Baldes & Smirk (1934) working with human subjects at University College, London. They were able to use the sensitive thermopiles that Hill (1931) had developed for measuring the heat production of muscle and nerve, and had also applied to determining the osmolarities of very small volumes of solutions by the depression of their vapour pressure. In one experiment the osmolarity of the blood fell 1% in a quarter of an hour after taking a litre of water by mouth, and was lowest, 3% below the initial value, after 1 hour. Meanwhile the water diuresis was only beginning 30 minutes after the water was ingested, reached its peak after 90 minutes, and began to decline rapidly 150 minutes from the start, after the osmolarity of the plasma had been rising steadily for more than an hour. Hence there was a delay of at least 30 minutes between changes in osmolarity of the blood and corresponding alterations in the rate of output of urine (Fig. 5.1). These observations have been confirmed many times; Smith (1951) quoted the average delay between maximal hydration and maximal diuresis as 15 to 20 minutes in dogs and rats, and about 40 minutes in man.

Verney found an explanation for this delay in the course of his work with the heart-lung-kidney preparation. Early attempts at perfusion showed that isolated kidneys could produce urine, but usually in large volumes and of low concentration, like the profuse urine formed during water diuresis. If, however, the animal's head, containing an intact pituitary gland, was included in the circuit, the urine was more concentrated and of smaller volume. The posterior lobe of the pituitary gland released something which could be carried to the kidney in the blood and suspend the water diuresis. The addition of extracts of the posterior lobe to the blood perfusing an isolated kidney reduced the volume of urine, with an approximately proportional increase in concentration. Because it could travel in the blood and switch the function of the kidney from water diuresis to conservation of water, Verney called this agent an antidiuretic hormone (ADH), and he was one of the first to demonstrate the antidiuretic activity of pituitary extracts, which had previously been supposed to exert a diuretic action and increase the volume of urine (Smith, 1937). This was probably because large doses were tested on anaesthetized animals which were dehydrated and in shock following surgical exposure of their kidneys, with low blood pressures and low rates of renal blood flow and glomerular filtration. Under these circumstances the pressor action of a large dose of pituitary extract might improve the perfusion of the kidneys and increase their capacity to produce urine. Water diuresis does not occur in anaesthetized animals, and the antidiuretic action of pituitary extracts

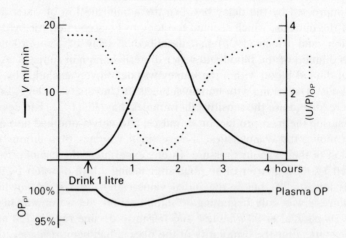

Fig. 5.1 Variations in urinary output, V (ml/min), urinary osmolarity with reference to plasma, $(U/P)_{OP}$ and osmolarity of plasma during a typical water diuresis.

was only revealed by Verney's classical work on physiological water diuresis in unanaesthetized, unrestrained and unconcerned dogs.

The antidiuretic effects of small doses and the pressor effects of larger doses of pituitary extracts are both due to an octapeptide with a molecular weight around 1100, which is still called vasopressin in recognition of the older established action and the fact that it is secreted in response to falling blood pressure. Most mammals, including man, produce arginine vasopressin (AVP), but the pig and hippopotamus have a lysine vasopressin, in which lysine replaces arginine in the side chain. Chemically, these both resemble mammalian oxytocin, which has little antidiuretic potency but a far greater action on plain muscle, especially of the uterus and the myoepithelial cells of the mammary gland, which it causes to contract and eject milk. Birds, reptiles and amphibia have an arginine vasotocin (with isoleucine in the ring as in oxytocin and arginine in the side chain). This is probably the most primitive of these related peptide hormones (Sawyer et al., 1960), and assists water balance in amphibia by promoting uptake of salt and water through the skin and reabsorption of water from hypotonic urine stored in the bladder. It has an antidiuretic action which is quite different from that of the mammalian hormones, depending upon glomerular vasoconstriction which reduces GFR. The structures and properties of these peptides are summarized in Table 5.1.

Vasopressin is no longer regarded as a hormone secreted by cells in the pituitary gland. It is synthesized in neurosecretory neurones, predominantly in the supraoptic and paraventricular nuclei of the hypothalamus, whose axons form the supraopticohypophyseal (SOH) tract which terminates in apposition to capillaries in the neural lobe of the neurohypophysis (formerly known as the posterior lobe of the pituitary gland). The peptide, combined with a carrier protein of larger molecular weight, moves down the axons in stainable granules, which accumulate at their endings or behind a cut if the SOH tract is divided (Zimmerman & Robertson, 1976). The nerve fibres of this tract, about 100 000 in man, transmit impulses which can be recorded electrically (Ishikawa et al., 1966), and which lead to the release of ADH from the terminals, much as neurotransmitters are released from other nerve endings. But instead of diffusing across a narrow synaptic cleft to act on the next cell, ADH is carried in the blood to its major target cells, in blood vessels or far away in the kidney, and therefore functions as a hormone rather than as a local transmitter.

Besides its vasoconstrictor action on the smooth muscle of blood vessels, vasopressin acts on the skin and the urinary bladder of amphibia, increasing their permeability to water so that water crosses more rapidly by osmosis under a given difference of osmolarity. Labelled ADH injected into the blood of mammals was shown by radioautography to be taken up by the collecting tubules and late distal tubules of the kidney (Darmady et al., 1960). It substantially increases the diffusional and the osmotic water permeabilities of isolated cortical collecting tubules from rabbits (Hebert et al., 1981) and

Table 5.1 Natural peptide hormones

	OXYTOCIN	ARGININE VASOTOCIN	VASOPRESSIN
		Birds, reptiles, amphibia: uterus, amphibian skin & kidney (water-balance principle)	

Structures:

OXYTOCIN:

```
          glyc (amide)
             |
           LEUC
             |
           prol
             |
cyst — asp   |
  S      \   |
  S       glut
  |         |
cyst — tyr — S — ISOLEUC
```

ARGININE VASOTOCIN:

```
          glyc (amide)
             |
           ARG
             |
           prol
             |
cyst — asp   |
  S      \   |
  S       glut
  |         |
cyst — tyr — S — ISOLEUC
```

VASOPRESSIN:

```
              glyc (amide)
                 |
(hog) LYS or ARG (most mammals)
                 |
               prol
                 |
cyst — asp       |
  S      \       |
  S       glut
  |         |
cyst — tyr — S — PHENYLAL
```

ACTIONS IN MAMMALS	OXYTOCIN	ARGININE VASOTOCIN	VASOPRESSIN
Antidiuretic	–	++	++++
Pressor	–	+++	++++
Uterine contraction	++++	++	–
Milk ejection	++++	+++	+

rats (Reif *et al.*, 1984) without increasing their permeability to small solute molecules, and without increasing the permeability of more proximal portions of the nephron. This action promotes the distal, facultative reabsorption of water without affecting the obligatory phase, and opposes water diuresis by allowing water to be reabsorbed passively under the osmotic gradient set up by accumulation of solutes in high concentration in the medulla (Section 5.5). The urine becomes more concentrated as it approaches the osmolarity of the interstitial fluid in the renal papilla, and its volume is reduced in proportion.

On the basis of investigations described in his mammoth Croonian Lecture on 'The Antidiuretic Hormone and the Factors Which Determine its Release', Verney (1947) proposed that the osmolarity of blood perfusing the hypothalamus is the most important single factor controlling the release of ADH. The hypothalamus is, however, an extremely busy region where neurone pools overlap and paths are intermingled, so that a large number of stimuli can activate the neurones which release ADH. Disturbing factors and some further homeostatic controls will be discussed in Section 7.2 on regulation of the volume of water in the body.

Verney's evidence was unavoidably indirect, for there was then no means of detecting AVP in the blood directly. He prepared trained dogs with loops of the common carotid artery brought outside the neck, wrapped in a tube fashioned from neighbouring skin, so that solutions differing in composition or osmolarity could be added to the blood perfusing the brain without disturbing the animals. Water was administered to establish water diuresis, and antidiuretic responses were presumed to be due to the release of amounts of endogenous ADH equal to test doses of exogenous hormone which produced the same antidiuretic effects. Injections of hypertonic solutions of sodium chloride, sodium sulphate or sucrose, to which cells are not readily permeable, elicited antidiuretic responses, whereas solutions of permeant solutes like urea and ethanol were quite ineffective. Solutions which produced profound antidiuretic responses when injected into carotid loops produced much smaller and delayed responses if they were injected into veins in the limbs (unless the internal carotid artery was tied off, when injections into carotid loops were no more effective than into peripheral veins). Arndt & Gauer (1965) later performed the converse experiment of infusing water into carotid loops in five dogs prepared like Verney's. Quantities which were too small to affect renal function when given by other routes evoked a typical water diuresis when injected into carotid loops. The brain therefore seemed to contain 'osmoreceptors', as Verney called them, which responded to effective rather than to total osmotic pressure. Jewell & Verney (1957) tried to localize these more precisely by observing responses to hypertonic injections into carotid loops after tying off more and more branches of the internal carotid artery. They later killed the dogs, fixed the brains *in situ* and injected them with coloured media through the carotid arteries. This narrowed the receptive region down to less than $100\,\mu$l of tissue which included the dorsomedial, ventromedial, supraoptic and paraventricular nuclei of the hypothalamus, but Verney was such a meticulous worker and so cautious in interpreting his results that he was never certain that he had identified the receptive cells. More recent work made possible by the development of radioimmunoassay techniques sensitive enough to measure the concentration of AVP in human and animal plasma confirmed that increasing osmolarity above a 'set point' of about 280 mosm is associated with increasing concentrations of AVP. Other things being equal, an increase of 1 mosm increases plasma AVP by 0.4 pg/ml, which is sufficient to increase the osmolarity of the urine by 100 mosm; 5 pg/ml of plasma yields a maximal antidiuretic effect in man (Robertson et al., 1976). In physiology, however, other things rarely are equal, and the effects of blood pressure, blood volume and some adventitious factors which modulate or override the response to osmolarity will be discussed in Section 7.2. There are also many unsolved problems about the osmoreceptive cells and their connections (Bie, 1980).

Meanwhile, the idea that dilution of the blood entering the hypothalamus suppressed the secretion of ADH provided Verney with an explanation for the phenomena of water diuresis, including the characteristic delay in its onset. After ingested water has been absorbed, the plasma diluted, and the release of ADH suppressed, there is a further delay while ADH already secreted is used up. Then the water diuresis can commence, and continue until the osmolarity of the blood increases enough for ADH to be secreted again to turn up the facultative reabsorption of water and terminate the diuresis. There is a disease, diabetes insipidus, in which the patients live in a state of perpetual water diuresis, being forced to drink up to 20 litres daily to avoid thirst and dehydration. A strain of rats genetically unable to secrete AVP (Brattleboro rats) provides a model; the condition can also be produced experimentally by hypothalamic lesions (Ranson et al., 1938), and treated with exogenous ADH, formerly as posterior pituitary extract, now as synthetic AVP. Verney was thus able to characterize water diuresis as a temporary, physiological state of diabetes insipidus.

5.4 THE DILUTING OPERATION

The change from antidiuresis to water diuresis requires the turning off or masking of the process which can make the urine more concentrated (Section 5.5), and also the turning on, unmasking or intensification of a diluting operation that can make the urine less concentrated than the plasma. Peters' (1944) statement; 'despite the extreme differences in composition of the contents of its various compartments, a uniform osmotic pressure prevails throughout the fluids of the body. It follows that the membranes between these compartments must universally permit the free passage of water...' can hardly apply without qualification to the kidneys, which produce, and must contain, fluids differing greatly in osmolarity from the body fluids in general. In so far as the renal tubule is continuous with the external environment, the urine and tubular fluids are not strictly body fluids; but no matter what the concentration of the final urine is to be, the mammalian kidney usually contains interstitial fluid that is more concentrated than the plasma as well as tubular fluid that may be either more concentrated or more dilute.

Beyond the proximal tubule the reabsorption of water becomes facultative and also ceases to be approximately isosmolal. Water and solutes are handled to some extent independently, so that the osmolality of the final urine may be varied, and with it the osmolality of the 'mirror-image' fluid that is returned to the plasma. Amphibian urine is always hypotonic, and the pioneers of micropuncture showed that the concentration of chloride and the osmolality both decreased with distance along the distal tubule (Walker et al., 1937). Mammals also produce hypotonic urine with a lower concentration of chloride than their plasma during water diuresis, though at other times the osmolality and the concentration of chloride may be far greater.

Early cryoscopic measurements on slices removed from kidneys chilled in liquid air (Wirz et al., 1951) suggested that the fluid in the lumina of all vessels and tubules in the cortex was isotonic with systemic plasma, but Wirz (1956b) made the striking observation that fluid entering distal tubules which were accessible to puncture on the surface of the rat's kidney was always hypotonic, even when the final urine was hypertonic. Later measurements showed that during water diuresis in rats and golden hamsters the fluid remained hyposmolal, and could become even more dilute as it continued along the remainder of the distal tubules and the collecting ducts (Hilger et al., 1958; Gottschalk, 1961). Clapp & Robinson (1966) first showed that distal tubules were accessible on the surface of the dog's kidney and that these also contained hypotonic fluid even when the urine was being maximally concentrated. Average distal tubular fluid/plasma ratios of osmolality were 0.41 during hydropenia and 0.24 during water diuresis. Then Bennett et al. (1968) found hypotonic fluid all along the distal segment even during antidiuresis in rhesus monkeys, and remarked that the epithelium must have a low permeability to water.

Since tubular fluid is already hypotonic when it emerges from the thick ascending limb of Henle's loop into the distal tubule, the process which makes it more dilute than the plasma must commence in the ascending limb, which should share this low permeability to water. Fluid in the thin ascending limb is also hypotonic to blood in adjacent vasa recta. The permeability to water was not detectably different from zero in the isolated, perfused thin and thick ascending limbs and the distal tubule both in the presence and absence of ADH (Kokko & Tisher, 1976), and the permeability of the collecting ducts was equally low except when ADH was present. Later measurements confirmed that permeability to water is very low, though not zero, in the distal tubule, ascending limb and collecting ducts; but in the collecting ducts ADH increases it by an order of magnitude (Hebert et al., 1981). This extremely low permeability in the absence of ADH allows these epithelia to conduct the hypotonic fluid they generate through the deep medulla (where the interstitial fluid is hypertonic to systemic plasma) without losing much water, so that it emerges into the renal pelvis as dilute urine.

This diluting mechanism, which is also present in the amphibian kidney, is presumably more primitive than the mammalian concentrating mechanism. It seems to have been retained in the mammalian kidney, and to be operating there all the time. It is responsible for the outflow of dilute urine during water diuresis, but it can be overlaid by a concentrating process downstream which the amphibia do not possess. The dilute fluid that enters the distal tubule has a low concentration of sodium, and both its low osmolality and the low concentration of sodium could be produced either by the addition of water or by the removal of salt through a membrane with a low permeability to water which precludes osmotic equilibration. After labelled inulin had been added to the blood entering the kidney, its concentration was greater in samples removed by micropipettes from the early part of the distal than from the proximal tubule, showing that water was removed, not added, on the way through the loop of Henle. The diluting process must therefore be a removal of solute without water, and this process can continue right through the distal tubules and the collecting system (Gottschalk, 1961). When solutes are reabsorbed, the water that carried them into the diluting segments is effectively trapped in the lumen.

The overall effect of the diluting operation can be measured by a free water clearance, defined by Smith (1956). The total amount of urinary solute excreted per minute can be expressed by an 'osmolar clearance', C_{osm}. Calculated as $V.OP_U/OP_P$, this is the volume of plasma containing the total amount of solute in osmoles excreted in unit time. With usual conventions it will be a number of ml per minute. If the urine were isosmolar with plasma ($OP_U/OP_P = 1.0$), the osmolar clearance would be equal to the urine volume per minute, V. Dilute urines contain more water per unit of solute than the plasma; they can be regarded as isotonic urines diluted with solute-free water provided by the diluting operation. The amount of such free water excreted in unit time will be simply $V - C_{osm}$. Hence the free water clearance, C_{H_2O}, $= V - C_{osm}$. This a measure of the amount of water left behind after the solute that brought it into the diluting segment as isotonic tubular fluid has been reabsorbed through the relatively water-impermeable epithelium. Since the diluting process begins beyond the end of the proximal tubules, organic solutes not destined for the urine have already been reabsorbed, and the approximately isosmolar fluid that remains contains approximately 90% of sodium salts and 10% of 'urea etc.' (Robinson, 1954, p. 72), where 'etc.' stands for creatinine and other urinary solutes. If obligatory reabsorption reclaimed five sixths of the glomerular filtrate, the human diluting segments would, in effect, be presented each minute with a mixture of 18 ml of isotonic saline and 2 ml of an isosmolar solution of 'urea etc.'. Removal of all the salt but no water would leave 20 ml of a one tenth isosmolar solution of urea and other urinary constituents. Since the most important solute which can be reabsorbed to leave osmolyte-free water is sodium, the amount of free water that can be generated is limited by the amount of salt delivered to the diluting segments. Maximal water diuresis can only be expected when sufficient sodium is left over from proximal 'obligatory' reabsorption and when its distal reabsorption is unimpaired. The free water clearance is therefore a measure of the amount of sodium that enters the diluting segments *and is reabsorbed from them.* As Smith pointed out, water diuresis may be impaired in sodium-depleted states when the urine contains almost no sodium. It may also be impaired by adrenal deficiency, and the impaired water diuresis has been used as a screening test in the diagnosis of Addison's disease. In the absence of aldosterone, less sodium is filtered because dehydration secondary to loss of sodium reduces GFR, and the smaller amount of sodium that reaches the diluting segment is poorly reabsorbed. The urine therefore contains sodium despite its low concentration in the plasma, and the capacity to generate solute-free water is impaired.

5.5 THE CONCENTRATING OPERATION

During water diuresis the low permeability to water of the collecting system in the absence of ADH protects dilute tubular fluid on its way through the medulla. With the change to antidiuresis, ADH in effect removes the water-proofing from the collecting tubules; but it remains to explain how the tubular fluid can then become so much more concentrated than the plasma before it emerges as urine. The difference in osmotic pressure across an ideally semipermeable membrane between plasma and maximally concentrated human urine, which is four times as concentrated, is of the order of 17 000 mmHg. This is no mean achievement for an organ whose cells contain 70 to 80% of water.

Morphological comparisons suggested that the loops of Henle, present only in the kidneys of animals which can make their urine hypertonic, might be the site of the concentrating operation. But the loops are a long way from the end of the nephron and it would seem better to minimize the length of tubule traversed by highly concentrated urine by keeping the concentrating process until the last. Moreover, the finding that fluid entering the distal tubules was hypotonic, even when the final urine was concentrated, excluded the loops from direct involvement in the concentrating process. Homer Smith (1951) once favoured some sort of active process in the distal tubules, because their taller, mitochondria-rich epithelium seemed better fitted than the thin, flat cells of the loops to generate and sustain large gradients. But he already had an inkling that the collecting ducts might be involved, and in a delightful later account (Smith, 1959) he was all but convinced.

Even though the loops do not themselves actively transport water, they still have a role in concentrating the urine and they point to the medulla, where they are located, as the site of that operation. Peter (1909) had noted that the width of the inner medullary zone is greatest in the kidneys of those animals which are best adapted to life in arid environments and produce the most concentrated urine. Schmidt-Nielsen & O'Dell (1961) ranked animals according to their capacity to concentrate the urine, and the order was about the same as for the relative thickness of medullary compared with cortical tissue. The depression of the freezing point of the most concentrated urine was least for the beaver (1°C) and pig (2°C); next came man (3°C), then rat, cat and dog (around 5°C), and desert rodents (10 to 12°C). The medulla is thinnest in the beaver; in desert rodents it forms a single, elongated papilla that protrudes into the upper end of the ureter.

5.5.1 The medullary osmotic gradient

There were early intimations of the presence of hypertonic tissue fluids in the renal medulla. In 1902 Filehne & Biberfeld noted that stronger solutions of sodium chloride were required to prevent the swelling of isolated fragments of medullary than of cortical tissue from rabbits. Ljungberg (1947) found that the concentration of chloride in the renal tissue fluids of rabbits increased with depth into the medulla to as much as three or four times that in the cortex, where it was similar to the concentration in the plasma. Progressively stronger saline solutions were required to prevent the swelling of slices cut from greater depths within the renal medulla of dogs, and chemical analysis showed that the increasing tonicity of the tissues was due chiefly to larger concentrations of sodium chloride and urea (Ullrich *et al.*, 1955; Ullrich & Jarausch, 1956). More precise localization of the concentrating process became possible when Hargitay *et al.* (1951) developed a method for determining the osmolality of very small samples of fluids by first freezing them in capillary tubes and then watching with a polarizing microscope for the last crystal of ice to disappear as they thawed in a bath of chilled alcohol, warmed slowly enough to maintain thermal equilibrium with the sample. Wirz *et al.* (1951) applied this method to the fluids in slices of renal tissue. Kidneys rapidly removed from rats which had been producing concentrated urine were immediately frozen in liquid air, and then allowed to warm to $-10°C$, when they could be cut into slices about 30 µm thick, at right angles to the axis of the renal papilla. These slices were then thawed very slowly in the microcryoscopic apparatus so that the melting points of the fluids in them could be determined.

The fluids in all tubular and vascular cross-sections within any slice had the same melting point. In the cortex this was the same as that of the plasma, so that the fluids in proximal and distal convoluted tubules appeared to be isosmolal with the plasma. In slices taken from increasing depths into the medulla, the fluids in all cross-sections were progressively more concentrated, up to four times as concentrated as the plasma in tubules and blood vessels at the papillary tips, comparable in osmolality with the urine that the kidneys were producing just before they were frozen. Lilien & Phillips (1966) cut frozen slices in a sagittal plane, to include cortex, outer and inner medulla, and renal papilla, and photographed the slices at regular intervals in the polarizing microscope as they were warmed. They confirmed that the fluids in the cortex were isosmolal with the plasma, and that the osmolality became greater at increasing depths into the medulla.

The conclusions drawn from these experiments were soon refined and largely confirmed in live, functioning kidneys. Wirz (1953) succeeded in withdrawing blood with micropipettes from capillary loops (vasa recta) near the tip of the golden hamster's single elongated renal papilla. The osmolality of these samples was far greater than that of systemic blood, and about the same as that of urine emerging at the papillary tip. A striking microphotograph published by Ullrich et al. (1961) showed shrunken, crenated erythrocytes in blood from vasa recta deep in the papilla; the osmolality was three times that of systemic blood and the PCV as low as 15 to 20%. Later microcryoscopic measurements by Wirz (1956b) confirmed with micropuncture samples that fluid from superficial proximal convoluted tubules of rats was always isosmolal with plasma during water diuresis or antidiuresis, but revealed that fluid from distal tubules was always hyposmolal. This had not been noted in the studies on frozen slices, possibly because the small amounts of distal tubular fluid present had somehow equilibrated with the far larger amounts of isosmolal fluid in proximal tubules, cortical blood vessels and interstitial spaces during preparation of the tissues. The observation was, however, soon confirmed on the living kidneys of several rodent species (Gottschalk & Mylle, 1959). In concentrating kidneys early distal tubular fluid was always dilute; fluids from the bend of the loop of Henle, from collecting ducts and from vasa recta were always hyperosmolal to systemic plasma, and to about the same extent at any depth below the cortex. Hence the medullary osmotic gradient first found in frozen slices was demonstrably present in living kidneys, and, as in dogs and rhesus monkeys (Clapp & Robinson, 1966; Bennett et al., 1968), the urine first became concentrated on its way along the collecting ducts.

Thus the accumulation of solutes, chiefly sodium chloride and urea, with greatly increasing osmolality in the depths of the medulla, is well established by many experimental observations. Although erythrocytes shrink as they pass through the inner medulla (Ullrich et al., 1961), the epithelial cells which reside there seem to avoid shrinking, and also the damaging effects of high concentrations of intracellular electrolytes, by synthesizing and retaining a variety of organic solutes (Balaban & Burg, 1987; cf. Section 7.3). It remains to explain how the accumulated extracellular solutes can remain relatively undisturbed by the circulation of blood through the medulla, how the medullary gradient is generated in the first place (Section 5.5.2) and how it is used to concentrate the urine (Section 5.5.3).

The persistence of the medullary osmotic gradient depends partly upon the fact that the medullary circulation is relatively slow compared with that in the cortex, but probably even more upon the anatomical arrangement of the blood vessels in the medulla. The rate of perfusion of the medulla is not inconsiderable by comparison with other tissues. It is similar in order of magnitude to the rate at which tubular fluid enters the loops of Henle, and so it should be sufficient to remove solutes as quickly as they can be delivered to the medullary interstitial fluid. If blood in the vasa recta approached diffusion equilibrium with interstitial fluid, and then flowed through the medulla as urine flows through the collecting ducts, it would carry away solutes that had been deposited in the medulla. The peculiar arrangement of the vasa recta, however, makes it possible to supply the medulla with blood without dispersing the solutes accumulated there.

Blood entering the medulla in the descending vasa recta does not continue in the same direction and leave after it has equilibrated with concentrated fluids in the depths of the medulla. The descending, or arterial, vasa recta end at different depths in the inner medulla by supplying a capillary plexus; this lies among the collecting ducts and the thin limbs of the loops of Henle and allows the capillary blood to equilibrate with local interstitial fluid. This plexus is drained by ascending, venous vasa recta which pick up capillary blood equilibrated with interstitial fluid at the levels where they commence and carry it up towards the cortex, allowing it to re-equilibrate partially with progressively less concentrated surroundings on the way. Constrained in this way to descend for different distances and then return, the blood flows through the inner medulla but tends to leave behind the solutes that are concentrated there. Further protection against loss of solute is provided by collecting the ascending and descending vasa recta together side by side in roughly conical vascular bundles which have their bases in the outer stripe of the outer medullary zone, extend through the inner stripe, and then become narrower as they tail off to apices near the tip of the papilla (Kriz, 1981). In the simpler type of medulla found in the kidneys of rabbit, guinea pig, cat, dog, rhesus monkey and man, the bundles consist exclusively of ascending and descending vasa recta. Rats, mice and desert rodents have more complex bundles which contain thin descending limbs of the loops of Henle as well as ascending and descending vasa recta. These arrangements appear well fitted to permit free exchange by diffusion between the ascending and descending streams moving alongside each other in the outer medulla. The vasa recta can therefore operate as a countercurrent exchanger, such as is employed in heating engineering, and found in the feet of seabirds and the flippers of marine animals, where it reduces heat loss to the surrounding water by exchange between arteries and veins which are in close contact with each other. The exchanger in the kidney may not be as efficient as the spectacular rete mirabile that protects the high concentration of oxygen built up in the swim-bladders of some deep-sea fish (Scholander, 1954); but it does probably constitute an effective diffusion trap guarding the solutes accumulated in the inner medulla.

5.5.2 The generation of the medullary osmotic gradient

Hargitay & Kuhn (1951) laid the foundations for much subsequent thinking about the renal concentrating mechanism in a mathematical paper in a German journal of electrochemistry and applied physical chemistry which was not immediately noticed by renal physiologists; one of the first accounts in English was presented by Robinson (1954). The underlying principle is extremely simple. If some water is moved across from the descending to the ascending limb of a U-shaped loop through which a solution is flowing, or if some solute is moved back from the ascending to the decending limb, the solution will be made more concentrated in the descending limb and diluted in the ascending limb. No matter whether some water is short-circuited or some solute recirculated, water molecules on average spend less time in the loop, and solute molecules which spend longer will accumulate in higher concentration towards the bend (Fig. 5.2). In the mechanism treated theoretically by Hargitay & Kuhn (1951) and illustrated by a working model, the limbs were side by side, separated by a semipermeable membrane, and a greater pressure was maintained in the descending limb to transfer water by ultrafiltration. In the absence of flow through the loop, equilibrium would be reached when the excess osmotic pressure due to the greater concentration of solute in the

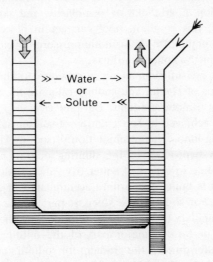

Fig. 5.2 Countercurrent flow in a loop with transfer of water from descending to ascending limb, or of solute from ascending to descending limb; and return of some effluent solution through a tube communicating with the ascending limb through a semipermeable membrane.

descending limb just balanced the applied hydrostatic pressure. With continuing flow, concentrated solution from the descending limb moves round the hairpin bend into the ascending limb, displacing the diluted solution onwards and allowing the solution in the descending limb to be concentrated further. The system acts as a countercurrent multiplier, which can amplify the small difference of osmolarity ('single effect') at any level to yield a much larger difference between either end of the loop and the bend. A more complicated mathematical treatment of transfer of solute from the ascending to the descending stream in the absence of a head of hydrostatic pressure predicted the generation of a similar difference in osmolarity along the loop (Kuhn & Ramel, 1959). The chief difference is that transfer of solute increases the concentration of the solute that is recirculated, whereas short-circuiting of water increases the concentrations of all solutes equally.

Hargitay & Kuhn (1951) pointed out that if a portion of the effluent from the loop was passed through a further descending tube communicating with the ascending limb through a semipermeable membrane, this portion should lose water to the more concentrated solution flowing past it and emerge with the concentration maintained at the bend of the loop. They suggested that their 'hairpin countercurrent diffusion system' might account for the production of concentrated urine in mammalian kidneys; the loops of Henle could serve as the multiplier, and collecting ducts made permeable by ADH could function as the additional tube running alongside in which some of the effluent was concentrated. In fact the limbs of the loops of Henle are not in contact with each other or with the collecting ducts. But the loops and the collecting ducts are all bathed in a common pool of interstitial fluid. If the loops can develop a gradient of osmolarity and communicate it to the intersititial fluid, this common pool can act in place of a semipermeable membrane to communicate the osmotic pressure developed by the multiplier to tubular fluid in the collecting ducts.

Since there is no sufficient head of pressure to shift water between the limbs of the loops of Henle, and sodium salts are the predominating solutes in the medullary osmotic gradient, Berliner et al. (1958) proposed that the single effect was achieved by recirculation of sodium salts from the ascending to the descending limb. The accumulation of sodium chloride in the medulla could thus be a byproduct of the diluting operation, which involves the abstraction of solute in excess of water from the tubule, while the medullary osmotic gradient is built up of solute accumulated in excess of water in the interstitial fluid. For sodium, the steepest part of the gradient between the cortex and the papillary tips is in the outer medulla, where the thick ascending limbs of Henle perform a major part of the diluting operation (Berliner, 1982). During water diuresis the gradient for sodium may be entirely confined to the outer medulla (Fig. 5.3); and it is rapidly abolished by loop diuretics like furosemide which inhibit reabsorption of sodium chloride from the thick ascending limbs (Jamison & Maffly, 1976).

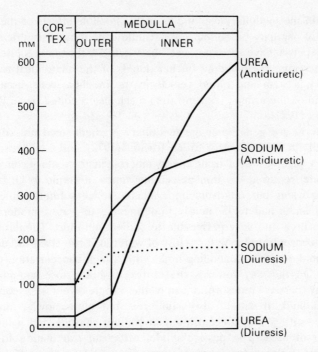

Fig. 5.3 Concentrations of sodium and of urea in tissue water of kidneys removed from dogs during antidiuresis and water diuresis. (Summarized and simplified from data of Ullrich & Jarausch, 1956, *Pflügers Archiv.* **262**, 537.)

Although it is steepest in the outer medulla, the gradient for sodium continues through the inner medulla. The question of whether this requires active transport by the thin limbs of the loops of Henle, or whether the medullary sodium gradient can be built up entirely by active transport in the thick ascending limbs, has been debated. A number of more or less complicated mathematical models have been advanced, but no proof that the kidney operates exactly like any of them. The models need not be discussed in detail here; they were well described by excellent reviewers (Jamison, 1974; Jamison & Robertson, 1979; Berliner, 1982) who accepted Stephenson's (1966) conclusion that no counterflow system in which all exchanges between the streams flowing past each other are purely passive could account for the medullary gradient without some further input of energy in the inner medulla itself. Later Stephenson (1987) concluded that existing models were still not quantitatively satisfactory, possibly because permeabilities measured in isolated tubular segments do not apply in the intact kidney, or because some important aspect of the concentrating mechanism has been overlooked. One factor might be the concentrated pelvic urine which bathes the papilla of a concentrating kidney; this may affect exchanges of water and urea with fluid in the collecting ducts and help to maintain the medullary osmotic gradient. Possible effects of the intermittent flow of papillary blood and tubular fluid caused by peristaltic activity of the renal pelvis have also not yet been defined (Schmidt-Nielsen, 1987). Many other aspects, including further details of the anatomical relations of the tubular system and blood vessels in the medulla were discussed in a symposium on the urinary concentrating mechanisms edited by de Rouffignac & Jamison (1987).

The energy for generating the medullary gradient need not come solely from local metabolism. Kokko & Rector (1972) and Stephenson (1972) proposed a 'passive model' using energy inherent in gradients of concentration. Their model required the thin descending limbs of Henle to be freely permeable to water but relatively impermeable to all solutes, while the thin ascending limbs had to be nearly impermeable to water, moderately permeable to urea and very permeable to sodium chloride. Tubular fluid that had been concentrated mainly by loss of water as it traversed the descending limbs should enter the ascending limbs with a high concentration of sodium chloride. On the way towards the cortex it should lose sodium chloride rapidly by passive reabsorption into the progressively less concentrated interstitial fluid. It should also gain urea, but more slowly, and end up hypotonic, with a low concentration of sodium chloride and a higher concentration of urea. The passive model offers an explanation for the enhancement of the kidney's concentrating power by urea, which helps to increase the concentration of sodium chloride in fluid entering the ascending limb by extracting water from the descending limb of the loop of Henle. This minimizes the back-leak of sodium chloride into the ascending limb from the interstitium and so enhances the net reabsorption of sodium chloride from the thin ascending limb (Jamison, 1976). Since a high concentration of urea in the inner medulla will also balance an equally high concentration in the collecting ducts, urea can be excreted in the urine in high concentration without the need for a urea-proof membrane to retain it (Section 4.2.1), and the whole of the medullary salt gradient is available to concentrate urinary solutes other than urea.

Isolated segments of ascending and descending limbs from rabbits appeared to have the permeabilities required to make the passive model feasible, and when a segment of ascending limb was perfused with a serum ultrafiltrate made hypertonic with 300 mosm sodium chloride in a bath made hypertonic with 300 mosm urea, the fluid emerged 200 to 300 mosmol/kg less concentrated than the bath, the salt having diffused out faster than urea diffused in (Rector, 1977). But there is some doubt about the working of the mechanism in intact rabbits. Gunther & Rabinowitz (1980) demonstrated augmentation of maximal urinary concentration following infusions of urea in hydropenic rats and dogs, but not in sheep, and they failed to do so with the same experimental protocol in calm, unanaesthetized, hydropenic rabbits receiving vasopressin. They added the teleological comment that this effect of urea might be more valuable for rats and dogs, which may eat large amounts of protein at long intervals, than for continuously grazing or nibbling herbivores. Moreover, although the rabbit's thin limbs appeared to have the permeabilities demanded by the passive model, other animals are less accommodating. The rat's thin ascending limb is no more permeable to urea than the descending limb, and only a quarter as permeable, instead of far more permeable, to sodium chloride. Berliner (1976) noted that the extent to which loss of water, gain of urea, and gain of salt contribute to the increase in osmolarity along the descending limb depends upon the species. The 'passive mechanism' may help to account for reabsorption of sodium from the thin ascending limb in the rabbit and the golden hamster, but active reabsorption of sodium chloride occurs in the rat, and seems most important in the sand rat *Psammomys obesus*. This remarkable animal lives on halophile plants and has a lot of salt to excrete. It can excrete urine with an osmolarity greater than 2000 mosm, but which contains only about 100 mm urea, and urea seems quite unimportant for its concentrating mechanism.

Apart from doubts about the role of the passive mechanism, there is independent evidence of active reabsorption of salt out of the thin ascending limb. In 1967 Jamison *et al.* sampled fluid from ascending and descending limbs in the surgically exposed papilla in rats. At any level, the contents of adjacent descending limbs had the same osmolality, and the osmolality of the contents of the thin ascending limbs was on average about 120 mosm less than in thin descending limbs, mainly because of a smaller concentration of sodium chloride. This would be expected if salt was transported out from thin ascending limbs into the interstitium, but Berliner (1982) still admitted that this reabsorption had not been proved without doubt to be active. However, reabsorption of salt without water from the whole of the ascending limb appears to be a major source of solute for the medullary gradient. Salt added in the first instance to the interstitial fluid will produce a local increase in concentration, from which it will tend to diffuse according to the available paths. The capillary plexuses offer the first option, and these do not appear to favour flow in any preferred direction. Ascending and descending vasa recta offer a choice of streams moving towards and away from the cortex, but in order to reach the cortex the vascular bundles have to be negotiated, and these seem designed to act as efficient solute traps, restricting the removal of solute from the medulla (Kriz, 1981). Ascending limbs of loops of Henle are presumably unavailable for net uptake because of outward transport of salt, but descending limbs offer access to streams directed deeper into the medulla. Hence salt reabsorbed from the ascending limbs of the loops of Henle is likely on balance to be carried into the inner medulla, simply because it has access to more streams leading in that direction than towards the cortex. The loop of Henle may therefore be more than a mere pumping device delivering sodium salts to the medulla (Berliner *et al.*, 1958). Active transport out of the ascending limbs and diffusion into the descending limbs could provide the single effect for a countercurrent multiplier in a way that ensures that the gradient is transmitted to the interstitial fluid as it is developed. Moreover, the employment of a common driving force for the concentrating and the diluting operations is a remarkable example of physiological economy.

Only about 14% of human nephrons (compared with 28% in rats and 100% in some desert rodents), possess long loops of Henle with thin ascending limbs. The thick ascending limbs of the more numerous cortical nephrons release their reabsorbed sodium chloride in the cortex and outer medulla. Consequently the long-looped, juxtamedullary nephrons take a disproportionate share in supplying salt to the inner medulla. All nephrons, however, are drained through collecting ducts, and these traverse the full depth of the inner medulla, where the common pool of hypertonic fluid allows those which have contributed less to make equal use of the medullary gradient for finally concentrating their urine. Species with larger proportions of long-looped nephrons can generally concentrate their urine more effectively than those with fewer nephrons contributing solute to the inner medulla.

The other principal component of the concentrated inner medullary fluid is urea. Unlike sodium, its concentration increases most steeply in the inner medulla (Fig. 5.3). It is believed to be reabsorbed passively from the papillary collecting ducts when the urine is concentrated by abstraction of water. Concentrated urine bathing the papilla in the renal pelvis is a possible additional source (Hogg & Kokko, 1979). Combined figures from several publications indicated that urea is concentrated in the deep inner medulla by recirculation in the countercurrent system (Ullrich et al., 1961a, Fig. 11). Of 100 molecules of urea in the glomerular filtrate of the rat during antidiuresis, 50 are typically reabsorbed from the proximal tubules and restored to the blood in the cortex. Yet 100 molecules enter the distal convoluted tubule, and only 20 of these will be excreted in the urine, the remaining 80 being reabsorbed from papillary collecting ducts. Thirty of these 80 will escape into the cortex in ascending vasa recta and join the 50 reabsorbed from the proximal tubules, while 50 must enter the descending or ascending thin limbs of the loops (both permeable to urea in the rat) and be added to the 50 left over from proximal reabsorption to make up the 100 entering the distal tubules. This is an oversimplified view of the mechanism, but there is no doubt that the urea is accumulated in high concentration in the deep inner medulla.

Although efficient countercurrent exchange in the outer medulla may prevent the loss of hypertonic fluid, it cannot totally prevent the removal of solute from the medulla. If the volume of the medulla is not to increase, a larger volume of blood must leave in the ascending vasa recta than the descending vasa recta deliver. This implies the loss of at least as much solute as would be contained in a volume of isotonic fluid equal to the total volume of water reabsorbed from the thin descending limbs and the collecting ducts. The loss of solute is minimized by the gradation of osmolality that keeps the interstitial fluid least concentrated near the cortico-medullary border. Descending vasa recta enter the medulla carrying blood with plasma proteins concentrated by the loss of glomerular filtrate. The high oncotic pressure of the protein-enriched plasma promotes the uptake of interstitial fluid into the vasa recta and the capillary plexuses they supply. This uptake is opposed as the external osmotic pressure increases in the inner medulla, and as at the same time oncotic pressure is depressed by the greater concentration of electrolyte. On the return journey toward the cortex, oncotic pressure increases again and the advancing blood takes up the more dilute interstitial fluid rather than the concentrated fluid from the deeper medulla. The outflow from the ascending vessels may be 30% greater than inflow through the descending ones (Zimmerhackl et al., 1985), thus removing water reabsorbed from the collecting ducts and descending limbs of Henle. Hence the vasa recta help to preserve the medullary osmolal gradient by trapping solute, while they also remove water from the medulla (Jamison & Maffly, 1976).

In a very small nutshell, sodium salts from the ascending limbs of the loops of Henle and urea from the papillary collecting ducts and perhaps also from pelvic urine are accumulated and trapped in the inner medulla, concentrated in the deeper parts because of a greater proportion of accessible inward-directed streams. The total concentration built up in the medullary osmotic gradient may reach many times that in systemic plasma, and it is available to concentrate the urine when ADH makes the collecting ducts permeable to water. The control and some limitations of this final concentrating operation are dealt with in Section 5.5.3.

5.5.3 Control and some limitations of the concentrating operation

Fig. 5.4 is an impressionistic diagram of conditions in the kidney of a fasting human subject who has not ingested any fluid since the previous evening. Experimental values have been adapted to human orders of magnitude for the osmolalities of plasma (300 mosm), and of very dilute and concentrated urines (30 and 1200 mosm). The thick ascending limbs of Henle and the distal convoluted tubules always deliver hypotonic tubular fluid (about 100 mosm) to the collecting ducts, which reabsorb about half the sodium chloride they receive (Schafer, 1979), and so can continue the work of earlier diluting segments while impermeability to water isolates their contents from the medullary osmotic gradient during water diuresis. Effective concentrations of vasopressin in the plasma (less than 10 pg/ml or 10 pm) increase the permeability of the collecting ducts and allow their contents to lose water to the medullary interstitial fluid and emerge as concentrated urine.

The antidiuretic hormone does not need to invoke an active transport of water as was once supposed; it need only permit passive reabsorption under the driving force of an osmotic gradient by providing access to the concentrated fluid stored in the inner medulla. Direct transport of water as such would be inefficient in solutions as dilute as the body fluids. Since a kilogram of pure water contains $1000/18 = 55.5$ mols, an isotonic solution (0.3 osm) contains $55.5/0.3 = 185$ molecules of water for each molecule of solute. Each molecule

CONTROL OF URINARY CONCENTRATION
Permeability of collecting ducts to water:

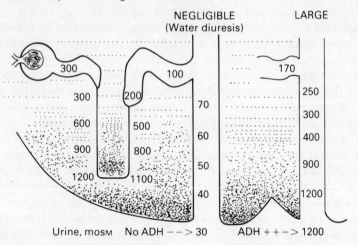

Fig. 5.4 Approximate osmolalities of tubular fluids and final urine in mosmol/kg. (Osmolality of medullary interstitial fluid similar to that in descending limbs of loops of Henle.)

of solute reabsorbed from the proximal convoluted tubule therefore takes 185 molecules of water with it, and each mosmol of solute stored in the inner medulla can abstract at least 46 mmol of water (0.83 ml) from tubular urine approaching 1200 mosm. Water taken up from the tubular fluid inevitably dilutes the medullary interstitial fluid unless more solute is added, and ADH, which increases the active transport of sodium by amphibian skins and urinary bladders (Macknight *et al.*, 1980), might be expected to assist by stimulating the processes which add solute to the medullary gradient. In rats and mice, but not in rabbits, ADH does enhance the reabsorption of salt from the medullary part of the thick ascending limb of the loop of Henle, without affecting that segment's extremely low permeability to water (Hebert & Andreoli, 1984). This would supply the outer medulla, where the gradient for sodium chloride is steepest, with more solute from the thick ascending limbs of cortical as well as of juxtamedullary nephrons.

It used to be taught that ADH increased the permeability of the distal convoluted tubules, so that a great deal of water was removed from the hypotonic fluid coming from the ascending limbs of the loops of Henle in the cortex, where there is a rich circulation of blood to carry it away. But although ADH may increase the permeability of the distal tubules in rats (Ullrich *et al.*, 1964) it does not seem to do so in all species. Clapp & Robinson (1966) found hypotonic fluid all along the distal convoluted tubule in dogs even when the urine was up to eight times as concentrated as the plasma; and Bennett *et al.* (1968) reported similar results in rhesus monkeys. Although ADH may not act on the distal or connecting tubules, it greatly increases the permeability of the cortical collecting ducts in rabbit, rat and man (Hebert *et al.*, 1981; Vanagawa *et al.*, 1981; Reif *et al.*, 1984). Water can therefore be removed from their contents in the cortex, and returned to the blood with sodium chloride reabsorbed from the thick ascending limbs of cortical nephrons. This importantly reduces the volume of water that has to be passed on to the medullary segments of the collecting ducts, where its reabsorption would dilute the medullary gradient.

The antidiuretic hormone reaches the kidney in the blood and must influence the cells through their basolateral membranes facing into the body. The permeability barrier that is opened is at the other poles of the cells, in the apical membranes, facing tubular fluid in the collecting ducts. Permeability for small solute molecules is not increased, and the activation energy for permeation of water itself is not altered, which suggests the opening up of more channels of the same selective kind as those already present in the membrane (Schafer, 1979). For many years it has been apparent that cAMP is a mediator of the cellular response. Antidiuretic hormone is believed to activate an adenyl cyclase in the basolateral membrane of responsive cells, leading to increased production of adenosine 3′, 5′-cyclic monophosphate (cAMP) which activates a protein kinase. Water-conducting particles are then somehow generated from cytoplasmic microtubular structures and carried towards the luminal pole of the cell to be incorporated into the apical cell membrane. Many details should be clarified as the problem becomes more amenable to ultrastructural as well as to biochemical studies (Hays, 1983; Hays *et al.*, 1987).

Maximal, or even supramaximal concentrations of ADH do not guarantee that maximally concentrated urine will be produced, for the highest attainable concentration depends upon other factors besides ADH. German pharmacologists in the 1890s had firmly established that hypertonic infusions were powerfully diuretic, even in dehydrated animals, and that the urine became much more dilute as its volume increased, even though the concentrated infusions increased the need to conserve water. Dreser (1892) was one of the first to advocate measurements of the freezing point to determine the osmotic pressure in physiological experiments. (He noted that the freezing point of his own urine when he got up in the morning was −2.3°C; he could reduce this to −0.2°C by drinking beer, but his blood serum froze at −0.56°C all the time.) He infused rabbits with 10% sodium chloride (11 times as concentrated as isotonic saline) and observed a profuse diuresis in which the concentration of the urine was greatly reduced. The observation was confirmed repeatedly in many laboratories using a variety of animals and solutes. Starling (1909) regarded the fact that concentrated infusions given to dehydrated animals provoked a copius flow of urine, far more dilute than the infusions and the previous urine, as so well-known that he gave no references. After that, not much more was heard until McCance (1945; Hervey *et al.*, 1946) found that healthy human subjects, dehydrated, and challenged with infusions of 5% sodium chloride or 25% sucrose, experienced a similar diuresis, with reduction in the maximal concentration of the urine. Sucrose, sodium chloride and urea contributed to the osmolality of the urine in varying proportions, and the extent to which it could be concentrated did not depend upon the nature of the solutes. The falling concentration means that the volume of urine must be increased more than in proportion to the total amount of solute excreted. Rapoport *et al.* (1949) repeated these studies with 11 different solutes and observed some of the largest urinary volumes ever recorded in human subjects, exceeding 20 ml/min per 1.73 m^2 of body surface. When its volume was small, the urine had about four times the osmolality of the plasma, but it became almost isosmolal at the highest rates of flow. The common pattern is shown in Fig. 5.5, with magnitudes appropriate for human subjects. This increase in volume of urine required to accommodate increased amounts of unreabsorbed solute is appropriately described as osmotic diuresis.

The phenomena of osmotic diuresis show that vasopressin is strictly an anti-water-diuretic hormone. It is unable to prevent osmotic diuresis, though it continues to be secreted, and indeed can be detected in the urine. It is also clear that the kidney can produce its most concentrated urine only in small quantities, such as are required to excrete normal amounts of urinary solutes. Extreme osmotic diuresis has yielded useful information about the concentrating mechanism and its limitations; even if some of the experiments are hardly 'physiological', they have practical applications. Fig. 5.5 explains why survivors at sea must not drink sea water. Human urine can match sea water in osmolality, but cannot exceed half its concentration of salt; far more water would be lost in excreting the salt than could be ingested with it. Diabetic ketosis offers a clinical example of osmotic diuresis which can cause dehydration through the loss of water with glucose and salts of ketoacids. Fig. 5.5 also explains the characteristic 'fixed specific gravity of 1010' (isosthenuria) of the urine of patients with chronic renal disease which has destroyed a large proportion of their nephrons. These patients still have a normal 600 mosmol or so of urinary solutes to excrete each day, and the greatly increased load per nephron provokes continuous osmotic diuresis in those that remain. If there are only 200 000 nephrons instead of 2 million, the flow through each nephron for a total urinary minute volume of 1.5 ml will be the same as through nephrons in normal kidneys at a minute volume of 15 ml, and the urine will be isosmolal with plasma. Incidentally, 1.5 ml/min = 2160 ml per day, which is approximately the volume required to remove 600 mosmol of solutes in 300 mosm urine.

Until the discovery of the medullary osmolal gradient and the advent of the countercurrent hypothesis there was no satisfactory explanation for the dilution of the urine during profuse osmotic diuresis. Rates of glomerular filtration were not increased, and were often reduced (Seely & Dirks, 1969). Some other possible explanations were examined by Robinson (1954) and discarded. The failure to maintain concentration did not seem to depend upon a limit to the kidneys' output of osmotic work. The possibility that tubular fluid had not time to reach diffusion equilibrium across the lumen was discounted. Moreover, the urine may become hypotonic (Zak *et al.*, 1954), which suggests that

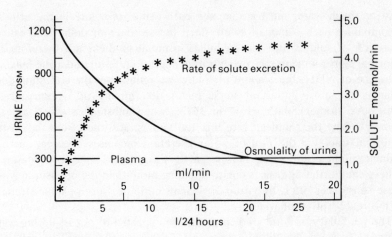

Fig. 5.5 Essential features of osmotic diuresis. Typical orders of magnitude for a dehydrated human subject.

hypotonic fluid leaving distal convoluted tubules does not equilibrate completely with the medullary gradient as it traverses the papillary collecting ducts. A limit to the rate at which water could be removed from fluid entering some late segment of the nephron against an osmotic gradient would have seemed plausible if water had to be transported actively out of the tubular fluid to leave it more concentrated. But if the movement of water out of the collecting system is passive, driven by the medullary osmotic gradient, the dilution of that gradient offers a better explanation for the falling concentration and the increasing volume of the urine.

Such a dilution or 'washing out' of the medullary gradient was demonstrated by Malvin & Wilde (1959). They established an osmotic diuresis by infusing dogs with hypertonic mannitol, and then removed the kidneys and found that the medullary hypertonicity had vanished. The concentrating mechanism can only work if sufficient solute is deposited in the medullary gradient and not too much dilute fluid enters the collecting ducts. All the salt from 6 ml of isotonic fluid entering the loop of Henle would have to be added to the medulla to reabsorb 1.5 ml of water and convert 2 ml of isotonic fluid entering the papillary collecting ducts into 0.5 ml of 1200 mosm urine. Mannitol, which cannot itself be reabsorbed, increases the rate of flow along the nephron and opposes reabsorption of sodium chloride by creating an unfavourable gradient of concentration (Wesson & Anslow, 1948). Consequently it gravely disrupts the concentrating mechanism because, however much the permeability of the collecting ducts is increased by ADH, there is no osmotic gradient to reabsorb water from the large flood of isotonic or hypotonic pre-urine. The final volume of the urine must always be at least equal to the number of osmoles of solute excreted divided by the attainable urinary osmolality. This cannot exceed the greatest osmolality maintained in the medullary gradient; hence at least as much water must accompany each osmol of solute in the urine as accompanies each osmol of solute deep in the inner medulla. The rate of excretion of solutes and the medullary osmolal gradient are therefore the principal constraints on the concentrating operation. Even under the maximal influence of ADH, the amount of solute emerging from the collecting ducts remains the most important single factor determining the volume of the urine. As Homer Smith wrote in 1937; 'when substances which are not reabsorbed by the tubules...are injected...or...absorbed from the gastro-intestinal tract, ...the rate of water excretion increases... urea, sucrose, sodium sulphate and other salts act in this manner. There is no reason to believe that...the diuresis is due to anything more than the opposition which these substances offer, by virtue of their osmotic pressure or ionic strength, to the reabsorption of water'.

The medullary osmotic gradient might be expected to persist during water diuresis, because the diluting segments, including the papillary collecting tubules, continue to reabsorb salt. However, unless these segments were completely impermeable in the absence of ADH, reabsorption of water from the extremely dilute tubular fluid under a greatly increased osmotic gradient would tend to dilute the inner medullary interstitial fluid. During water diuresis in dogs the increase in concentration of sodium chloride with depth below the cortex was halved, and mostly limited to the outer medulla (Ullrich & Jarausch, 1956; Fig. 5.3). However, although the osmolality (990 mosm) and the concentration of sodium (230 mM) had been similar in the papillary tip and the urine during antidiuresis, substantial differences of 400 to 500 mosm and 60 to 100 mM sodium appeared at the peak of water diuresis, when the osmolality and the sodium concentration at the papillary tip were approximately halved and the urine became very dilute (Boylan & Asshauer, 1962). The medullary gradient can therefore be washed out by prolonged water diuresis, and does not remain in reserve for restarting the concentrating operation quickly.

Water diuresis largely eliminates the contribution of urea, which accounts for nearly a half of the hyperosmolality of the inner medulla (Fig. 5.3). Urea leaves the medulla passively when its concentration in the fluid in the collecting ducts falls during either water diuresis or osmotic diuresis due to salt (Haas *et al.*, 1965). This extra urea is excreted before the peak of the diuresis and accounts for the 'exaltation' of the clearance (Section 4.2.1). In 19 experiments on two human subjects the amount of urea thus washed out averaged 250 mg. This could have been accommodated in a conical gradient, with the concentration of urea in the urine at its apex and the concentration in the cortex at its base; the calculated volume of the cone was about 50 ml, and gave a very rough estimate of twice the volume of the inner medulla in each human kidney. When urea itself was used as the osmotic diuretic, its concentration in the urine did not fall and no extra urea was excreted to exalt the clearance, suggesting that urea was not washed out from the medulla because there was no gradient of concentration to drive net diffusion from the interstitial fluid into the collecting ducts.

About as much urea as had been washed out of the kidney early in water or saline diuresis re-accumulated during the next hour or two, while the output of urine fell and the urinary concentration of urea was increasing to prediuretic values. During this period there was an 'abatement of the clearance' as the rate of excretion of urea fell far below the initial value, to which it returned after the inner medullary store had been refilled (Haas *et al.*, 1965). In dogs after one kidney was removed at the height of water diuresis, the papillary osmolality and sodium concentration in the remaining kidney returned to their prediuretic values after a few hours. It took from 30 minutes to 3 hours to restore the medullary gradient in rats after water diuresis and a little longer for the maximum response to ADH to be established (Atherton *et al.*, 1969; Hai & Thomas, 1969). These time relations are consistent with the countercurrent hypothesis of the concentrating mechanism. If ADH switched on an active epithelial transport of water, the transition from diluting to concentrating the urine should be much more rapid; and if the high concentration in the inner medulla was due to previously concentrated fluid flowing through the papillary collecting ducts, the formation of concentrated urine would have to precede the restoration of medullary osmolality by some hours (Robinson, 1954).

5.5.4 Osmoregulation by ADH

When the urine is not already maximally concentrated, additional ADH reaching the kidneys can reduce its volume and increase its concentration in proportion. In a healthy person producing 1 litre of urine daily, additional ADH could reduce the volume to 500 ml and double the concentration. Adult human subjects ordinarily have about 600 mosmol of mixed urinary solutes to excrete every day. With a maximal concentration of 1200 mosm this requires a minimal urinary volume of 500 ml/day. The same solutes could be excreted in 1000 ml of 600 mosm urine, in 2 litres of isotonic (300 mosm) urine, or, during sustained water diuresis or in diabetes insipidus, in 20 litres of very dilute (30 mosm) urine. Persons with diseased kidneys unable to generate hypertonic urine have to live with a minimal urine volume of 2 litres per day which no amount of ADH can reduce.

The excretion of water in hypotonic urine increases the osmolality of the plasma and the kidneys can eliminate excess water very briskly; their defence against hypertonicity is slower and more limited. The excretion of hypertonic urine removes solute from the body in excess of water and dilutes the plasma, but the kidneys cannot manufacture water, apart maybe from 30 to 50 ml daily from oxidation of hydrogen in their metabolic fuels; and the amount they can recover from the tubular fluid is limited by the amount of solute in the urine. Within these limitations the kidneys can be directed by ADH to vary the excretion of water so as to stabilize the osmolality of the plasma and of other body fluids in equilibrium with it. Vasopressin may have an extrarenal role in controlling systemic arterial pressure, but subpressor doses can slow the excretion of water, and the likeliest everyday role for ADH is in controlling the kidneys' contribution to osmoregulation. The integration of this osmotic control with nonosmotic factors related to the homeostasis of volume, and with some other factors which are not primarily homeostatic, will be deferred to Section 7.2 on the kidneys' role in regulating the volume of water in the body.

The common statement in textbooks and elsewhere that ADH can control the osmolality of the blood within about 1% does less than justice to the precision and sensitivity of the osmoregulatory mechanism. The full range of concentrating and diluting capacity is called forth by a range of plasma ADH concentrations from 0.5 to 5.0 pg/ml (0.5 to 5 pM), and healthy adults normally have plasma concentrations between 2 and 2.5 pM, in the middle of this range (Robertson *et al.*, 1976). An alteration of 1 mosM in the plasma (which is only about 0.3% of the prevailing osmolality, and would be hard to detect with a laboratory osmometer) changes plasma ADH concentration by about 0.4 pM and urinary osmolality by 100 mosM. Hence the adjustment to urinary osmolality is 100 times larger than the change in the plasma which provokes it.

After reviewing arguments about whether the secretion of ADH is controlled by hypothalamic osmoreceptors or by receptors sensitive to the concentration of sodium chloride in ventricular cerebrospinal fluid, Schrier *et al.* (1979) concluded in favour of Verney's original view that the most important single factor that stimulates the release of ADH is an increase in the effective osmolality of blood perfusing the hypothalamus. Intracarotid infusions of hypertonic saline, sucrose or urea in dogs all increase sodium chloride concentration in the cerebrospinal fluid; but only saline and sucrose, which shrink cells, are powerful stimuli for the release of ADH, while urea, which enters cells though it does not readily cross the blood–brain barrier, is not. (See Section 7.2 for further discussion.)

Since the cell membranes are permeable to water, the osmoregulatory action of the kidneys, exerted directly on the plasma passing through them, sets the osmolality in cellular as well as extracellular fluids throughout the body. This osmolality fixes the volume of water associated with each unit quantity of solute in every major compartment (the renal inner medulla is a nonconforming minor compartment). Since the total volume in the extracellular compartments depends on the amount of sodium they contain (also under renal control; Section 7.4), osmoregulation under the influence of ADH may be regarded as a mechanism which serves primarily to defend the volume of the cells. Animals in the wild tend to take no more water than they need, and secrete ADH rather constantly to keep their urine concentrated, thereby reducing the times when they must risk attack from predators as they drink or void. Humans, who are erratic drinkers, often far in excess of homeostatic needs, seem to rely more on water diuresis to protect them against incidental water intoxication.

Cells throughout the body shrink when extracellular osmolality increases, and swell if the plasma is suddenly diluted; but the vast majority of them have no access to effectors which might correct these aberrations. Osmolality is one of several intensive properties which are transmitted through cell membranes; others are temperature and the partial pressures of respiratory gases. In each case a few specialized cells, strategically placed in or in relation to the central nervous system, experience changes in the common environment which affects all cells and initiate action which will help to restore optimal conditions not only for themselves but also for other cells all over the body (Robinson, 1978). For osmoregulation, the principal initiating cells are the hypothalamic osmoreceptors and the neurosecretory neurones they control; these secrete more ADH when increasing osmolality shrinks cells bodywide, and reduce or cease secretion when the body is overloaded with water.

About 300 mosm is often taken as a round figure which the mammalian osmoreceptor−ADH mechanism is set to maintain; but since there are considerable variations between individuals and between species, it is more accurate to speak of a range from 265 to 295 mosm. American and European citizens average about 280 mosm, with individual variations between 276 and 291 mosm for the threshold above which plasma ADH increases; this threshold has been reported as low as 265 mosm in Japan. Mammals other than man fall in the higher part of the range, with thresholds for rats, dogs and monkeys close to 290 mosm (Robertson *et al.*, 1977; Schrier *et al.*, 1979).

The great antidiuretic potency of vasopressin merits a final comment. Verney once commented that it took remarkably few molecules per cell to produce its maximal physiological effect; and a dose−response curve for rats showed that 1 μu of ADH led to the reabsorption of 5 ml of water (Gauer & Tata, 1968). At 400 u to the milligram, and a molecular weight of 1084; 1 μu would weigh 2.5 pg and contain about 2.5×10^{-15} mol. Since 5 ml of water contains 5/18 or about 0.28 mol, it follows that each molecule of ADH would be responsible for the reabsorption of $0.28 \div 2.5 \times 10^{-15} = 10^{14}$ molecules of water! Alternatively, Kleeman (1972) estimated that healthy people would need to secrete between 1 and 2 u of ADH daily to maintain maximal concentration of their urine. With lower rates of secretion to accommodate drinking in the daytime, the daily requirement would rarely be more than 1 unit, or 2.5 μg. Hence 1 mg would be more than most people would need to maintain their water balance for a year!

CHAPTER 6
Renal control of acid−base balance

6.1 INTRODUCTION

By making the urine acid or alkaline the kidneys help to maintain the normal reaction (pH) of the body fluids, which is important because the functions of the cells, especially of excitable cells in the neuromuscular and nervous systems, are impaired if the pH of the surrounding fluid is not kept close to 7.4. At mammalian body temperatures pH 6.8 signifies neutrality, because the concentrations of hydrogen ions and of hydroxyl ions are then equal and 160 nM; at pH 7.4, hydrogen ion concentration is 40 nM and hydroxyl ion concentration is 640 nM. Mammalian ECFs were therefore felicitously characterized by Pitts *et al.* (1954) as 'blandly alkaline'. Strictly, it is activity rather than concentration of hydrogen ions that influences cellular functions and that pH meters measure, but the distinction may be ignored in very dilute solutions. Bland alkalinity has to be maintained although acid and alkaline substances are ingested and produced in metabolism. Meat and most mixed diets yield sulphuric and phosphoric acids derived from dietary proteins and phospholipids, vegetarian diets yield bicarbonate after their organic anions have been oxidized, achlorhydric patients may drink dilute hydrochloric acid, and most indigestion remedies contain alkalis. The kidneys, however, can excrete bicarbonate when the plasma is too alkaline, or counter inroads made by acids into the body's stores of bicarbonate by excreting acid urine and replenishing the plasma with freshly made bicarbonate.

The reaction of the body fluids is determined by the buffer ratio of the principal buffer pair, bicarbonate and carbonic acid. In terms of the Henderson−Hasselbalch equation

$$pH = pK'_a + \log \frac{[HCO_3^-]}{0.03 P_{CO_2}} \qquad (6.1)$$

where pK'_a is 6.1 at 38°C and the partial pressure of carbon dioxide is in mmHg. (The numerical factor in the denominator is 0.225 for partial pressures in kilopascals, KPa.) Oxidation of metabolic substrates produces carbon dioxide continuously, and the respiratory centres, which are sensitive to pH as well as to the partial pressure of carbon dioxide, regulate its partial pressure in the body fluids briskly, from minute to minute, by controlling the rate at which the lungs excrete it. The kidneys control the concentration of bicarbonate more sedately, from day to day, by adding more bicarbonate to the plasma than the glomeruli filter, or by allowing some filtered bicarbonate to escape reabsorption and be excreted in the urine. Thus the respiratory system adjusts the denominator of the Henderson—Hasselbalch equation while the kidneys stabilize the numerator.

When the first *'Reflections on Renal Function'* was written, many physicians and physiologists regarded the cations in the body fluids as bases, so the kidneys had to excrete 'fixed acids without losing the fixed base that accompanied them into the glomerular filtrate' (Robinson, 1954). Newer conceptions of acids and bases have made it proper to think of bicarbonate directly as the principal base that keeps the plasma alkaline, where Pitts spoke of the accompanying cations as 'bicarbonate-bound base'. Information on the chemical background, on extrarenal mechanisms, and on the integrated control of the reaction of the body fluids, may be found in textbooks and monographs, and in a small introductory book (Robinson, 1975c). The present account concentrates on the kidneys' contribution.

Secretion of hydrogen ions used to 'reabsorb' bicarbonate was dealt with in Section 4.3.2. When all the filtered bicarbonate has been reabsorbed the body's acid—base state (whether this is normal, acidotic or alkalotic) is unchanged. No hydrogen ion has been excreted in the urine, and no more bicarbonate has been added to the plasma than was present in the glomerular filtrate. Only hydrogen ions secreted into the tubular fluid after all bicarbonate has been reabsorbed are excreted in the urine and matched by extra bicarbonate added to the plasma to prevent or mitigate acidosis. If, however, insufficient hydrogen ion is secreted to deal with the whole filtered load of bicarbonate, its reabsorption is incomplete, and bicarbonate is excreted in alkaline urine.

6.2 RENAL DISPOSAL OF ACIDS

By far the most abundant acid product of metabolism is carbonic acid. Human adults generate around 13 000 mmol of carbon dioxide every day. This could in principle yield 26 000 mmol of hydrogen ions, but there is hardly any carbonate in body fluids and 13 000 mmol of sodium hydroxide would be enough to convert the day's carbon dioxide to bicarbonate at pH 7.4 if it were not removed. Fortunately this large daily quota of potential acid does not have to be disposed of by the kidneys. The lungs remove carbon dioxide so effectively that, instead of posing a threat to neutrality, it is an important source of bicarbonate, which is the body's principal buffer base.

The kidneys' common task is to protect the body against nonvolatile acids which cannot be destroyed by further metabolism or breathed out like carbon dioxide. The most important of these is sulphuric acid, formed by the oxidation of sulphur from the amino acids cysteine and methionine. Nearly 140 mmol of hydrochloric acid arises each day from the metabolism of cationic amino acids which were electrically balanced by chloride ions in the plasma; but this is more than compensated for by bicarbonate produced from the metabolism of glutamate, aspartate and other organic anions (Halperin & Jungas, 1983). About 15 mmol/day of phosphoric acid is generated from the metabolism of phospholipids. Much of the phosphoric acid excreted is not, however, formed by oxidation of phosphorus in the body, but released from phosphoproteins and phospholipids which already contained it in the oxidized form. People on mixed diets ordinarily excrete 50 to 80 mmol of urinary acid each day, mostly sulphuric and phosphoric acids and ammonium. The total amount depends mainly upon how much sulphur is oxidized; it can be greatly increased when more acid is generated or ingested, and it may include lactic acid during shock or anaerobic exercise, or ketoacids during ketosis (cf. Robinson, 1975c).

There is something paradoxical about the manner of the kidneys' elimination of acids from the body. Strong acids in solution are ionized to hydrogen ions (protons) and the anions which are their weak conjugate bases. The threat to normal alkalinity comes not from the bases (which used to be called 'fixed acids') but from the protons, and while the anionic bases remain in the plasma and can be easily excreted by simply not reabsorbing them from the glomerular filtrate, the protons present more of a problem. Protons from strong acids are taken up by buffer bases (the stronger conjugate bases of weaker 'buffer acids'), especially bicarbonate in the plasma. Taking sulphuric acid as an example,

$$\begin{aligned} H_2SO_4 &\rightarrow SO_4^{2-} + 2H^+ \\ 2H^+ + 2HCO_3^- &\rightarrow 2H_2CO_3 \rightarrow 2H_2O + 2CO_2 \end{aligned} \quad (6.2)$$

Two molecules of bicarbonate have been lost from the plasma in exchange for one of sulphate. The weak buffer acid, carbonic, has been formed, and the fall in pH is limited because more carbon dioxide is removed in the expired air and this reduces its partial pressure to match the reduction in bicarbonate. The kidneys cannot excrete the protons which posed a threat to the plasma's reaction, because these no longer exist; they have become hydrogen atoms in two molecules of body water. But although the fall in pH has been minimized, the loss of bicarbonate impairs the body's capacity to buffer protons from further additions of acid. To restore the normal state of acid−base balance it is not sufficient for the kidneys merely to excrete sulphate; the depleted stores of bicarbonate must also be replenished.

The kidneys do this in a subtle way, employing the same mechanism by which bicarbonate is 'reabsorbed' without having to enter the cells through their rather impermeable apical membranes. Renal epithelial cells, in proximal and distal convoluted tubules and also in the collecting ducts, contain carbonic anhydrase (CA in the equation), and can generate carbonic acid rapidly from metabolic carbon dioxide. The acid immediately ionizes:

$$CO_2 + H_2O \overset{CA}{\rightarrow} H_2CO_3 \rightarrow HCO_3^- + H^+ \quad (6.3)$$

and releases bicarbonate and hydrogen ions in equal numbers. The protons are secreted into the tubular fluid, while the bicarbonate ions pass through the basolateral cell membranes and enter the plasma together with reabsorbed sodium ions. Figure 6.1 illustrates the common mechanism. In the proximal convoluted tubules, where the epithelium is extremely leaky, with transepithelial pds no greater than 1 or 2 mV, and there is ample bicarbonate in the lumen, much of the secretion of hydrogen ions can be achieved passively. The step of about 60 mV from cell interior to lumen is uphill, but a neutral sodium/hydrogen antiporter in the apical cell membrane enables it to be driven by the steep electrochemical gradient for sodium maintained by the basolateral pumps (Rector, 1983). In the distal nephron little or no bicarbonate remains to take up hydrogen ions, and the epithelium is tight. Passive net transfer of hydrogen ions from plasma at pH 7.4 to urine at pH 4.4 (i.e. with a ratio of $[H^+]_U/[H^+]_P = 1000{:}1$) would require a transepithelial pd of 183 mV, lumen-negative, according to Nernst's equation (Robinson, 1975b); and no pds as large as this have been recorded. Active secretion of protons therefore becomes increasingly necessary as the tubular fluid gets more acid, and a booster pump is required at least in the collecting ducts.

The acidification of the urine is thus an extension of the process which initially replaces filtered bicarbonate in the plasma. The new bicarbonate added to the plasma is generated from carbonic acid which is also the source of hydrogen ions secreted into the tubular fluid and excreted in the acid urine. It is pointless to ask whether the bicarbonate added to the plasma is merely a byproduct of the generation of hydrogen ions to acidify the urine, or whether the urinary hydrogen ions are byproducts of the generation of bicarbonate for the plasma. However, the fact that the body's cells live in the plasma and not in the urine might suggest the manufacture of bicarbonate as the primary aim; the two processes are inseparable, and nothing would be gained by secreting hydrogen ions into the urine if bicarbonate were not

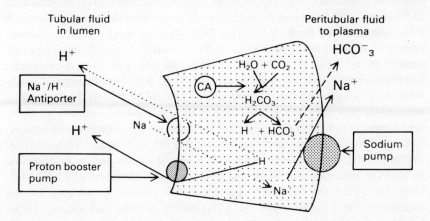

Fig. 6.1 Generation of hydrogen and bicarbonate ions in renal tubular cells; secretion of hydrogen ions into tubular fluid and addition of equal amount of bicarbonate to plasma via peritubular fluid. Booster pump at lower left required chiefly in collecting ducts; basolateral sodium pump in all segments. Solid lines denote active, dotted lines passive transport.

added to the plasma. The simple stoichiometry of the reactions ensures that when all bicarbonate that was used up in buffering protons in the body has been restored, precisely as many hydrogen ions will have been excreted in the urine as were originally released and buffered. This can be seen most clearly by following the fate of hydrogen ions secreted into the renal tubules.

6.3 HYDROGEN IONS IN THE TUBULAR FLUID

Although it is convenient to describe three important consequences of the addition of hydrogen ions to the tubular fluid as though they occurred in successive segments of the nephron, it is important to realize that the processes overlap and are not associated with particular anatomical segments.

6.3.1 Reabsorption of filtered bicarbonate

So long as bicarbonate remains in the tubule it takes up hydrogen ions and is destroyed by conversion to carbonic acid, which then breaks down to carbon dioxide and water. Meanwhile an equal amount of bicarbonate is added to the plasma. Some of the evidence for this way of recovering filtered bicarbonate was outlined in Section 4.3.2, and few additional comments are required here. The daily filtered load of bicarbonate in man is about $25 \times 180 = 4500$ mmol, so that the rate of reabsorption must be about 3 mmol/min. One tenth of the body's resting oxygen consumption, about 24 ml or 1 mmol per minute, could provide no more than 1 mmol of carbon dioxide per minute. Reabsorption of more than a third of the filtered bicarbonate in this indirect manner would therefore require more hydrogen ions than the kidneys' metabolic carbon dioxide could supply, and some of the carbon dioxide used as a source of hydrogen ions would have to come from the blood or be taken back into the cells from the tubular fluid. Recirculation of carbon dioxide (indicated by the dotted line in Fig. 6.2, 1a) is facilitated by carbonic anhydrase located in the brush borders of proximal tubular cells in several species including man (Lönnerholm & Wistrand, 1984). Rapid breakdown of newly formed carbonic acid raises the tension of carbon dioxide in the lumen and encourages it to diffuse into the cells; at the same time it removes carbonic acid which would otherwise lower pH and oppose the secretion of hydrogen ions. As an alterative to recirculation of carbon dioxide, Rector (1973) suggested that carbonic acid might diffuse into the cells, and there dissociate to provide hydrogen and bicarbonate ions in equal numbers (Fig. 6.2, 1b). Since the ionization does not require catalysis, this could account for unexpectedly rapid rates of hydrogen ion secretion with carbonic anhydrase inhibited.

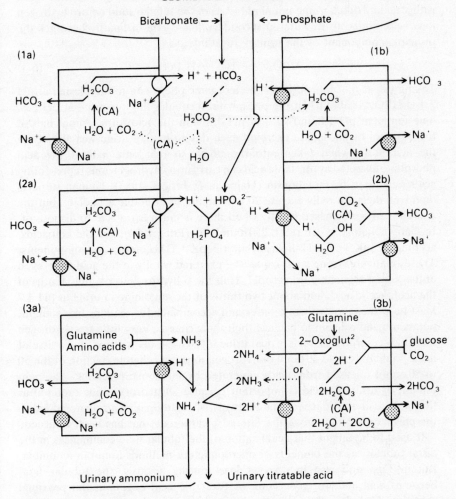

GLOMERULAR FILTRATE

Fig. 6.2 1 Reabsorption of filtered bicarbonate. Dotted lines show recycling of carbon dioxide (**a**) or of carbonic acid (**b**).
2 Generation of titratable acid, protons derived from water through carbonic acid (**a**) or directly (**b**).
3 Secretion of ammonium; (**a**) traditional scheme; (**b**) as envisaged by Halperin and Jungas (1983).

6.3.2 Generation of titratable acid

As bicarbonate disappears, other buffer bases in the glomerular filtrate take up hydrogen ions, and the pH of the tubular fluid falls as their conjugate buffer acids accumulate and contribute to the titratable acid excreted in the urine. The total amount excreted is discovered by titrating the urine back with standard alkali to the initial pH (7.4) of the tubular fluid before hydrogen ions were added to it. Filtered secondary phosphate ordinarily becomes the principal component of the urinary titratable acid:

$$HPO_4^{2-} + H^+ \rightarrow H_2PO_4^- \qquad (6.4)$$

Taking pK as 6.8, four fifths of the inorganic phosphate in the plasma at pH 7.4 is HPO_4^{2-}; about half the phosphate in tubular fluid or urine at pH 6.8, nine tenths at pH 5.8 and 99% at pH 4.8 is in the acid form. About half of the 30 mmol of phosphate excreted each day in human urine was already in the acid form when taken into the body, so that only half of the acid phosphate excreted as titratable acid can carry away hydrogen ions representing acids generated by metabolism (Halperin & Jungas, 1983). Human subjects on mixed diets normally excrete 20 to 30 mmol of titratable acid daily, but the amount can be increased greatly when there is much extra acid to dispose of. In diabetic ketosis it can reach 250 mmol/day (Pitts, 1974), and the ketoacids, acetoacetic (pK 3.6) and β-hydroxybutyric (pK 4.7) become major components. These relatively strong acids cannot be excreted wholly in the acid form even at the lowest attainable urinary pH. Half the β-hydroxybutyric, nine tenths of the acetoacetic acid, and about two thirds of the creatinine in urine at pH 4.7 must be present as conjugate bases and accompanied by cations like sodium, potassium and calcium to balance their ionic charge. Very little free hydrogen ion can be excreted as such in acid urine; at pH 4.4, cH is 40 μM, and a litre of urine could only hold 40 μmol of hydrogen ions, a negligible fraction of the 50 to 80 mmol released from acids generated by metabolic reactions. The generation of titratable acid is important because all hydrogen ions excreted as titratable acid are matched quantitatively by additional bicarbonate added to the plasma over and above the filtered bicarbonate that has been returned.

It used to be taught that acidification of the tubular fluid commences in the distal tubules, as the pioneers of micropuncture methods found in amphibia. But in rats, and also in dogs at least during acidosis, the tubular fluid becomes acid and the generation of titratable acid begins in the proximal convoluted tubules. The majority of the filtered bicarbonate is removed very early in the proximal tubules; by the middle third its concentration in the remaining tubular fluid has been reduced to 5 to 8 mM in rats, 10 mM in rhesus monkeys and 16 mM in dogs (Malnic, 1974; Steinmetz, 1974). Rats generate most if not all of their urinary titratable acid in the proximal tubules, and lose some further downstream, for more titratable acid leaves the late proximal tubules than enters the early distal tubules and continues into the urine (Karlmark et al., 1983). Hence there seems to be need for active secretion of hydrogen ions in the proximal as well as in the distal nephron. Bichara et al. (1983) claimed that three quarters of the proton secretion by isolated segments of rabbits' proximal convoluted tubules was attributable to sodium/hydrogen countertransport, while one quarter depended upon primary proton pumping.

To make the tubular fluid 0.6 to 0.7 pH units more acid than the plasma by passive transport of protons would need a transepithelial pd of the order of 40 mV, which is at least 10 times greater than occurs in proximal tubules. Steinmetz (1974) stated that pH can fall as low as 6.0 in proximal tubules, and this would require a pd greater than 80 mV.

Evidence that the secretion of protons could be dissociated from reabsorption of sodium led Giebisch & Malnic (1976) to propose an alternative mechanism for primary active secretion of hydrogen ions which were to be derived directly from water, without the intermediate formation and ionization of carbonic acid:

$$H_2O \rightarrow OH^- + H^+ \qquad (6.5)$$

The hydroxyl ions left behind in the cells were neutralized by combining with carbon dioxide, to make one molecule of bicarbonate for every proton secreted;

$$OH^- + CO_2 \xrightarrow{\text{CA}} HCO_3^- \qquad (6.6)$$

This reaction is catalysed by carbonic anhydrase which would then play a dual role; it would both accelerate the neutralization of hydroxyl ions in the cells and the breakdown of carbonic acid in the tubular lumen. The alternative mechanism is shown on the right hand side in Fig. 6.2 (2b). Since further work provided stronger evidence for coupling the secretion of protons with the reabsorption of sodium, Rector (1983) accepted the earlier mechanism shown in Fig. 6.1. Aronson (1983) reviewed these and other possible mechanisms for active secretion of hydrogen ions in the kidney. The capacity to extrude protons appears to be a property shared by many cells. A typical membrane potential of about 60 mV would require the negatively charged cytoplasm to be 1 pH unit more acid than the surroundings if hydrogen ions were distributed passively at equilibrium across their membranes.

The renal tubules show the asymmetry, or polarity, characteristic of epithelial cells which live between two worlds (the external environment and the plasma) by, among other things, extruding protons across their apical membranes and sodium across their basolateral membranes. These functions appear to be independent of each other in segments of the collecting ducts where secretion of protons and provision of bicarbonate for the plasma are not impaired by removing sodium or inhibiting its transport with ouabain. A lumen-positive pd is maintained here by electrogenic proton pumps in the apical membranes of special intercalated cells rich in carbonic anhydrase. The secretory activity of these cells is increased by acidity, low concentrations of bicarbonate and high partial pressures of carbon dioxide in peritubular blood; and aldosterone promotes it independently of its effects upon the transport of sodium or potassium (Levine & Jacobson, 1986).

Members of another population of cells may act in the opposite direction by secreting bicarbonate into the lumen. In his Homer Smith Award Lecture,

Steinmetz (1986) described, in addition to the predominant granular cells which actively transport sodium and have their oxygen consumption reduced by ouabain, some 20% of intercalated, carbonic anhydrase-rich, acid-secreting cells which were discovered in the urinary bladder of the fresh-water turtle *Pseudemys scripta*. These cells actively transport protons, and their oxygen consumption is reduced by inhibitors of carbonic anhydrase. They are of two kinds: the α-type has an apical membrane rich in rod-shaped particles, and secretes protons into the lumen, both the number of the particles and the area of the apical membrane are increased by carbon dioxide; the β-type has less numerous rod-shaped particles, located at the basolateral membrane, and secretes bicarbonate into the lumen in exchange for chloride. The turtle's bladder may be a good model for acid-secreting parts of the mammalian distal nephron, for the cortical collecting ducts of the rabbit have similar intercalated cells. Rabbits are ordinarily herbivorous; they produce alkaline urine containing bicarbonate and their intercalated cells are mostly of the β-type. Loading with acid, however, increases the proportion of cells of the α-type (cf. Section 8.3)

6.3.3 Secretion of ammonium

Ammonium and ammonia constitute an acid−base pair. The cation, ammonium, is a weak Brønsted acid:

$$NH_4^+ \longleftrightarrow NH_3 + H^+ \tag{6.7}$$

Both the cation and the uncharged base are present in all solutions in proportions determined by the pH, as the Henderson−Hasselbalch equation predicts:

$$pH = pK' + \log([NH_3]/[NH_4^+]) \tag{6.8}$$

Since pK' is close to 9 in body fluids, no more than 1% of the buffer mixture is ammonia at pH 7, 0.1% at pH 6 and 0.01% at pH 5. The mixture is therefore more appropriately described as ammonium than as ammonia. Biological membranes have been supposed to be freely permeable to the uncharged base and almost impermeable to the cation. Passive transport of the mixture across these membranes was believed to occur by 'non-ionic diffusion' of the base. This readily accounted for what was known as the trapping of ammonia in acid solutions. The ratio of [ammonia]/[ammonium] would be about 1/100 at pH 7 and 1/1000 at pH 6. Hence with equal total concentrations on both sides of a membrane permeable only to ammonia, ammonia should diffuse 10 times as fast from the neutral to the acid solution as from the acid to the neutral. The total concentration would have to be 10 times greater on the acid side to equalize the rates of diffusion of ammonia in the two directions, and ammonium would accumulate on the more acid side of the membrane against a concentration gradient. Good & Knepper (1985) pointed out that the hydrated ammonium ion has about the same radius as potassium, to which biological membranes are appreciably permeable; hence, although no comparative values are available, ammonium may be expected to cross membranes as such as well as indirectly by non-ionic diffusion of ammonia.

Pitts (1974) established that about 70% of the ammonium in the urine was formed in the kidney — 60% from glutamine and 10% from amino acids; 30% was derived from the arterial blood, but even this portion probably came from the kidneys in the first place, for there is more ammonium in renal venous than in arterial blood. The tubular fluid is usually more acid than the plasma, and takes up ammonium in higher concentration, but the volume of plasma flowing through the kidney is so much greater than the flow of tubular fluid that the blood takes away more ammonia than the urine unless the urine is strongly acid. The traditional view, illustrated on the left in Fig. 6.2 (3a), was that the urine begins to be acidified in the distal convoluted tubules, and that the acid fluid encouraged ammonia to diffuse from the cells and be trapped in the lumen as ammonium ions. The production of ammonia thus allows the tubular fluid to take up more hydrogen ions without further lowering its pH, which would increase the gradient against which hydrogen ions had to be secreted. Additional bicarbonate, equivalent in quantity to the hydrogen ions taken up and excreted as ammonium, is added to the plasma; the ammonium is an expendable cation, manufactured by the kidney, which can replace sodium or other essential cations and allow these to be reabsorbed from the acid tubular fluid in the distal tubules and collecting ducts.

Human subjects on mixed diets ordinarily excrete 30 to 50 mmol of hydrogen ions daily in the form of ammonium; this, together with 20 to 30 mmol excreted as titratable acid corresponds to the 50 to 80 mmol of nonvolatile acid produced by metabolic activities. The total output of urinary acid (= titratable acid + ammonium) removed from body is precisely matched by new bicarbonate added to the plasma to regenerate buffer systems which had temporarily harboured protons from nonvolatile acids that were ingested or produced in metabolism. The amount of ammonium excreted can be increased to as much as 500 mmol when severe acidosis is sustained for a week or more; but there is still no satisfactory explanation for the slow adaptive increase (Tannen, 1978). Moreover, this traditional account which is found in most textbooks (including Robinson, 1975c) requires some modification in the light of more recent views about the site of secretion of ammonium and about the form in which it is secreted.

The urinary ammonium is a product of metabolizing cells, and the bulk of the kidney's cells lie in the cortex, the majority lining proximal convoluted tubules. The cortex has a very rich blood supply which might be expected to carry off most of the ammonium, and yet human subjects excrete more than half the amount of ammonium they produce under normal conditions and about three quarters when they are mildly acidotic (Good & Knepper, 1985). In rats there is as much ammonium in the tubular fluid at the end of the

proximal convoluted tubule as will appear in the final urine, and non-ionic
diffusion of ammonia hardly seems enough to account for so much being
secreted into the tubular lumen rather than lost into the blood. There may be
a selective transport, possibly of ammonium itself into the proximal tubules.
From there it seems to reach the urine without following round the whole
length of the nephron. A great deal is reabsorbed from the loop of Henle,
especially from the thick ascending limb, and added to the medullary interstitial fluid. Being a cation, ammonium, unlike ammonia, is affected by electrical
as well as by concentration gradients. It is similar in size to potassium, and
might be reabsorbed from the thick ascending limb of the loop of Henle
where other cations, like potassium, calcium and magnesium (the last two
considerably larger than potassium or ammonium) are reabsorbed under the
influence of a transepithelial pd of the order of 10 mV, lumen-positive. After
being reabsorbed ammonium appears to diffuse into the thin descending
limbs of the loops and be carried deeper into the inner medulla. When Stern
et al. (1985) washed out the cortico-medullary gradient by mannitol diuresis,
the rate of excretion of ammonium during mild acidosis in Sprague–Dawley
rats was reduced, though the rate of production was not. The increase in
concentration of ammonium along the inner medullary collecting ducts was
also greatly diminished. It thus appears that much of the ammonium generated
in the proximal tubular epithelium is selectively secreted into the tubular
fluid, reabsorbed from the ascending limb, concentrated in the medullary
gradient, and then resecreted into acid tubular fluid in the medullary collecting
ducts.

Halperin & Jungas (1983) insisted that the catabolism of glutamine by
glutaminase yields ammonium, not ammonia; and even if ammonia were first
released, the mixture would contain predominantly ammonium at the pH
prevailing in the cells. They further insisted that what is secreted into the
tubular lumen is also ammonium, not ammonia, possibly transported across
the membrane directly as ammonium, perhaps by a dual path, as ammonia
(diffusing) and hydrogen ions by way of the proton pump. If what is added to
the tubular fluid is already ammonium, it cannot take up protons as ammonia
was formerly supposed to do. How then can it help with the excretion of
protons to balance protons which had been formed and buffered in the body?
The answer seems to be that each molecule of glutamine yields two molecules
of ammonium and one of 2-oxoglutarate, which, when it is oxidized or
converted to glucose, yields two molecules of bicarbonate. Hence one molecule
of bicarbonate is still made available to the plasma for each molecule of
ammonium excreted, but this occurs when the ammonium is generated rather
than when a proton is generated and secreted to combine with ammonia in
the tubular fluid (Fig. 6.2 (3b)). The sum of the urinary titratable acid and
ammonium still measures the kidneys' activity in defence of the plasma's
bland alkalinity; the ammonium still replaces essential cations which might
otherwise be lost if their charge was needed to match the charge on anions

which are the weak conjugate bases of nonvolatile acids in the urine. Moreover, the excretion of ammonium performs a further service by preventing that ammonium from going to the liver and being converted to urea, where the production of a molecule of urea would take the ammonia from two molecules of ammonium, and release two protons:

$$2\,NH_4^+ \rightarrow 2\,NH_3 + 2H^+$$
$$2\,NH_3 + CO_2 \rightarrow CO(NH_2)_2 + H_2O \tag{6.9}$$

However, there is considerable argument about the role of urea formation by the liver (Walser, 1986). What is clear is that the overlapping of the three major processes outlined in Fig. 6.2 now looks far more extensive than it did; the proximal convoluted tubule has come to appear the principal site for them all, and it is no longer possible even to say when, let alone where, (1) passes into (2) or (2) into (3)!

Although acidification of tubular fluid begins in the proximal convoluted tubules, even during acidosis as much as 10% of filtered bicarbonate may remain to enter the distal convoluted tubules (Malnic, 1974). The absence of luminal carbonic anhydrase in this segment permits carbonic acid formed by the combination of hydrogen ions with bicarbonate to persist for several seconds, during which its behaviour as a fairly strong acid (pK' c.3.6) temporarily makes the pH of the tubular fluid lower by up to 0.8 unit than it will become after the carbonic acid has decomposed. The difference, known as a disequilibrium pH, can be measured by comparing pH readings made with a rapidly responding microelectode in the tubular fluid and with an external pH electrode on a sample of the fluid which has been withdrawn and has had time to come to equilibrium. This acid disequilibrium pH can be abolished by infusing carbonic anhydrase so that the enzyme is present in the tubular fluid. It may enhance the secretion of ammonium by encouraging diffusion from the cells before the tubular fluid passes on into the renal pelvis. A similar acid disequilibrium pH of up to 0.7 unit which appears in proximal convoluted tubules when carbonic anhydrase is inhibited provides part of the evidence that the reabsorption of filtered bicarbonate is achieved largely through secretion of hydrogen ions (Du Bose, 1983).

6.4 CONTROLLING FACTORS

If all filtered bicarbonate is 'reabsorbed' indirectly by reacting with hydrogen ions in the tubules and being replaced by new bicarbonate from the cells, only 1 or 2% of the hydrogen ions which are secreted are destined to be excreted in the urine in the form of titratable acid and ammonium. Even if half the filtered bicarbonate were reabsorbed as such, less than 5% of the hydrogen ions secreted would ordinarily be excreted in the urine. Whether the urine is to be acid or alkaline depends upon the relation between the filtered load of bicarbonate and the rate of secretion of hydrogen ions. If the filtered load exceeds the total rate of secretion of hydrogen ions, residual bicarbonate will be excreted in alkaline urine; whereas a smaller filtered load of bicarbonate will take up less hydrogen ion and leave more to be excreted as titratable acid and ammonium in acid urine. The principal factors which determine whether the urine shall be acid or alkaline, and the rate of excretion of urinary acid or bicarbonate, are therefore the filtered load of bicarbonate and the rate of secretion of hydrogen ions. Moreover, so long as GFR remains constant, the filtered load is proportional to the concentration of bicarbonate in the plasma.

6.4.1 The concentration of bicarbonate in the plasma

The effect of bicarbonate concentration in isolation from other factors can be illustrated on the assumption that the rates of glomerular filtration and of tubular secretion of hydrogen ions do not change. With a typical human GFR of 125 ml/min, and a plasma bicarbonate concentration of 24 mM, the filtered load of bicarbonate is 3 mmol/min. The urine is normally acid and titratable acid and ammonium amount to 50 to 80 mmol/day. If the rate of secretion of hydrogen ions is constant and 3.05 mmol/min, this will suffice to reabsorb all filtered bicarbonate and leave 0.05 mmol/min or $0.05 \times 1440 = 72$ mmol/day to be excreted as titratable acid and ammonium, with the addition of a further 72 mmol/day of bicarbonate to the plasma after all that was filtered has been replaced. These figures are shown in the third row of Table 6.1.

If GFR and hydrogen ion secretion were constant, variations in the concentration of bicarbonate in the plasma would provide an automatic renal compensation for metabolic alkalosis and acidosis. When the concentration of bicarbonate is greater than the normal, reabsorption of filtered bicarbonate is incomplete; bicarbonate is excreted in alkaline urine, and the concentration of bicarbonate is lowered because less is replaced in the plasma than is removed by glomerular filtration. In metabolic acidosis, when the body's stores have

Table 6.1 Effect of plasma bicarbonate concentration; hydrogen ion secretion and GFR (125 ml/min) constant (Robinson, 1975c)

Plasma [bicarbonate] mM	Bicarbonate filtered mmol/min	H ion secreted* mmol/min	Urine reaction	Urine contents	mmol/min
48	6.0	3.05	Alkaline	Bicarbonate	2.95
36	4.5	3.05	Alkaline	Bicarbonate	1.45
24	3.0	3.05	Acid	Titr. acid + ammonium	0.05
18	2.25	3.05	Acid	Titr. acid + ammonium	0.80
12	1.5	3.05	Acid	Titr. acid + ammonium	1.55

* Bicarbonate added to plasma.

been depleted and the concentration of bicarbonate in the plasma is subnormal, reabsorption is complete, the urine is acid, and additional bicarbonate equal to the total amount of titratable acid plus ammonum in the urine is added to the plasma to raise its concentration towards normal. Table 6.1 correctly shows the directions of change, but the rates of removal and addition of bicarbonate to the plasma have been exaggerated because of the assumption that the rate of secretion of hydrogen ions was constant. The hypothetical figures in the table show excretion of total urinary acid at a rate of 0.80 mmol/min, or 1152 mmol/ day, which is far too great a response to a moderately severe metabolic acidosis which reduces the plasma bicarbonate concentration by 25% to 18 mM. The rates shown for excretion of bicarbonate in alkaline urines when the concentration of bicarbonate in the plasma is abnormally large are also exaggerated. In fact the rate of secretion of hydrogen ions is decreased during metabolic acidosis and increased during alkalosis, so that the actual rates of excretion of acid or alkali are perhaps one third those shown in the table, and it takes correspondingly longer to repair the disturbances. These points are illustrated by rather more realistic figures in Table 6.2.

Table 6.2 Hydrogen ion secretion and excretion of urinary acid; GFR 180 l/day

	Acid−base status		
	Metabolic alkalosis	Normal	Metabolic acidosis
Plasma [bicarbonate] mM	33	25	17
Bicarbonate filtered mmol/day	6000	4500	3000
Total hydrogen ion secreted mmol/day	5600	4580	3400
Bicarbonate reabsorbed mmol/day	5600	4500	3000
Bicarbonate excreted mmol/day	400	0	0
Urinary titratable acid mmol/day	0	30	100
Urinary ammonium mmol/day	0	50	300
Total urinary acid excretion	0	80	400

These figures illustrate how nearly twice as much hydrogen ion is secreted during metabolic alkalosis as during metabolic acidosis, but against no gradient, for the urine is alkaline and no hydrogen ion is excreted. Normally 80/4580, less than 2% of the hydrogen ion secreted into the tubular fluid is excreted in the urine; but this is increased to 400/3400, almost 12%, and against a steep gradient, during acidosis when the urine is strongly acid. The assumption underlying the different rates of secretion of hydrogen ions in Table 6.2 was that these were roughly proportional to the partial pressure of carbon dioxide in the blood, which was reduced when respiration was stimulated by the lowered pH of the plasma in metabolic acidosis, and increased when pulmonary ventilation was slowed by the raised pH of the plasma during alkalosis. These alterations in carbon dioxide tension, which result from the combined sensitivity of the respiratory centres to carbon dioxide and to pH have the effect of minimizing the displacement of the pH of the plasma from 7.4; but by slowing the kidneys' response to the excess or deficiency of bicarbonate, they delay restoration of normal amounts in the body's stores of buffers. Since the functioning of the nervous system is more liable to be disturbed by alterations in pH than by changes of the amount of buffer in the body, this delay is of no great consequence. The view that the rate of hydrogen ion secretion is simply proportional to the tension of carbon dioxide is, however, oversimplified and requires further consideration (Section 6.4.2).

It has been known for several decades that the partial pressure of carbon dioxide in alkaline urines is often far greater than that in the body fluids, and this is not merely a reflection of the higher carbon dioxide tension in the blood during metabolic alkalosis (Pitts & Lotspeich, 1946). Tensions may exceed 100 mmHg, and were for some time regarded as evidence that bicarbonate that did not escape into the urine was 'reabsorbed' indirectly by secretion of hydrogen ions into the tubular fluid; and that, in the absence of carbonic anhydrase, fluid was carried on into the renal pelvis before carbonic acid formed from the reaction of hydrogen ions with bicarbonate had time to break down to carbon dioxide and water. If this reaction continued in the lower urinary tract from which carbon dioxide could less easily diffuse into the blood, its presence would be revealed by an increased partial pressure. The elevation of the carbon dioxide tension in alkaline urine can be reduced by injecting carbonic anhydrase intravenously so that it reaches the tubular fluid (Ochwadt & Pitts, 1956). But an elevation of carbon dioxide tension may also develop along the inner medullary collecting ducts before a tubular fluid reaches the renal pelvis, and, though reduced, it is not abolished by infusing carbonic anhydrase (Graber *et al.*, 1982). The inference that the high partial pressure of carbon dioxide in alkaline urines implies that hydrogen ions have been added to the tubular fluid may only be valid when the urine is reasonably dilute and contains other buffers besides bicarbonate. Bicarbonate solutions more concentrated than 100 mM or so develop high carbon dioxide tensions without the addition of hydrogen ions, because the concentration of carbon dioxide at equilibrium is about 1% of the concentration of bicarbonate (Maren, 1978; Malnic, 1980). This whole complicated topic was admirably reviewed by Berliner (1985).

6.4.2 The rate of secretion of hydrogen ions

For a given filtered load of bicarbonate, the urinary excretion of acid or alkali should be determined by the rate of secretion of hydrogen ions. The urine should be acid when more than enough hydrogen ion is secreted to restore all the filtered bicarbonate to the plasma, and alkaline when the filtered load of bicarbonate exceeds the rate of secretion of hydrogen ions. Classical studies using elevated concentrations of filtered bicarbonate to encourage the secretion of hydrogen ions indicated that the rate was proportional to the partial pressure of carbon dioxide in the renal arterial blood (Pitts *et al.*, 1954). Later studies confirmed this, whether carbonic anhydrase was active or inhibited, and suggested that the partial pressure of carbon dioxide is the most important single factor determining the rate of seretion of hydrogen ions (cf. Robinson, 1975c). Increasing the partial pressure should improve the supply of carbon dioxide for generating hydrogen ions from carbonic acid or for removing hydroxyl ions left in secreting cells. It should also reduce the gradient against which hydrogen ions must be secreted by lowering intracellular pH.

Tubular secretion of hydrogen ions at a rate proportional to the partial pressure of carbon dioxide can provide a slow automatic renal compensation for disturbances of plasma pH of respiratory origin. Retention of carbon dioxide causes respiratory acidaemia; but the associated high partial pressure enhances renal tubular secretion of hydrogen ions. This makes the urine acid and adds more bicarbonate to the plasma, gradually increasing its concentration to match the elevated concentration of carbon dioxide and returning the buffer ratio towards normal. The renal response to respiratory alkalaemia resulting from loss of carbon dioxide through hyperventilation assists acclimatization at high altitudes. Increased ventilation provoked by the peripheral (carotid body) chemoreceptors' response to hypoxia lowers the partial pressure of carbon dioxide and makes the plasma and cerebrospinal fluid alkaline, so that both the central and the peripheral chemoreceptors at first oppose the hypoxic drive to increase respiratory exchange. The lowered partial pressure of carbon dioxide, however, reduces the rate of renal hydrogen ion secretion, so that some filtered bicarbonate escapes in alkaline urine, and the concentration of bicarbonate in the plasma is gradually reduced. Freshly formed cerebrospinal fluid also has a lower concentration of bicarbonate (Severinghaus *et al.*, 1963). After a week or so, when the concentrations of bicarbonate in the plasma and cerebrospinal fluid have fallen to match the low partial pressure of carbon dioxide, pH is lowered towards normal, the chemoreceptors no longer oppose the response to the low partial pressure of oxygen, and the release of oxygen from oxyhaemoglobin, which had been impaired while the plasma was alkaline, is restored. The 'lowered bicarbonate threshold' which underlies the kidneys' contribution to acclimatization may now be explained by diminished renal secretion of hydrogen ions. Instead of being puzzled by the excretion of bicarbonate despite its low concentration in the plasma, we attribute the low concentration to continued excretion of bicarbonate because too little hydrogen ion is secreted to complete its reabsorption. Finally, after renal compensation has occurred, hypercapnic states end up with an increased concentration of bicarbonate in the plasma, and hypocapnia is matched by a lowered concentration of bicarbonate, so that these disturbances might be better described as respiratory acidaemia and respiratory alkalaemia than as acidosis and alkalosis.

6.4.3 Some modifying factors

The neat picture of automatic renal compensation for altered concentrations of bicarbonate and of carbon dioxide in the plasma has to be modified to take account of a number of other factors, some homeostatic and some interfering. These include the volume of extracellular fluid (ECFV), the amount of potassium in the renal tubular cells, aldosterone, PTH and the effects of drugs which inhibit carbonic anhydrase.

A. The volume of extracellular fluid

The interactions of changes in the volume of extracellular fluid with the kidneys' control over acid–base balance are too complicated to deal with in detail here. Seldin & Rector (1972) set the stage admirably, and a brief review by Sabatini & Kurtzman (1984) highlighted most of the current problems.

Although many details of the underlying mechanisms are still undisclosed, it has been established that depletion of the ECFV stimulates the renal secretion of hydrogen ions and the addition of bicarbonate to the plasma, whereas expansion of ECFV inhibits these processes. Depletion of ECFV leading to the excretion of acid urine and the addition of excessive amounts of bicarbonate to the plasma plays an important role in the generation and maintenance of metabolic alkalosis, both experimentally and in clinical situations. This may include stimulation of the secretion of hydrogen ions into distal parts of the nephrons where little or no bicarbonate remains and the tubular fluid is most strongly acidified. Micropuncture techniques applied to single nephrons have shown that the rate of secretion by the proton pump in these distal regions depends importantly upon the gradient from cell to lumen (Al-Awqati, 1978). The much greater bulk of hydrogen ion secretion which subserves proximal reabsorption of filtered bicarbonate is less subject to this limitation, but appears to be particularly sensitive to expansion of the ECFV.

Classical attempts to define an upper limit to the rate of secretion of hydrogen ions, by measuring the reabsorption of bicarbonate as its concentration in the plasma was elevated, unwittingly revealed the inhibitory effects of increasing the ECFV. Maximal rates of about 25, 28 and 45 mmol per litre of glomerular filtrate in dogs, men and rats respectively, were a few mmol/l higher than plasma thresholds below which no bicarbonate appeared in the urine and above which it was excreted increasingly freely. But the large infusions used to increase the concentration of bicarbonate in the plasma for the clearance studies substantially expanded the ECFV, and if this expansion was avoided, by infusing smaller volumes of hypertonic bicarbonate solutions, no upper limit was found, even above 60 mmol/l. Stopped-flow microperfusion of single nephrons in rats also showed no upper limit at least up to 100 mmol/l (Malnic, 1974), though the inhibitory effect of expanding the ECFV was first directly demonstrated by micropuncture studies during free flow. Thus the apparent Tm values derived from the earlier clearances did not indicate true maximal rates of hydrogen ion secretion under normal conditions, but rates inhibited by expansion of ECFV.

After the classical studies by Pitts' group (Pitts & Lotspeich, 1946; Pitts *et al.*, 1949) showed that absolute rates of reabsorption of bicarbonate were proportional to the filtered load, it became usual to express rates in mmol per litre of glomerular filtrate instead of in mmol per unit time. If absolute rates of transport of bicarbonate were limited like those of glucose, the thresholds would be inversely proportional to GFR. Increases in filtration rate would then lead to acidosis from the loss of bicarbonate in the urine, and reductions in filtration rate would make the urine acid and establish a metabolic alkalosis by the addition of excessive amounts of bicarbonate to the plasma. It is therefore of practical importance as well as of academic interest that the rate of hydrogen ion secretion that determines the renal threshold for excretion of bicarbonate should be independent of GFR. A maximal rate per unit volume of glomerular filtrate protects the body's acid−base status from fluctuations in filtration rate. Moreover, since most of the filtered water is reabsorbed, and the reabsorbed fluid is added to the blood and becomes ECF, the amount of bicarbonate reabsorbed from each unit volume of glomerular filtrate determines the concentration of bicarbonate maintained in the plasma.

The rate of excretion of sodium is also largely protected from fluctuations in GFR, with more than 99% of filtered sodium normally reabsorbed as well as more than 99% of filtered bicarbonate. Larger volumes of glomerular filtrate deliver proportionately larger amounts of sodium as well as of bicarbonate into the proximal tubules; hence the proximal reabsorption of sodium helps to provide secreted hydrogen ions (through the hydrogen/sodium antiporter) to effect reabsorption of the bicarbonate. To the extent that the reabsorption of bicarbonate is thus secondary to reabsorption of sodium, it is not surprising that what has been called glomerulotubular balance (GTB) applies to bicarbonate as well as to sodium. Both ions are reabsorbed at rates proportional to GFR; rates per unit volume of glomerular filtrate of about 25 mmol/l for bicarbonate and 150 mmol/l for sodium serve to maintain the normal composition of the plasma.

Great expansion of the ECFV profoundly depresses reabsorption of sodium in the proximal tubules (cf. 'third factors' in Section 7.4.4). This could be expected to be accompanied by reductions in proximal hydrogen ion secretion and in the rate of reabsorption of bicarbonate. It is not, however, clear whether expansion of ECFV inhibits the secretion of hydrogen ions or reduces net reabsorption of bicarbonate by increasing leakage back into the tubule. Expansion of ECFV with saline could upset the balance of Starling forces across the peritubular membranes by increasing hydrostatic pressure or reducing oncotic pressure in the peritubular capillaries. Either of these would oppose the uptake of reabsorbed fluid into the capillaries, and increased pressure in the interstitial fluid could dilate the lateral intercellular spaces between proximal tubular cells and increase the permeability of the paracellular pathways available for diffusion back into the tubular lumen. Rector (1983) pointed out that since passive back-diffusion depends upon concentration or electrochemical gradients, the only ion whose back-diffusion would be much increased would be bicarbonate; the gradient for sodium is small and that for chloride would more likely favour reabsorption. Since bicarbonate in the tubular fluid would have to be accompanied by cations to preserve electro-neutrality, a reduced net reabsorption of bicarbonate resulting from back-diffusion might be added to the list of 'third factors' opposing the proximal tubular reabsorption of sodium!

B. Potassium stores, especially in renal tubular cells

Depletion of body potassium is well recognized clinically as a cause of metabolic alkalosis. Potassium lost from cells is only partially replaced by sodium, and the cells become more acid. Potassium-depleted renal tubular cells, with their lowered pH, tend to secrete more hydrogen ions into the tubular fluid for a given carbon dioxide tension. They make the urine more acid and add bicarbonate to the plasma, so that the overall intracellular acidosis is masked by alkalosis in the ECFs (cf. Robinson, 1975c). Alkalinity of the plasma tends to depress respiration, causing retention of carbon dioxide and an increase in its partial pressure which also promotes the addition of hydrogen ions to the urine and of bicarbonate to the plasma. Against this, the high concentration of bicarbonate in the plasma increases the filtered load; this might be expected to counteract the effect of the accelerated hydrogen ion secretion, but potassium depletion leads to vasoconstriction in the kidney which may reduce GFR enough to compensate for the increased concentration of bicarbonate. Moreover, many clinical examples of hypochloraemic alkalosis accompanying potassium depletion occur when sodium is also depleted, with a reduction in the ECFV which itself reduces GFR.

Potassium depletion is an important cause of alkalosis and, paradoxically, sustained alkalosis may be a cause of potassium depletion. Hydrogen ions displace potassium from cells, and, conversely, alkalosis tends to shift potassium from extracellular fluids into cells all over the body. But while most cells are bathed in extracellular fluid, the cells lining the renal tubules open on their apical sides onto the tubular lumen, which leads out of the body; and factors which tend to shift potassium into cells elsewhere tend to shift it through renal tubular cells into the urine.

C. Aldosterone

Aldosterone has long been known to promote the tubular reabsorption of sodium and the secretion of potassium and of hydrogen ions; when potassium is deficient it promotes acidification of the urine and the addition of new bicarbonate to the plasma. More recently it has been shown to stimulate both sodium-dependent secretion of hydrogen ions in cortical collecting tubules and sodium-independent hydrogen ion secretion in medullary collecting tubules (Sabatini & Kurtzman, 1984). A deficiency of ECFV, signalled by a reduction in the volume of blood, is a major physiological cause of increased secretion of aldosterone (Section 7.4.3); but the capacity to acidify the urine despite serious depletion of ECFV is impaired in Addison's disease when aldosterone is lacking. Aldosterone helps to promote the acidification of the urine and the addition of bicarbonate to the plasma in some clinical forms of metabolic alkalosis, especially with concomitant depletion of sodium and ECFV. Huth *et al.* (1959) did not observe the characteristic renal alkalosis during experimental human potassium deficiency unless adrenal steroids were administered. Moreover aldosterone, mobilized by a dwindling ECFV as large quantities of conjugate bases such as those of the ketoacids carry cations, mainly sodium, away in the urine, might contribute to the adaptive increase in excretion of titratable acid and ammonium during prolonged acidosis.

D. Parathormone

The hormone of the parathyroid glands affects and may partly control the kidneys' handling of hydrogen and bicarbonate ions. But the effects, which depend upon dose, duration and species, are often contradictory and poorly understood. For example, patients with spontaneous hyperparathyroidism usually have a metabolic acidosis, and acute dosing reduces renal generation of bicarbonate for 1 to 2 days; but prolonged (3 to 12 days) infusions of PTH produce metabolic alkalosis in human subjects, as they do in dogs and rats. The whole confusing picture was surveyed in an editorical review by Hulter (1985).

E. Carbonic anhydrase

The puzzling metabolic acidosis that complicated treatment with the early sulphonamides ceased to be mysterious when it was realized that the drugs inhibited carbonic anhydrase (Berliner & Orloff, 1956). More specific and effective inhibitors were used as tools for the investigation of renal function, and their ability to reduce the rate of secretion of hydrogen ions for a given partial pressure of carbon dioxide helped to elucidate the link between secretion of hydrogen ions into the urine and addition of bicarbonate to the plasma. They also began to be used as diuretics, because their inhibition of renal tubular secretion of hydrogen ions led to a loss of filtered bicarbonate in the urine. The removal of sodium and water with this bicarbonate in approximately isotonic urine offered the prospect of treating oedematous patients without assaulting their kidneys with toxic mercurial diuretics. But the diuretic action is transient and self-limiting. When the concentration of bicarbonate in the plasma becomes low enough for uncatalysed secretion of hydrogen ions to cope with the filtered load, no more bicarbonate is excreted; the diuresis and the removal of excess sodium also cease. The concentration of plasma bicarbonate is maintained at a new, lower level and the intensity of the acidosis does not increase further. As when the renal secretion of hydrogen ions is reduced by a lowered partial pressure of carbon dioxide at high altitudes, metabolic acids can be dealt with as before, but with a lower set point for the concentration of bicarbonate in the plasma.

6.5 CONCLUSION

If GFR, cellular potassium content and the ECFV are all normal, renal defence of acid–base balance in the extracellular compartment is adjusted automatically by the partial pressure of carbon dioxide and the concentration of bicarbonate in the plasma. Some other physiological factors modify this intrinsic regulation as illustrated in Fig. 6.3.

Overall control of acid–base balance depends upon centres in the brain. Alterations in carbon dioxide tension are all-pervading; they spread through cellular and transcellular fluids (of which the cerebrospinal fluid is particularly important) as well as the plasma and ECF. Concentrations of bicarbonate, in contrast, are private to each individual cell and transcellular fluid. Changes in carbon dioxide tension quickly alter pH in the same direction in all the fluids of the body, but the actual magnitudes of the changes following a common alteration in carbon dioxide tension depend upon the local concentrations of bicarbonate. The kidneys operate directly on the plasma but slow alterations they make in its concentration of bicarbonate affect plasma pH and so may lead to alterations in carbon dioxide tension which affect pH in the cells and in the cerebrospinal fluid. If the partial pressure of carbon dioxide determines the concentration of bicarbonate in each cell and transcellular fluid as it does (via renal tubular hydrogen ion secretion) in the plasma, it can serve as an integrating factor for the control of pH throughout the body. Alterations in carbon dioxide tension should lead to rapid changes in pH in all compartments, followed, if the new levels are sustained, by slower compensating changes in the local concentrations of bicarbonate.

Until these local, private adjustments in concentration of bicarbonate have been made, pH changes in the cells and in the cerebrospinal fluid tend to be opposite in direction to pH changes in the plasma. An increased concentration of bicarbonate which raises pH in the plasma will affect the peripheral chemoreceptors and slow respiratory exchange, leading to retention of carbon dioxide which will tend to make the cells more acid. This initial tendency will, however, be resisted, because the increased partial pressure of carbon dioxide will also make the cerebrospinal fluid more acid and stimulate respiration through the central chemoreceptors. The partial pressure of carbon dioxide, which controls the kidneys and may also ultimately set the concentrations of

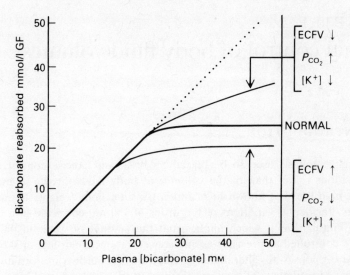

Fig. 6.3 Effects of extracellular fluid volume (ECFV), carbon dioxide tension and plasma potassium concentration upon the rate of bicarbonate reabsorption (= renal tubular hydrogen ion secretion). (Composite impression of three diagrams in Batlle & Kurtzman, 1985.)

bicarbonate in all the fluids of the body, depends upon the rate of respiratory exchange called by neurones in the respiratory centres. If their rate of discharge is determined by the effect of their own intracellular pH on the state of ionization of imidazole groups, pH throughout the body will be controlled by the ionization of imidazole groups in a few strategically placed cells! For a fuller discussion of the manner in which the central chemoreceptors which monitor the pH of the cerebrospinal fluid might act on behalf of the cells to stabilize their pH, while the peripheral chemoreceptors primarily guard the body's supplies of oxygen and the bland alkalinity of the ECFs, see Robinson (1978).

CHAPTER 7
Renal control of body fluid volumes

7.1 INTRODUCTION

Although emphasis used to be placed on brisk and precise control of the compositions rather than of the volumes of body fluids, grown animals including man are well known to maintain constant body weights for months or years. Incidental variations of the order of 1% are corrected in a day or two (Elkinton, 1960), which implies that the amount of water in the body must be controlled as precisely as any concentration, albeit less briskly. The quickest responses to alterations in intensive properties are variations in pulmonary ventilation following alterations in pH or the partial pressure of carbon dioxide; these occur in minutes. Water diuresis in response to a load of water is established in less than an hour. The removal of water corrects volume as well as concentration, but this should probably be regarded as a typically brisk response to disturbance of an intensive property (osmolality) rather than as a rapid response to change in an extensive property (volume). It takes several days to eliminate excess water and salt ingested as an isotonic saline solution.

So long as the amount of solute in the body is unaltered, adjustments of the gain or loss of water that keep osmolality constant also keep the total amount of water in the body (TBW) constant by matching the amount of water to the amount of solute. The expression

$$TBW = (Total\ body\ solute)/osmolality$$

strictly yields the amount of body water in kilograms; but with dilute aqueous solutions like the body fluids the common practice of stating the result in litres involves a negligible error. A typical individual weighing 70 kg, whose body contains 12.6 osmoles of solute and whose kidneys set the osmolality to 300 mosm, will have a total of $12.6 \div 0.3 = 42$ litres of body water.

The chemical anatomy of the body fluids, together with the capacity to handle water and solutes independently, enables the kidneys to regulate the distribution of water between the major compartments as well as the total amount in the body. The body water is not a single, homogeneous solution that fills two thirds of a curiously shaped skin bag. The ICF and ECF are both electrolyte solutions, their principal cations being potassium in the cells and sodium outside the cells. The accompanying anions in the ICF are mostly organic, especially phosphoric esters, while the anions of the ECF are almost all inorganic, mostly chloride and bicarbonate. Sodium chloride and sodium bicarbonate together contribute about 95% of the osmolality of the ECF, and the concentrations of the remaining solutes are well controlled. Consequently, the osmolality maintained throughout the body fixes the concentration of sodium in the ECFs, and their combined volume is determined by the amount of sodium they contain. It follows that the retention of enough water to make osmolality normal is not sufficient in itself to preserve the normal ECFV; it leads to expansion of the ECFV (oedema) if excessive amounts of salt are retained, and to gross depletion of the ECFV if large amounts of salt are lost in intestinal fluid (e.g. diarrhoea, vomiting, aspiration) or by copious sweating. But so long as intake is greater than extrarenal losses, the kidneys can control the amount of salt in the body. This control over the amount as well as of the concentration of extracellular solute involves them more directly in regulating the volume of extracellular than of intracellular fluid. By adjusting the excretion of water and fixing osmolality they stabilize the volume of the cells; at the same they set the stage for regulating the ECFV by controlling the excretion of salt.

After a brief outline of some other factors involved in regulating the TBW, and a little about the kidneys' part in controlling the volume of intracellular fluid, the remainder of this chapter will be devoted to a more detailed consideration of the ways in which renal excretion of sodium is adjusted to regulate the ECFV.

7.2 THE KIDNEYS AND THE TOTAL VOLUME OF BODY WATER

Maintenance of a normal amount of body water is achieved by balancing voluntary intake plus metabolic production (about 0.3 l/day in man) against losses. Daily voluntary intake includes about a litre of water in 'solid' food; additional amounts consumed in beverages depend upon habitual drinking patterns, augmented by thirst as a reminder in case too little is ingested. Absorption of water from the intestinal tract is controlled only by the amount placed in it. The kidneys (subject to restrictions outlined in Section 5.5.3) can control urinary output over and above extrarenal losses.

Some losses of water from the body are inevitable. Evaporation removes about 500 ml of water daily from the surface of the skin, which has to be kept moist to remain flexible. The lining of the pulmonary alveoli has to be moist to permit exchanges of oxygen and carbon dioxide in solution, and the expired air is saturated with water vapour at the temperature of the respiratory passages no matter how dry the inspired air may be. A person at rest at sea level loses about 500 ml/day in expired air; the loss increases in proportion when high altitude, or exercise, or both, require greater rates of ventilation. A further 500 ml has to be lost every day as a vehicle for solutes excreted in the urine (Section 5.5.3), even when healthy kidneys are induced by ADH to conserve water. These minimal losses may be greatly exceeded when sweat is secreted in response to rising body temperature. Faecal losses are normally small, and approximately isotonic with body fluids. But insensible losses of pure water as vapour and the secretion of hypotonic sweat remove water in excess of solute, and increase the osmolality of the body fluids. The kidneys alone cannot prevent this, but increasing osmolality evokes thirst as well as the secretion of ADH to promote retention of water in the body.

If intake plus production exceeds losses, the body fluids are expanded and diluted; thirst is absent and the secretion of ADH is reduced or suppressed until water diuresis has removed the surplus water. When intake and production fail to match inevitable losses, the body fluids shrink; and osmolality increases if more water is lost than would be needed to make an isotonic solution of any solute lost. Thirst is evoked, and secretion of ADH encourages the kidneys to retain ingested water. Section 5.5.3 dealt only with the osmotic stimulus to secrete ADH. A more complete list of factors increasing the secretion of ADH includes some that are related to volume regardless of osmolality (Table 7.1). Moreover, the hypothalamic neurone pools concerned with thirst overlap those controlling the release of ADH, and the factors which increase thirst also stimulate the release of ADH.

Table 7.1 Factors evoking thirst and secretion of ADH

	Factor	Receptors	Comment
1	Blood osmolality +	Hypothalamic osmoreceptor in or around supraoptic nucleus	Loss of pure water would increase both osmolality and cerebrospinal fluid [NaCl]
2	[NaCl] in cerebrospinal fluid +	Lining of third ventricle	? auxiliary osmoreceptors
3	Angiotensin II	Not applicable: see text	Formed in blood when renin is released from kidney
4	Arterial BP −	Carotid sinus baroreceptors	Reduced rate of discharge
5	Central venous volume −	Stretch receptors in walls of heart (volume receptors)	Reduced rate of discharge

1, 2 The hypothalamic osmoreceptors were postulated by Verney (1947) on the basis of a lifetime of meticulous experimentation on dogs and cats. Andersson (1978) who worked exclusively with goats, and on drinking rather than on urinary excretion, proposed that the primary receptors are situated in the ependymal lining of the third cerebral ventricles and are stimulated by an increased concentration of sodium chloride in the cerebrospinal fluid rather than by increased osmolality. But this cannot by itself account for drinking by sheep (McKinley et al., 1978); and Schrier et al. (1979) argued against it being primary factor controlling the secretion of ADH (cf. 5.5.3).

Both receptors might exist and reinforce one another; the loss of water without solute would increase both the osmolality of the blood and the concentration of sodium chloride in the cerebrospinal fluid, causing Andersson's receptor to function as an auxiliary osmoreceptor. Robertson (1984) considered that both thirst and the release of ADH are triggered by neurones close to each other and to the hypothalamic neurosecretory cells; that effective osmotic pressure is the most important stimulus; and that secretion of ADH has a lower threshold — occurring when plasma osmolality exceeds 280 mosm, while over 290 mosm is required to elicit thirst. Hence the kidneys should begin conserving supplies of body water before thirst calls for increased input. This would minimize the daily turnover of water, and would also be in line with Fitzsimons' (1976) view that drinking is normally in excess of immediate needs and related to anticipated future requirements, leaving thirst in reserve to be called on in emergencies. Thompson *et al.* (1986), however, were not convinced that the thresholds differ appreciably.

3 Renin released from the renal juxtaglomerular apparatus splits off the decapeptide, angiotensin I (AT I) from angiotensinogen in the plasma, and a converting enzyme which is most abundant in the lungs releases the octapeptide AT II from AT I. Angiotensin II stimulates the secretion of aldosterone by the zona glomerulosa of the suprarenal glands, and this may be its most important action. The stimuli which cause renin to be released from the kidney will be discussed later (7.4.3) in relation to the role of aldosterone in controlling the renal excretion of sodium; they are mostly activated by reductions in the volume of circulating blood. Angiotensin II is also a powerful vasoconstrictor, and, when injected into the ventricular cerebrospinal fluid, it augments thirst and stimulates the secretion of ADH. The antidiuretic hormone, like AT II, is a powerful vasoconstrictor which may be directly involved in the homeostasis of blood pressure (Rascher, 1985; cf. Bennett & Gardner, 1986). But since blood pressure cannot be sustained without a sufficient volume in the vessels, it is appropriate that AT II and ADH should help to maintain the volume in the vessels as well as the tension in their walls.

4 The rate of discharge from the carotid sinus and aortic baroreceptors reflexly controls sympathetic tone. The reflex response to reduced discharge when arterial pressure falls includes increased activity of vasoconstrictor nerves and of the renal sympathetic nerves which mediate secretion of renin. This would lead indirectly to thirst and increase secretion of ADH; Schrier *et al.* (1979) reviewed evidence that the baroreceptors modulate the release of ADH directly. Increased discharge inhibits it, while reduced discharge, or denervation of the baroreceptors, increases the output of ADH. The extreme thirst of victims of trauma whose blood pressure is low is well known.

5 About three quarters of the blood is in the venous system and the heart; and stretch receptors on the low-pressure side of the circulation — in the walls of the large intrathoracic veins and the chambers of the heart, might be expected to monitor changes in volume. Observations that while systemic

arterial pressure was maintained following small losses of blood, the circulating concentration of ADH increased in parallel with tone in resistance
vessels and a decline in rate of discharge from the cardiac receptors, suggested
that the low pressure receptors responded to the falling blood volume. They
were probably more important modulators of ADH release than the arterial
baroreceptors, whose rate of discharge was reduced by larger losses of blood
that caused arterial pressure to fall (Gauer & Henry, 1963). The role of the
cardiac receptors will be discussed further in Section 7.4 in relation to the
control of the excretion of sodium. It has been confirmed that they mediate
effects of changing volume on secretion of arginine vasopressin (AVP) in
dogs; but the sino-aortic baroreceptors appear to be more important in
monkeys and men (Menninger, 1985). See also the critical discussion by
Goetz et al. (1975).

The development of a sufficiently sensitive radioimmunoassay to measure
the concentrations of ADH in human plasma under physiological conditions
made it possible to demonstrate the effects of signals derived from alterations
in blood volume and blood pressure impinging on the primarily osmoregulatory
mechanism. The solid line in Fig. 7.1, based upon a figure published by
Robertson et al. (1976) shows the relation between plasma ADH concentration
and osmolality when both blood pressure and blood volume are normal. The
dotted lines show how increased blood pressure and blood volume reduce the
response of plasma ADH concentration to rising osmolality, and how reductions in the pressure or volume of blood lead to greater concentrations of
ADH in the plasma even when osmolality is normal. This one diagram shows
in man the combined effects of the principal osmotic and nonosmotic stimuli
for secretion of ADH and reveals effects of deficient volume independent of
associated changes in osmolality.

The osmotic and volume-related factors in Table 7.1 and Fig. 7.1 may be
supposed to guard the body's water balance from day to day. But other
factors interact with these, and may override them in the short term. Blair-
West et al. (1985) kept sheep on a low intake of water for a week before
rehydrating them in three ways — allowing them to drink water, or 0.9%
sodium chloride solution, or supplying water through a stomach tube. The
amount of water or of saline ingested voluntarily was equivalent to the deficit
in body weight. The osmolality of the plasma increased slowly after the
saline, and decreased slowly after intake of water. But after all three treatments the concentration of AVP in the plasma fell very rapidly from about
15 to 5 pg/ml, before the osmolality had time to change. Gebruers et al.
(1985) pointed out that hypotonic diuresis after drinking isotonic saline solutions had been known in human subjects since 1916, and Borst (1954)
reported that the response to drinking 1.5 litres of a model ECF might begin
with a typical water diuresis that continued for several hours, even though the
concentration of sodium in the plasma was rising. Gebruers' human subjects
drank 0.5 to 2 litres of water, or isotonic saline, or isotonic mannitol (this

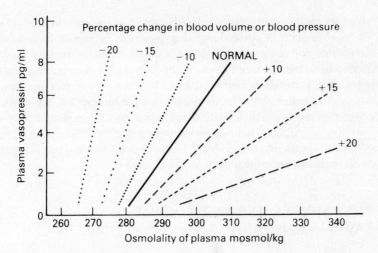

Fig. 7.1 The effects of alterations in blood volume and blood pressure upon the response of plasma vasopressin concentration to osmolality. (Based on a scheme by Robertson *et al.*, 1976.)

solute was not absorbed and always caused diarrhoea). Antidiuretic hormone was not assayed in the plasma, but there was always a typical water diuresis during the first hour, with approximately the same increase in volume and decrease in osmolality of the urine. Only after the mannitol solution had been ingested did the volume of the urine decline and its osmolality increase during the second hour. Water diuresis following rapid intravenous infusions of isotonic saline in recumbent, well-hydrated human subjects (Strauss *et al.*, 1951) might be attributed to expansion of the volume of plasma or ECF; but little expansion can have occurred in the first hour of Gebruers' experiments, and ECFV was probably contracting after the mannitol. In later experiments (Cotter *et al.*, 1986) plasma volume did not expand, but plasma AVP fell after drinking the isotonic mannitol. The initial diuresis might have been associated with the act of swallowing, or triggered by liquid passing some receptor high in the alimentary tract. The urinary response was much smaller if the isotonic solutions were introduced through a nasogastric tube, and the authors pointed out that in the classical experiments of Verney's group, which set the pattern of much subsequent thinking, fluid loads were always given by stomach tube, so that no complications associated with swallowing could arise.

Some items from an annotated list of a dozen miscellaneous factors which affect the release of ADH in ways which do not always appear to subserve homeostasis (Robinson, 1954) may be briefly recapitulated here. Hypnosis, cold and alcohol inhibit the release of ADH; conditioned reflexes and emotional disturbances may inhibit or stimulate. Standing usually stimulates the release of ADH, and lying down inhibits it; but this postural effect is overridden by sleep. Most anaesthetics also increase the secretion of ADH, and Valtin *et al.* (1982) pointed out that their effects persist so long that results reported for conscious or 'awake' animals following surgery may be complicated by effects of anaesthesia. If the supraoptico-hypophyseal tract is a final common path which can be activated by impulses converging from a diversity of sites within the nervous system, a large number of factors which need not be related to homeostatic mechanisms may be expected to affect the secretion of ADH. Then, after disturbing factors have exerted their effects, the receptors listed in Table 7.1 can respond to what has happened and direct such further adjustments as are required.

7.3 THE KIDNEYS AND THE VOLUME OF INTRACELLULAR FLUID

Animal cells have nonrigid membranes, but their volumes are well controlled. Swelling, even if it does not break essential contacts, moves intracellular structures apart and increases the distances that metabolites must traverse by diffusion to sustain metabolic sequences. The principal solutes in the cells are potassium salts of organic acids. Potassium is taken into the cells by the ion pumps that extrude sodium, using energy derived from metabolism and applied in the form of ATP. The pattern of accompanying anions also depends upon metabolic processes, so that the solute content of each cell is determined by its own on-going metabolic activity. So long as the cells and the ECF remain in osmotic equilibrium, the common osmolality maintained throughout the body fluids then determines how much water accompanies the solutes inside the cells as well as outside them. The total amount of intracellular solute that ultimately determines the volume of each cell must depend upon genetic factors. There usually seems to be enough to sustain a volume of about $100\,\mu m^3$ for each pg of DNA; but just how this comes about is not known (Kregenow, 1977). For any given solute content the cells will swell if extracellular osmolality falls and will shrink if it rises. Hence the kidneys' primary contribution to regulating the total volume of intracellular fluid is made by setting the osmolality within all the body fluids. As stated in Section 5.5.3, renal osmoregulation acts essentially to stabilize the volume of the cells. The kidneys also conserve potassium for the cells to take up, or excrete potassium which the cells reject.

The cells can, however, alter their solute content to restore normal volume when alterations in osmolality are not corrected. Cells in isolated tissues placed in hypotonic solutions first swell and then slowly regain their normal volume by allowing potassium to escape without being replaced by sodium (Macknight & Leaf, 1977). Avoidance of swelling is particularly important for the brain which is enclosed within the rigid bony cranium so that swelling of the cells leaves less room for ECFs including blood, and may dangerously

impair the circulation. In some chronic illnesses the concentration of intracellular potassium is low, and so are the concentration of extracellular sodium
and the osmolality set by the thirst–ADH mechanism. These have been
called 'tired cell syndromes'; the primary cause of the low osmolality throughout the body might be a failure of the osmoreceptor cells to maintain their
own normal content of potassium, causing them to shrink and release ADH
at abnormally low values of osmolality (Elkinton, 1956). But there are many
other possible causes of what has been called 'inappropriate secretion of
ADH' (Martinez-Maldonado, 1980).

Measures to prevent shrinking are required when osmolality increases, and
cells in the brain may increase their solute contents by the addition of amino
acids and non-electrolytes, rather than by increasing concentrations of the
major inorganic cations, which might impair neural function (Pollock &
Arieff, 1980). Mammals cannot live with increments of systemic osmolality
much greater than 100 mosm; but when their kidneys are producing maximally
concentrated urine, cells in the inner medulla are subjected to increments
approaching 1000 mosm. Erythrocytes in the vasa recta shrink greatly, and
presumably increase their internal concentrations of electrolytes to match the
surroundings; but the epithelial cells would be expected to be less tolerant of
shrinkage, and of high concentrations of electrolytes which would damage
their enzymes. The cells of osmotically conforming marine animals avoid
shrinkage in osmolalities comparable with those attained in the renal medulla
by maintaining large intracellular concentrations of organic osmolytes such
as polyhydric alcohols, amino acids and their derivatives, and urea — accompanied by methylamines which neutralize its denaturant effect on proteins
(Yancey et al., 1982). Inner medullary cells in kidneys producing concentrated
urine probably employ the same expedient, and so avoid shrinking without
risking large increments in the intracellular concentration of electrolytes.
Cultured papillary epithelial cells from rabbits synthesized and accumulated
large concentrations of sorbitol after adaptation to growth in hypertonic
media; cells from other species accumulated betaine, glycerophosphoryl
choline and inositol (Bagnasco et al., 1986). Substantial concentrations of
these compounds have also been found in renal inner medullary tissue of rats,
rabbits and dogs (Balaban & Burg, 1987).

7.4 THE KIDNEYS AND THE VOLUME OF EXTRACELLULAR FLUID

7.4.1 Introduction: the excretion of sodium

Having fixed the osmolality (and hence the concentration of sodium) in the
sodium-rich ECF by controlling the excretion of water, the kidneys can
regulate the volume of ECF by controlling the excretion of sodium. Provided
intake exceeds losses by other routes, the kidneys control the body's sodium

balance, and most of the rapidly variable portion of the body's sodium is in solution in the ECF.

Chemical analyses of a few whole corpses suggested that adult human bodies contain between 4000 and 5000 mmol of sodium; but dilution of radioactively labelled sodium in living subjects yielded substantially smaller values, around 40 mmol/kg of body weight, for sodium exchangeable with the marker in up to 24 hours (Edelman & Leibman, 1959; Forbes, 1962). Whole-body counting after neutron activation in 80 healthy subjects aged between 30 and 90 gave intermediate results, averaging between 43 mmol/kg for women and 48 mmol/kg for men (Ellis *et al.*, 1976). The discrepancy between this estimate and the older chemical analyses is unexplained, but there seems no doubt that some sodium in the bone mineral is too far from the surface of the crystallites to exchange with markers in the plasma. The exchangeable fraction includes sodium on the surfaces of bone crystallites, about 100 mmol in cells, and about 2500 mmol in solution in the ECF, which is more rapidly variable in amount than the sodium in the skeleton and the cells, and may be characterized as 'mobile' sodium. Rapid variations in sodium balance represent changes in the amount of mobile sodium, and reflect changes in the volume of ECF. If osmoregulation sets the concentration of sodium in the plasma at 150 mM, there will be about 140 mmol in a litre of ultrafiltrate, and the volume of ECF will be 1 litre for each 140 mmol of mobile sodium.

The volume of ECF required to accommodate 2500 mmol of mobile sodium at 140 mmol/l is 18 litres. The figure of 15 litres, copied from textbook to textbook for many years, rests on early measurements of the volume of distribution of inulin, which, with a molecular weight of 5000 is too large to penetrate into the interstices of dense connective tissues like cartilage, or enter transcellular fluids like the cerebrospinal, ocular and synovial fluids which are separated from the main mass of ECF by complete layers of cells. Its volume of distribution therefore underestimates the volume of ECF and overestimates the ICFV calculated by subtracting the ECFV from the TBW (Elkinton & Danowski, 1955; Edelman & Leibman, 1959).

A realistic rough distribution for a 70 kg man would be, in litres: TBW, 42, made up of ICF, 23; ECF, 18; and transcellular fluids, 1. ECF comprises 3 in plasma; 12 in interstitial fluid and lymph (including 3 in bone); and 3 in dense connective tissues not penetrated by inulin.

Ordinary human diets supply between 100 and 200 mmol of sodium each day. A litre of lost intestinal fluid would remove about 150 mmol and a litre of sweat would remove about 50 mmol. In the absence of intestinal losses and copious sweating, the kidneys' capacity to vary the daily rate of urinary excretion between a few mmol and several hundred mmol enables them to hold the balance with a wide margin of safety. Homer Smith's remark (1937) that the composition of the internal environment depends not so much on what the mouth takes in as upon what the kidneys keep applies particularly well to sodium.

The central role of the kidneys in regulating the distribution as well as the total amount of water in the body can be summarized very briefly in a simple diagram:

$$\pm \text{ EXCR OF WATER} \rightarrow \text{EC OP} \quad \begin{array}{l} \nearrow \text{ICOP} \rightarrow \text{ICFV} \approx \text{K content} \\ \\ \searrow \text{EC [Na]} \\ \qquad \searrow \rightarrow \text{ECFV} \approx \text{Na content} \end{array}$$

$$\text{(ADH)}$$

$$\pm \text{ EXCR OF Na} \rightarrow \text{Na content} \underline{\hspace{3cm}}$$

$$\text{(X?)}$$

The rate of excretion of water is rather simply controlled by ADH; but there is no corresponding single factor which can account for alterations in the rate of excretion of sodium. A number of factors conspire to increase the rate of excretion when the volume of blood or of ECF is increased, and to reduce excretion and promote retention of sodium in the body when it is in short supply or when the volume of blood or of ECF is diminished. Evidence (Robinson, 1954) that loss of blood through trauma; or redistribution of blood away from the central veins, lungs and heart, by changed posture, by trapping it in the limbs behind tourniquets; or interference with venous return by abdominal compression or obstruction of the vena cava, were all followed by retention of sodium, while manoeuvres directed to increasing the central, intrathoracic volume of blood were followed by increased rates of excretion of sodium, need not be repeated here in detail. These alterations in the rate of excretion of sodium, together with the dramatic increase when the ECFV is expanded with saline, and the virtual disappearance of sodium from the urine during states of deficiency, are appropriate in direction to keep the ECFV normal. It remains to consider how they are brought about.

The rate of excretion of sodium, which is easily measured as $V \times [\text{Na}]_U$, is determined by the difference between the filtered load and the rate of reabsorption of sodium by the tubules. The filtered load, $\text{GFR} \times [\text{Na}]_P$, is proportional both to the rate of glomerular filtration and to the concentration of sodium in the plasma. Alterations in plasma concentration are usually ignored, for this is taken to be held constant by osmoregulatory mechanisms; but if these allow variations of $\pm 1\%$ in osmolality, variations of the same order in $[\text{Na}]_P$ may occur. However, rapid changes in GFR are more to be expected than rapid changes in the concentration of sodium in the plasma.

The sodium in the urine is a small unreabsorbed residue from the much larger amount delivered into the tubules by glomerular filtration. Under ordinary conditions the filtered load of sodium is about 25 000 mmol/day, and the rate of excretion is around 100 mmol/day, so that the tubules reabsorb

24 900 mmol/day. Hence if GFR increased by 0.4% to 25 100 and tubular reabsorption did not alter, the rate of excretion would be doubled. Likewise an increase of 0.4% in the rate of reabsorption with no alteration in GFR would reduce the rate of excretion of sodium to zero. From this it follows that:

1 The rate of excretion of sodium is exquisitely sensitive to alterations in either GFR or tubular reabsorption.

2 The rate of excretion, all other things being equal, should be equally sensitive to variations in the concentration of sodium in the plasma.

3 All ordinary alterations in the rate of excretion of sodium could be produced by alterations in GFR or in tubular reabsorption (the other being assumed constant) that would fall within limits of experimental error and would therefore be extremely difficult to demonstrate. Hence it is not surprising that the literature contains contradictions and controversial interpretations. Rates of tubular reabsorption can only be determined by subtracting measured rates of excretion from estimates of filtered load, and are therefore no more accurate than the measurements of GFR that are used to calculate the filtered loads.

4 The rate of reabsorption of sodium is nearly always approximately equal to the filtered load. When the difference is not significant statistically, the sodium in the urine proclaims its physiological significance. Reductions in GFR must be accompanied by smaller rates of reabsorption, if only because there is no more sodium to reabsorb; and increases in filtered load are usually matched by increased reabsorption. This close correspondence between filtered load and rate of reabsorption is referred to as 'glomerulotubular balance' (GTB). Its possible mechanisms have been intensively investigated (Gertz & Boylan, 1973), and some of them will be mentioned briefly. Routine GTB is clearly important for the maintenance of sodium balance and the ECFV, which would otherwise tend to fluctuate with incidental alterations in GFR. It is also important that GTB is not invariable; it can be overridden or adjusted to permit fine control of the rate of excretion of sodium.

If we continue to ignore the concentration of sodium in the plasma, which might be called the 'zeroth factor' in sodium excretion, the first and second factors are readily identified as GFR and tubular reabsorption. The importance attached to these two factors has tended to vary from time to time. When GFR was accepted as a physiological constant, variations in the excretion of sodium were attributed to alterations in tubular reabsorption. Then, after aldosterone had been identified and its action established, the second factor was accepted as the control of distal tubular reabsorption by aldosterone and as being of paramount importance. But the effect of aldosterone is delayed about an hour; and with the realization that the glomerular circulation is subject to reflexes arising in the cardiovascular system, the first factor — variations in GFR — appeared as a more immediate mechanism for bringing about rapid adjustments in sodium excretion. At all events it is now recognized that neither GFR nor tubular reabsorption is constant, and that both factors are adjusted to regulate the excretion of sodium.

The demonstration that large infusions which expand the ECFV produced dramatic effects, which could not be explained by changes in GFR or by changes in tubular reabsorption mediated by aldosterone, led to the recognition that there must be another, so-called 'third factor', capable of overriding GTB, at least in emergency. The hunt for possible mechanisms has suggested that there may be more than one 'third factor'. The three chief factors and their interaction may now be sketched in a little more detail.

7.4.2 The first factor: glomerular filtration rate

The rate of glomerular filtration is reduced when sympathetic tone is increased reflexly to maintain systemic arterial blood pressure (Section 3.3.4.3A). This occurs with upright postures and exercise, and also when blood is lost or when the volumes of plasma and ECF are reduced because of dehydration or deficiencies of sodium. The sensitivity of glomerular filtration to vasomotor nerve impulses would apparently permit homeostatic control of the excretion of sodium to begin very rapidly and very early in the nephron. Although large increases in GFR were observed in rather heroic experiments involving massive infusions of saline in dogs, this did not establish that far smaller loads or deficiencies in other animals including man would lead to proportional alterations in GFR. Renal denervation when tone is already minimal does not increase GFR (Section 3.3.4.2A), and moderate increases in sympathetic constrictor tone act preferentially on the efferent glomerular arterioles, and reduce RPF with little effect on GFR. Moreover, reflexes arising from the carotid baroreceptors seem less effective than emotional stresses, which are not associated with disturbances of volume (Section 3.3.5). Karim et al. (1984) reported reductions of about 40% in RBF and 70% in GFR in dogs when pressure in an isolated, perfused carotid sinus was lowered from about 180 to 60 mmHg. But the magnitudes of the changes were outside the physiological range, and the renal vasoconstriction (which was abolished by dividing or tying the renal sympathetic nerves) appeared to affect the afferent more than the efferent glomerular arterioles. Reflexes from atrial receptors, which might be specifically concerned with monitoring plasma volume, have not been proved to produce any consistent effect on GFR (Linden & Kappagoda, 1982; Skorecki & Brenner, 1981).

There is nevertheless evidence that GFR varies in parallel with moderate changes in ECFV following infusions. For example, increases of up to 30% in the volume of plasma or ECF after slow infusions of saline in rats, and decreases of 13% after infusions of polyethylene glycol, were accompanied by comparable percentage alterations in whole-kidney GFR and in SNGFR measured by micropuncture methods; and the rate of excretion of sodium varied in parallel with GFR (Brenner & Berliner, 1969). O'Connor &

Summerill (1979) gave dogs influsions of saline which increased ECFV up to 9% and observed increases in GFR up to 12%. When they compared their results with others in the literature, including some for sodium depleted human subjects with low GFR and elevated concentrations of plasma protein, it appeared that GFR usually increased about 2% for each fall of 1 g/l in the concentration of protein in the plasma. A wider comparison had led O'Connor (1977) to conclude that the effects of smaller and larger infusions could all be fitted to this same linear relation. Small alterations in plasma volume should therefore be accompanied by homeostatically appropriate changes in GFR, though these would usually be too small to measure. Although O'Connor believed that such changes alone were sufficient to control the excretion of sodium to regulate ECFV, at least in dogs, he admitted that human diurnal variations of 15% in GFR, a magnitude that could be produced by 1 to 2 litres of saline, occur without a change in concentration of plasma protein, and indeed without any other known cause.

Other reviewers have been more sceptical. Both Earley & Daugherty (1969) and Klahr & Slatopolski (1973) emphasized that GTB (see Section 3.3.5.4) is so effective that even quite large alterations in GFR may occur with only minimal changes in excretion of sodium. The adjustments that maintain GTB are so brisk (they act in minutes or even seconds) that they must depend upon intrarenal mechanisms. Thus compensation was as complete in less than 1 minute as in over 5 minutes (Brenner et al., 1968), which would exclude any humoral or neurohumoral loop involving aldosterone. Knox & Haas (1982) concluded that although GFR and SNGFR increase, this is not the chief cause of the faster excretion of sodium after volume expansion; the excretion of sodium can be accelerated even if an increase in GFR is prevented. Skorecki & Brenner (1981) recognized that GFR varied with ECFV, but did not accept alterations in GFR or redistribution of blood flow between superficial and deeper nephrons as important regulators of the excretion of sodium. There is often little change in excretion of sodium when GFR increases from causes other than expansion of ECF, which suggests that control of the rate of excretion of sodium is largely postglomerular. De Wardener (1978) regarded GFR as relatively unimportant compared with variations in reabsorption, especially from the collecting ducts.

It was proposed in Section 3.3.5.4 that reflexes which affect the kidneys' share of the cardiac output incidentally affect GFR, but do not primarily control it. It is immaterial that changes in GFR do not directly determine the excretion of sodium, because by no means all changes in GFR result from disturbances of the volume of plasma or of ECF as such. Physical activities and postural changes from recumbency to standing, which reduce GFR reflexly, are not initially accompanied by reductions in the volume of blood or of ECF. Reflexes concerned with homeostasis of pressure and distribution of blood must deliver a flickering barrage of impulses that cause the rate of glomerular filtration to fluctuate continually. Since a change of 0.4% in GFR lasting 24 hours would alter the rate of excretion of sodium by 100% if there were no change in reabsorption, a change of 0.4% lasting 1 hour could alter the day's output of sodium by 100/24 or about 4%. Reductions in GFR of 4% for an hour's walking or of 20% during half an hour's jogging would reduce the day's output of sodium by 40% and by 100% respectively if GTB did not prevent this. However, many changes in GFR which are thus largely prevented from dominating the excretion of sodium would not be appropriate for volume homeostasis. Walking and jogging mimic loss of blood in so far as they reduce the volume in the large intrathoracic veins and the heart. But changes in GFR with exercise cannot be regarded as primarily volume-homeostatic in the same sense as the similar changes that accompany haem-orrhage or reductions in the volume of ECF and plasma.

The somewhat disappointing conclusion seems to be that the 'first factor' controlling the excretion of sodium is first in time, and also in location in the nephron, but not foremost in importance for preventing or correcting dis-turbances in the ECFV. How much filtered sodium shall remain to be excreted is determined downstream.

7.4.3 The second factor: tubular reabsorption and aldosterone

The rate of reabsorption by the renal tubules determines how much of the filtered sodium shall be excreted, and the first established regulator of this rate is the salt-retaining hormone, aldosterone, secreted by cells in the zona glomerulosa of the adrenal cortex. The most important known factor which stimulates these cells to secrete is angiotensin II, normally generated in the plasma by renin released from the kidney. The modified arteriolar smooth muscle cells which synthesize and release renin are part of the kidney's vascular organ (Section 1.3), and secretion of renin into the renal venous blood can be increased reflexly from the cardiovascular system through the renal sympathetic nerves. But although renin can be released reflexly as quickly as glomerular filtration can be controlled, and the adrenal cortical cells respond in minutes to circulating angiotensin II, the humoral control of tubular reabsorption by aldosterone is subject to a long delay, because aldosterone takes up to an hour to exert its characteristic action in the distal nephron. This hormonal control therefore acts too slowly to play a part in GTB, but aldosterone is important because it can modify GTB and effect long-term adjustments in the proportion of filtered sodium that is reabsorbed.

The suprarenal glands were believed to produce salt-retaining hormones long before aldosterone was known. Homer Smith (1957) remarked in a memorable review that, after approximately 14 598 papers on the suprarenal glands had been published in 1951, 1952 and 1953, 'we still do not know anything much about them except that they somehow promote the tubular reabsorption of some fraction of the filtered sodium and that, in their absence, as Loeb and his colleagues showed many years ago,' (early in the 1930s) 'excessive loss of sodium in the urine leads to depletion of the extracellular fluid'. There were early indications that only a small fraction of the filtered sodium was involved. Patients with Addison's disease who lacked adrenal cortical function and suffered chronic depletion of sodium and ECFV could be kept in sodium balance by the daily addition of a few hundred mmol of extra salt to the diet; hence the amount of sodium whose loss the adrenal cortical hormones could prevent was no more than 1 or 2% of the normal filtered load.

Aldosterone was identified as the most active adrenal cortical salt-retaining factor by Simpson *et al.* (1953). Its action is not confined to the renal tubule; it also had direct physiological actions on the amphibian urinary bladder, on mammalian salivary and sweat glands, and on the intestinal mucosa, reducing the secretion of sodium and promoting its retention in the body (Leaf & Sharp, 1971; Pelletier *et al.*, 1972). Because patients with Addison's disease, like adrenalectomized animals, showed impairments of the secretion of hydrogen ions and of potassium, as well as deficient reabsorption of sodium, aldosterone was presumed to act in a small segment of the distal convoluted tubules where sodium was avidly reabsorbed and potassium and hydrogen ions were secreted. Recent investigations using perfused segments of isolated nephrons have shown, however, that the most likely site is the cortical collecting tubule, where aldosterone promotes both the reabsorption of sodium and the development of the normal lumen-negative transepithelial pd. This pd and the reabsorption of sodium, are both minimal or zero in adrenalectomized animals (Kokko, 1985). Aldosterone is believed not to stimulate the sodium pump directly, but to increase the permeability of apical cell membranes so that sodium is more readily taken up from the lumen and the concentration in the cells increases. Because sodium is one of the three essential substrates for the basolateral Na-K-ATPase, an increase in its intracellular concentration increases the rate of the pump reaction and the transfer of sodium across the cells into the peritubular fluid.

One of the most striking features of the renal action of aldosterone is its characteristic delay. Direct injection into one renal artery of a normal dog was followed by an increased excretion of potassium in comparison with the other kidney, but there was no change in excretion of sodium unless the dog had previously been adrenalectomized. Then there was also a reduction in the rate of excretion of sodium; but both this and the increased excretion of potassium were delayed about an hour after the injection (Barger *et al.*, 1958). The delay had nothing to do with the structural complexity the kidney, for there was a similar delay between the application of aldosterone and enhanced transport of sodium by isolated sheets of amphibian urinary bladder *in vitro* (Crabbé, 1961). The latent period is believed to be required for the production of a specific protein which becomes incorporated into sodium channels in the apical cell membranes. Actinomycin D, which blocks the synthesis of RNA, and puromycin, which blocks the synthesis of protein, both inhibit the action of aldosterone. According to the induction hypothesis, aldosterone is taken up into the cell and conveyed to the nucleus combined with a receptor. There it induces the synthesis of a messenger RNA which directs the synthesis of the specific protein. This hypothesis is attractive, even though the evidence for it is largely circumstantial (Leaf & Sharp, 1971). Whatever its mechanism, the delay has the important consequence that rapid adjustments to the rate of tubular reabsorption of sodium cannot be attributed to changes in the concentration of circulating aldosterone.

Even though aldosterone may only control the reabsorption of 1 or 2% of the filtered load, this amounts to 250 to 500 mmol of sodium each day, and is enough to compensate for all ordinary variations in intake. Hence the action of aldosterone alone could provide all adjustments required to regulate the body's sodium balance and to stabilize the ECFV. O'Connor (1962) pointed out, however, that variations in the concentration of aldosterone normally fall on the rather flat, upper part of the dose–response curve, and consequently produce much smaller changes than might be expected from the profound effects of small doses given to adrenalectomized animals and patients with Addison's disease. No store of preformed aldosterone is held in the cortex; its secretion reflects the rate of biosynthesis, so that renal tubular reabsorption of sodium is ultimately controlled by the factors which determine the rate at which the cells of the zona glomerulosa produce aldosterone. The best recognized of these factors are (1) the adenohypophysial adrenocorticotrophic hormone, ACTH; (2) the concentrations of sodium and potassium in the blood supplying the suprarenal glands; and (3) angiotensin II, which is generally regarded as the most important. These factors are now briefly discussed. Reviews by Coghlan et al. (1971) and by Fraser et al. (1979) provide further detail and background information. The recently characterized atrial natriuretic factors (ANF, atriopeptins), formed in mammalian cardiac atria and released when these are distended, promote the excretion of sodium by direct actions in the kidney which will be discussed in Section 7.4.4.4. They are mentioned here because they may be important inhibitors of the secretion of aldosterone (Needleman & Greenwald, 1986).

A. Adrenocorticotrophin, ACTH

The adrenocorticotrophic hormone, ACTH, supports the growth and healthy functioning of the suprarenal cortex. It also regulates the rate of secretion of the glucocorticoid hormones, which, in turn inhibit its own secretion from the adenohypophysis. Such a reciprocal relation is not seen with ACTH and aldosterone, however, and the zona glomerulosa does not atrophy when ACTH is lacking. Stimulation of the cortex as a whole by ACTH results in a temporary increase in the rate of secretion of aldosterone, but this is not maintained. Diurnal fluctuations in the secretion of aldosterone persist after parallel fluctuations in secretion of cortisol are abolished by suppressing the secretion of ACTH. However, secretion of aldosterone responds less briskly to its 'normal' stimulus of salt depletion if ACTH is lacking and salt depletion increases the extent to which ACTH boosts the secretion of aldosterone. Adrenocorticotrophin therefore influences, though it does not definitively regulate, the production of aldosterone. The action seems to be permissive or supportive, and is possibly limited to maintaining the general metabolism of the cells and their supply of metabolites, without controlling the rates at which specific metabolites are used for biosynthesis.

B. The concentrations of sodium and potassium

The great loss of sodium and the increased concentration of potassium in the plasma in Addison's disease are important consequences of failure to secrete aldosterone, and a low sodium status is an important cause of increased secretion from a normal adrenal gland. The discovery that the concentrations of sodium and potassium in the perfusing blood affected the gland directly followed the development in Australia of a technique for transplanting the adrenal glands of sheep into the neck, where they were supplied with blood from the carotid artery and drained into the jugular vein (Denton *et al.*, 1959). The vessels were enclosed in a sleeve of skin so that they could be punctured without disturbing the animals. Agents which might influence secretion could then be introduced directly into the arterial blood, and the whole venous effluent from the gland could be collected. Sheep were also useful experimental animals because controlled depletion of the body's store of sodium could be produced by salivary fistulas, while the sodium/potassium ratio of the saliva could be used conveniently for biological assay of mineral-ocorticoid activity by an important nonrenal action. This pioneering work showed that the secretion of aldosterone was directly stimulated by lower concentrations of sodium or higher concentrations of potassium in the gland's arterial plasma, but it was not at first apparent whether fluctuations within the physiological range were effective.

Blair-West *et al.* (1963) soon showed that lowering of sodium concentration alone was less effective than raising potassium concentration, but that a lowered sodium concentration enhanced the effect of a raised potassium concentration. The relatively small importance of the concentration of sodium in sheep was indicated by the finding that increasing sodium concentration in the adrenal arterial blood had little effect upon the secretion of aldosterone in sodium-deficient animals. Increased concentrations of potassium were, however, very potent stimuli; changes of less than 0.5 mM, well within the physiological range of variation, were effective (Funder *et al.*, 1969).

Potassium increases the production of aldosterone and of its immediate precursor, corticosterone, by adrenal tissue *in vitro*. Large concentrations act on the early step from cholesterol to pregnenolone, which is promoted by ACTH and stimulated by angiotensin. The great sensitivity of the secretion of aldosterone to potassium has been confirmed in many species *in vivo*. Even infusions which are too small to increase potassium concentration detectably in systemic plasma may increase the secretion of aldosterone; indeed, potassium ranks in importance with angiotensin as a major physiological stimulus, and the renin−angiotensin system is not essential for potassium to exert its action. Rising concentrations of potassium in the plasma of anephric patients maintained in a stable condition by haemodialysis increased the secretion of aldosterone, which, in the absence of kidneys, could still promote the excretion of potassium in the faeces. A reported absence of increased secretion during severe hyperkalaemia in human subjects may be explained by the observation that production of aldosterone was maximally stimulated by 8.4 mM potassium, while greater concentrations (which are life-threatening) were inhibitory. Substantial deficiencies of sodium act indirectly on the early steps leading to secretion of aldosterone, so that the dose−response curve of aldosterone production with increasing potassium concentration in the plasma in dogs is made steeper by sodium depletion and flatter by loading with sodium.

Low concentrations of sodium in the plasma appear to act directly on the last step in the biosynthetic pathway, between 18-OH-corticosterone and aldosterone, but the effects of a low sodium status are probably mainly indirect. Deficiency of sodium does not necessarily lead to correspondingly low concentrations in the plasma. The maximally depleted human subjects of McCance's (1937) classical experiments had their serum sodium concentration diminished by only about 10% after they had lost about a third (more than 800 mmol) of their exchangeable sodium. Smaller losses, during the first few days of depletion before the subjects ceased to lose weight, probably left the sodium concentration practically unchanged, and the presumed strong stimulation of their adrenal secretion must have had other causes.

The direct effect of sodium concentration on the adrenal cortex appears to be quite unimportant in human subjects. There was no evidence of a stimulatory effect from falling concentrations of sodium in anephric patients maintained by haemodialysis. In one instance the concentration of aldosterone in the plasma actually increased 10-fold while sodium was being retained. Moreover, even with an intact renin−angiotensin system, the secretion of aldosterone may be minimal despite concentrations of sodium in the plasma as low as 115 mM in patients with inappropriate secretion of ADH (Walker & Cooke, 1973). In short, the capacity of sodium status to modulate the responses to angiotensin and to the direct action of potassium is probably much more important than any direct influence of the concentration of sodium upon the secretion of aldosterone.

C. Angiotensin II (and renin)

Angiotensin II is the most powerful known agent stimulating the cells of the adrenal zona glomerulosa to secrete aldosterone. The octapeptide reaches the adrenal cortex in arterial blood after renin released from the kidney has split off AT I from its precursor in the plasma, and then the converting enzyme, mainly in the lungs, has removed two more amino acids to yield AT II. Fraser *et al.* (1979) summarized the claims of AT II to be considered the controller of the secretion of aldosterone. It stimulates the production of aldosterone both by adrenal cortical cells in culture and by the adrenal gland *in situ*. There is usually a good correlation between concentrations of aldosterone in the plasma and those of AT II and/or renin. The minimal secretion of aldosterone by patients unable to secrete renin is increased by exogenous AT II. Inhibitors of AT II or of the converting enzyme depress plasma aldosterone concentration. Plasma renin and AT II are increased by depletion and reduced by loading with sodium. Clinically, oversecretion of renin leads to hyperaldosteronism; and excessive secretion of aldosterone by tumours is accompanied by low concentrations of renin and of AT II. The stimulating action of AT II is specific; physiological doses increase the secretion of aldosterone (but not of other corticoid hormones) in normal human subjects regardless of their sodium status, though the dose−response curve becomes steeper with deficiency and less steep with abundance of sodium. The precise mechanisms of the action of AT, and of its interaction with sodium status and potassium, are not established.

Despite its specificity as a stimulus, AT alone cannot fully account for the adrenal response to alterations in sodium status (Coghlan *et al.*, 1971). It does not have the same effects as depletion of sodium, and it cannot sustain increased rates of secretion of aldosterone or increase them further during moderate sodium deficiency. When sodium is supplied to sodium-deficient sheep, the rate of secretion of aldosterone falls, but several hours before, not after, the concentrations of renin and AT fall in the plasma. Hence it appears that additional facts or unknown interactions between known factors are necessary to account for the rate of secretion of aldosterone. One such factor might be the heptapeptide, [des-Asp[1]] AT II (AT III), which is present in plasma (especially in rats) and has similar actions to AT II (Peart, 1978). But the combined effects of AT II and AT III could not account completely for the increased secretion of aldosterone in sodium-depleted sheep (Blair-West *et al.*, 1979). Carey & Sen (1986) reviewed other possible factors.

To the extent that AT II determines the secretion of aldosterone, the factors that control the release of renin from the kidney must play an important part in regulating the tubular reabsorption of sodium. Coghlan *et al.* (1971) recognized three major systems which cooperate to control the release of renin, and these were reviewed in greater detail by Davis & Freeman (1976). One of these is extrinsic, the efferent renal sympathetic nerves; the other two are within the kidney — a postulated renal vascular receptor and the macula densa.

D. The renal nerves

The juxtaglomerular cells are richly innervated by efferent fibres from the sympathetic nerves supplying the kidney, and several workers have shown that stimulation of these nerves increases the output of renin in the renal venous blood, even when precautions are taken to prevent alterations in perfusion pressure or glomerular filtration. The increased secretion of renin in response to haemorrhage or depletion of sodium is reduced by dividing the nerves or blocking transmission in them with local anaesthetics; it is not abolished, however, showing that the renal nerves are not the sole channels of control. In chronic experiments other mechanisms compensate for the lack of sympathetic innervation, and the renin responses become normal in a few weeks. Increased concentrations of renin in the plasma following postural change in human recipients of transplanted (and hence denervated) kidneys provide further evidence that mechanisms independent of the renal nerves can increase the secretion of renin. The action of the renal sympathetic nerves on the juxtaglomerular cells is mediated through β-receptors; and circulating catecholamines may augment the effect of transmitters from sympathetic nerve endings. Besides their direct action on the juxtaglomerular cells, the renal nerves may influence the release of renin by vasomotor actions which affect renal vascular receptors; they may also alter the rate of glomerular filtration and so change the load of salt presented to the macula densa. When adrenaline and noradrenaline mimic the effects of sympathetic stimulation, they too may presumably act indirectly by altering renal hae-modynamics as well as directly on the renin-secreting cells.

Other circulating humoral agents which can affect the juxtaglomerular cells include angiotensin and AVP. These vasocontrictors inhibit the release of renin directly; and AT II, which is a very potent inhibitor, is probably responsible for an important negative feedback restricting the output of renin. Effects of potassium are contradictory and probably include actions on vessels as well as direct actions on juxtaglomerular cells. Davis & Freeman (1976) remarked that the responses to increased concentrations of sodium and potassium in the plasma cannot be demonstrated in nonfiltering kidneys. They both depend upon a functioning tubular system, and are probably brought about indirectly through the macula densa. Plasma renin activity increases much more steeply with falling renal arterial pressure in dogs when their intake of sodium is low than when it is normal (Gibbons et al., 1984), but low dietary intakes do not affect the concentration in the plasma significantly, and presumably act in other ways. Inhibitory effects of loading with sodium are probably indirect through the macula densa. The inhibitory effects of increased concentrations of circulating aldosterone on secretion of renin are also probably indirect.

E. A renal vascular receptor?

There appears to be a rather direct action on secretion from the juxtamedullary cells arising from some effect of perfusing pressure in the glomerular arterioles themselves. Reductions in perfusing pressure in dogs elicit increased secretion of renin from denervated kidneys even when no glomerular filtrate is being formed, and signals cannot be expected to arise from the macula densa. The postulated vascular receptor has not been clearly identified. Relaxation of elements in the walls of the afferent glomerular arterioles may directly release renin from granules in the juxtaglomerular cells. The fact that the vascular receptor appears able to release renin when the arterioles are dilated as well as when they are constricted has suggested that the effective stimulus might be stretching of sensitive elements in the walls of the vessels. All elements would presumably be stretched when the vessels were relaxed and dilated. Less actively contractile elements would also be stretched when vasoconstrictor nerve impulses or circulating vasoconstrictors caused muscular elements arranged in series to contract and the modified muscle cells containing renin granules could be expected to be less actively contractile than ordinary arteriolar muscle cells.

F. The macula densa

Apart from these direct, mechanical effects, a reduction in systemic arterial pressure with consequent slowing of glomerular filtration should reduce the amount of sodium chloride reaching the macula densa and the distal nephron. There has been controversy over whether the effective stimulus to the macula densa is a reduction or an increase in the amount of sodium chloride delivered into the distal tubule. Early theories of autoregulation of glomerular filtration and RPF by tubuloglomerular feedback (TGFB) assumed that the delivery of too much salt caused renin to be released locally, and to reduce filtration rates in individual glomeruli. This became less probable with the realization that locally generated AT II would most likely constrict glomerular efferent arterioles and increase the filtration fraction if not GFR itself (see Sections 2.2.7 and 3.3.5.3). It now seems more probable that a reduction in the load of sodium chloride delivered to the macula densa leads to release of renin from the kidney into general circulation and this may be of greater physiological importance than a possible contribution of renin to autoregulation without the kidney.

Jackson *et al.* (1985) proposed a simpler scheme in which the release of renin is controlled by two major mechanisms — stimulation through β-adrenergic receptors, and increased biosynthesis of prostaglandins, which act as mediators for the renal baroreceptors as well as for the macula densa.

Although the medulla is a major source of renal PGs, some, particularly

PGI_2 and PGE_2 are synthesized by cortical arteries and arterioles, as well as by glomerular arterioles and mesangial cells (Schlondorff & Ardaillou, 1986). Heinrich (1981) reviewed early evidence that PGs can stimulate the juxta-glomerular cells to release renin. In dogs they appear to mediate the function of the renal baroreceptor, which is most important for controlling release of renin at perfusion pressures within the autoregulatory range. They may also mediate the action of the macula densa, which becomes more important when GFR is more variable at pressures below the autoregulatory range (but still large enough to maintain filtration, without which there would be no flow past the macula densa). Increases in secretion of renin in response to intrarenal infusions of arachidonic acid, or to activation of the renal baro-receptors by clamping the aorta above the renal arteries, in dogs with denervated, β-blocked and nonfiltering kidneys, were totally abolished when biosynthesis of PGs was suppressed with indomethacin (Gerber et al., 1981). These nonfiltering kidneys were, however, far from normal, because sup-pression of glomerular filtration while perfusion pressures were still in the normal range was achieved by ureteral ligation and 2 hours of total ischaemia, which left the tubules degenerated and blocked with casts. With a denervated but filtering kidney whose baroreceptors were inactivated by maximal vaso-dilatation with papaverine, the increase in release of renin after reducing delivery of fluid to the macula densa by aortic constriction was also abolished by cyclo-oxygenase inhibitors. Prostaglandins were therefore claimed to be the sole mediators of renin release secondary to stimulation of either the baroreceptors or the macula densa.

Prostaglandins, especially PGI_2, and, to a lesser extent, PGE_2, stimulate the release of renin from renal cortical slices of several species, and from intact kidneys of dogs following injection into the renal artery (Jackson et al., 1985). The precursor, arachidonic acid, also increases secretion of renin when it is injected into the renal artery of rabbits, rats and dogs (even in the vasodilated, nonfiltering kidney with β-adrenergic receptors blocked); and indomethacin prevents this stimulation. Inhibitors of PG synthesis also reduce basal plasma renin activity in rabbit, rat and man, and diminish the increased secretion of renin which normally occurs in a variety of circumstances in-cluding sodium depletion, inhibition of converting enzyme (which reduces inhibition of renin release by AT II) and adrenalectomy (which eliminates inhibition by circulating aldosterone). Moreover, renal synthesis of PGs is increased by sodium depletion and by procedures like reduction of renal perfusion pressure which stimulate the release of renin when the biosynthesis of PGs is not inhibited. Jackson et al. (1985) accordingly accepted that synthesis of PGs is required for nonadrenergic release of renin, and spoke of a 'prostaglandin—renin axis' within the kidney which can be activated either by the intrarenal baroreceptors or from the macula densa.

7.4.3.1 INTEGRATION OF THE PRINCIPAL MECHANISMS
CONTROLLING SECRETION OF ALDOSTERONE

The manner in which the various mechanisms cooperate may be illustrated by considering a gradually increasing depletion of sodium with consequent reductions in the volumes of ECF and circulating blood. As blood volume begins to shrink, the initial loss will be almost entirely from the venous system; less atriopeptin (which would inhibit the secretion of aldosterone) may be released into the circulation, and the rate of discharge of the low-pressure mechanoreceptors in the great veins and the chambers of the heart will diminish. Since one of the chief effects of impulses from these receptors appears to be the central inhibition of sympathetic tone, there should be increased sympathetic activity, initially in venomotor nerves; this should keep up the venous return to the heart by reducing the volume of the venous system so that it still fits snugly round the smaller volume of blood. As long as acceleration of the heart and constriction of arterioles can maintain systemic arterial pressure, the initial effect on the kidney will be greater activity in the sympathetic nerves; this will increase the secretion of renin from the juxtaglomerular cells and reduce RBF somewhat, with minimal effects on glomerular filtration. Greater sympathetic activity with further depletion may be augmented by secretion of adrenaline and noradrenaline from the suprarenal medulla. Glomerular filtration will be slowed as RBF is further reduced, so that less sodium chloride enters the nephrons and reaches the macula densa. When the loss of blood volume becomes too large for systemic arterial pressure to be maintained, falling renal perfusion pressure will add signals from the renal baroreceptors to those from the macula densa. Any reduction in the concentration of sodium in the plasma with severe depletion will further reduce the filtered load so that still less sodium chloride reaches the macula densa.

As the various factors stimulating secretion are gradually recruited by postural change, progressive loss of blood, sodium depletion or dehydration, more and more renin is released into the blood. The AT II that it generates is a powerful vasoconstrictor, and may have a direct role in maintaining systemic arterial pressure. Circulating AT II acts centrally to enhance sympathetic tone, to stimulate thirst, and possibly (cf. Heinrich *et al.*, 1986) to release ADH. It may itself promote the tubular reabsorption of sodium, but its most important action is probably to stimulate the synthesis of aldosterone in the adrenal cortex. There are certainly other factors yet to be discovered. The mobilization of aldosterone to conserve sodium by enhancing its renal tubular reabsorption is a good example of a process of which the whole is more than the sum of the parts! The best known parts of this process are summarized in Figure 7.2.

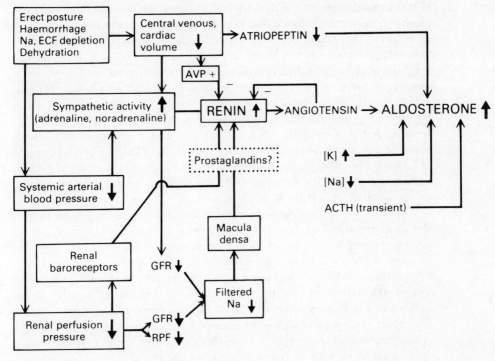

Fig. 7.2 Summary of the principal known factors which increase the secretion of aldosterone during sodium depletion or loss of blood.

7.4.4 'Third' and some other factors

7.4.4.1 INTRODUCTION

The rate of glomerular filtration and the concentration of sodium in the plasma determine how much sodium enters each renal tubule, while aldosterone controls the reabsorption of up to 2% of the normal filtered load from a short segment of the cortical collecting tubule. If aldosterone were to increase reabsorption from the proximal tubule, it would reduce the amount of sodium chloride reaching the macula densa, and stimulate the secretion of more aldosterone, with the possibility of a positive feedback. The removal of the bulk of the filtered load by the the proximal tubules and the ascending limbs of the loops of Henle provides for fine tuning of the kidney's handling of sodium by nice adjustments to the reabsorption of the small remaining fraction (de Wardener, 1978). Control of the routine, aldosterone-insensitive reabsorption of 98% or more of the normal filtered load of sodium must depend upon factors operating in other parts of the tubular system.

The existence of other factors besides variations in filtered load and tubular reabsorption controlled by aldosterone became clear when de Wardener *et al.*

(1961) expanded the ECFV of anaesthetized dogs rapidly with large infusions of isotonic saline and observed an impressive increase in the rate of excretion of sodium. This could not be attributed to a reduced rate of secretion of aldosterone because it was immediate, and because the dogs had received large doses of 9α-fluorohydrocortisone. Moreover, it could not be due to an increase in GFR, such as often occurs in dogs infused with saline, because the increased urinary excretion of sodium occurred in experiments in which the rate of glomerular filtration actually fell. These important observations were amply confirmed in other laboratories and micropuncture methods revealed a dramatic inhibition (by more than 30%) of the rate of reabsorption of sodium from the proximal tubules, so that a greater fraction of filtered sodium was excreted, even when GFR was reduced substantially by a clamp on the renal artery (Dirks et al., 1965).

Whatever was responsible soon came to be spoken of as the 'third factor'. But its nature is still uncertain. The impressive natriuresis might represent an emergency response to the challenge of an unnaturally large and rapid expansion of the ECF created by enthusiastic experimenters. Bricker (1967), however, claimed that a third factor, independent alike of glomerular filtration and of aldosterone, modulates the excretion of sodium, at least when the number of functioning nephrons is reduced, and might also contribute to the day to day regulation of sodium balance under normal circumstances. Since it is improbable that one single mechanism can account for all that happens, it may be better to refer to 'third factor(s)' in the plural.

De Wardener et al. (1961) attributed the inhibition of tubular reabsorption to a change in the quality of the blood, probably the presence of a natriuretic hormone (a kind of physiological diuretic, promoting the excretion of sodium by inhibiting its tubular reabsorption), because the excretion of sodium increased in a recipient dog linked in cross-circulation with the animal whose ECFV was expanded. Earley & Daugharty (1969) accepted that the phenomenon was well established in dogs and rats, and that it probably occurred in man. They dismissed the evidence for a hormone inhibiting tubular reabsorption as circumstantial and conflicting, and considered 'physical factors' which might increase the excretion of sodium independently of total GFR and aldosterone. One possibility was a redistribution of blood flow and glomerular filtration away from the deeper, juxtamedullary nephrons with long loops of Henle towards superficial nephrons with short loops and a smaller capacity to reabsorb sodium. No proof of such a redistribution of blood flow has been presented (Section 2.3.2), and there is no convincing evidence that it plays an important part in regulating the excretion of sodium (Skorecki & Brenner, 1981). More plausible alternatives are alterations in haemodynamic factors such as perfusion pressure or renal venous pressure, and variations in the balance of forces between the tubules and the peritubular capillaries. These 'Starling forces' depend upon the difference in hydrostatic pressure between tubular lumina and peritubular capillaries, and upon the oncotic (colloid osmotic) pressure of postglomerular plasma in the peritubular capillaries (assuming the tubular fluid to be protein-free). They also depend upon the composition of the blood, because the PCV (haematocrit) affects viscosity, and the concentration of protein in the plasma determines its oncotic pressure. Some of the physical factors will be considered briefly after an attempt to evaluate the status of possible natriuretic hormones.

7.4.4.2 NATRIURETIC HORMONES?

Johnston & Davies (1966) confirmed the observations of de Wardener's group that the rate of excretion of sodium increased in a recipient dog in cross-circulation with a donor which had received an infusion of saline. By constricting the aorta of the recipient animals they replaced the increase in GFR which accompanied diuresis in some of de Wardener's experiments with a decrease, and the natriuresis still occurred despite the smaller filtered load. It was confirmed that the diuresis and natriuresis were much smaller in the recipient than in the donor dogs, but the donors had been given a litre of saline 'as rapidly as possible' — actually at about 9 ml/min — so that their blood was diluted, GFR was increased and the filtered load of sodium was far greater. The dogs had been pretreated with deoxycorticosterone acetate, and the smaller diuresis in the recipients, whose own plasma had not been expanded, was attributed to a humoral agent other than aldosterone conveyed in the donor's blood. Many circulating natriuretic substances were reported in the next decade; Dirks et al. (1976) tabulated nine, believed to vary in molecular weight from 500 to 50000, but not isolated or clearly identified.

De Wardener (1977, 1982) reviewed the quest for the natriuretic hormone over 20 years, which had become one of his major interests. A number of groups using different experimental procedures demonstrated natriuretic activity (assayed in cross-circulated recipient animals or by denervated or isolated, perfused kidneys) in the plasma of animals after rather large and rapid expansion of the ECF with saline. It was often necessary to re-infuse the urine or supply saline to the recipient animals because otherwise the natriuresis failed (possibly through an increasing concentration of plasma protein) unless the lost sodium and water were replaced. Some promising initial claims to have obtained natriuretic agents from plasma by dialysis or ultrafiltration could not be confirmed. Those who sought natriuretic material in the urine of salt-loaded animals and humans were more successful, and their results were more repeatable. There appeared to be at least two active materials; one, larger, with a molecular weight greater than 30000, had a prolonged action which developed slowly, the other (conceivably derived from the first) was smaller, molecular weight less than 500, and had a quicker, shorter action. There was no agreement about their chemical nature, how they acted or where they came from. In 1977 de Wardener concluded modestly that the elusive natriuretic hormone was still hypothetical, yet well worth looking for.

The next 8 years saw important progress (de Wardener & Clarkson, 1985).

A natural inhibitor of renal Na-K-ATPase, active *in vitro*, was extracted from the plasma of rats, dogs and human subjects, in amounts which increased greatly with increased intakes of salt or expansion of ECF and blood volume by infusions. The inhibitor in human plasma had been greatly concentrated but not isolated or completely identified. It appeared to have a molecular weight around 350; it behaved as a polar compound, soluble in water, 95% acetone, and organic solvents with high dielectric constants. It was not a catecholamine and might be a peptide. It inhibits intracellular Na-K-ATPase about 1000 times as strongly as ouabain, but its action is much briefer. Its site of origin was still undetermined, but an inhibitor could be extracted from the brain. It is possible that the active substances from plasma, urine and brain might be the same; but inhibitory substances derived from the urine and brain appeared less likely to be peptides than the one from the plasma. Plenty remained to be clarified, and despite de Wardener's long sustained enthusiasm, de Wardener & Clarkson (1985) did not go beyond the cautious statement that 'it has sometimes been assumed that the natriuretic activity of the plasma and its increased capacity to inhibit sodium transport' (after the volume of blood has been expanded) 'are due to a change in the concentration of the same circulating substance'.

A hormone which is only released in response to a large and rapid increase in the volume of blood might have some value in an emergency, but its physiological role in the day to day regulation of sodium balance and extra-cellular fluid volume would be harder to defend. The more recently isolated atrial natriuretic peptides (see later), which have been precisely characterized through the application of molecular biological techniques, might appear more credible as natriuretic hormones. But they cannot be regarded as 'third factors' controlling the tubular reabsorption of sodium, because they do not inhibit the Na-K-ATPase; they relax smooth muscles and seem to increase the excretion of sodium haemodynamically, mainly be increasing the rate of glomerular filtration.

De Wardener (1977, 1982) insisted that the activity of the natriuretic hormone can only be convincingly demonstrated by experimental procedures in which a rat's or a dog's blood volume is expanded rapidly and substantially with blood in equilibrium with that already circulating, so that neither the PCV nor the concentration of plasma protein is altered. Experiments in which fluid volume is expanded with saline, Ringer's solution or various concentrations of albumin are quite unsuitable because the associated hae-modilution masks effects which could indicate the presence of a humoral agent. This requirement is tantamount to an admission that the effects of postulated natriuretic hormones are relatively insignificant by comparison with those of the physical factors which the rigorous experimental design is intended to avoid.

7.4.4.3 PHYSICAL FACTORS

Increases in renal perfusion pressure, or in renal venous pressure, and the reduction of renal vascular resistance with vasodilator drugs, as well as intravenous infusions, have often been found to increase the rate of excretion of sodium, even when the rate of glomerular filtration was unchanged or diminished (Dirks *et al.*, 1976). Many of these procedures must modify the hydrostatic and oncotic pressure of blood in the peritubular capillaries. The changes in protein concentration which determine oncotic pressure have actually been measured in Munich Wistar rats (for a tabular summary see Brenner *et al.*, 1974). Infusions of isoncotic fluids like plasma or equilibrated blood increase peritubular capillary hydrostatic pressure without affecting oncotic pressure. Hyperoncotic infusions which increase the uptake of interstitial fluid into the circulation should expand the blood volume by more than the volume infused, and must also reduce the PCV; increased systemic oncotic pressure should oppose an increase in glomerular filtration rate and the increase in oncotic pressure resulting from loss of the filtrate, leaving a substantial increase in hydrostatic pressure in the peritubular capillaries as the principal effect. Infusions of isotonic or hypertonic saline, which profoundly depress proximal tubular reabsorption of sodium and water, should reduce the oncotic pressure of postglomerular plasma as well as increasing peritubular capillary pressure. If, therefore, the Starling forces were to control the transfer of fluid from tubular lumen to peritubular capillary plasma, alterations in the hydrostatic pressure and oncotic pressure of plasma in the peritubular capillaries might serve as a final common path for the various physical factors affecting tubular reabsorption.

The difference in hydrostatic pressure across the walls of the peritubular capillaries is small, and the oncotic pressure of the postglomerular plasma is greater than that of systemic plasma because of the loss of the glomerular filtrate. Hence a combined difference ($\Delta\pi - \Delta P$) of the order of $10\,\text{mmHg}$ should be available to effect the uptake of protein-free reabsorbate into the peritubular capillaries (Schafer, 1982). If the glomerular capillaries correspond to the arteriolar ends of systemic capillaries, where the head of pressure favouring efflux exceeds the difference of oncotic pressure favouring influx, the peritubular capillaries are roughly analogous to the venular ends, where these conditions are reversed and fluid returns into the capillaries under the influence of the Starling forces. An important difference is that, in order to be reabsorbed, the tubular fluid must cross not only the capillary wall, but the tubular epithelium and the intersitital space as well. Although Ludwig (1844) believed that the head of oncotic pressure was sufficient for reabsorption of the glomerular filtrate, we now believe that the reabsorbate must first be actively transported from the tubular lumen into the interstitial spaces before the Starling forces can effect its uptake into the peritubular capillaries. These forces provide no more than a small fraction of the total driving force necessary for tubular reabsorption, for metabolic inhibitors abolish net transport of sodium from proximal tubules even when the oncotic driving force is unimpaired (Giebisch, 1978). But the Starling forces do appear to influence the rate of reabsorption. Green *et al.* (1974) showed that though the rate of reabsorption from tubules perfused with cyanide was minimal, and hardly affected by the concentration of protein in peritubular capillary plasma, removal of protein depressed the maximal rate of reabsorption by as much as 50% when active transport was not inhibited. Giebisch (1978) concluded that the Starling forces, though acting mainly on fluid already transferred into the interspaces following actively transported sodium, make an important contribution to GTB. If fluid is transferred from the tubules faster than the peritubular capillaries take it up, the lateral intercellular spaces between the epithelial cells are distended, and this promotes back-diffusion through the paracellular pathway of sodium which has been transported out through the cells (Fig. 7.3); the sodium pump is not directly inhibited, but the net rate of reabsorption is slowed (Windhager & Giebisch, 1976). Conversely, an increase in filtration rate (and therefore in FF) with a given rate of glomerular blood flow should increase the oncotic pressure of postglomerular plasma and promote reabsorption of the extra filtrate.

This attractive conception of the mechanism of tubular reabsorption offers a plausible hypothesis to account for the action of the physical factors when they disturb the normal state of GTB and alter the rate of excretion of sodium. For example, when expansion of the ECF with saline reduces the concentration of protein in the postglomerular blood and increases pressure in the peritubular capillaries, both of these should weaken the local Starling forces and inhibit reabsorption. But although the explanation is attractive, the relative importance of differences in hydrostatic and oncotic pressure is debated, and not all are even agreed that the experimental support for the hypothesis is convincing. Because many of the arguments are inconclusive, no elaborate discussion (which would be lengthy) is warranted here. Details may be traced through reviews which give access to a large and often contradictory literature.

Brenner *et al.* (1971b) showed that the inhibition of proximal tubular reabsorption in rats infused with isotonic saline could be prevented by perfusing the peritubular capillaries with albumin solutions having the same oncotic pressure as that of postglomerular plasma before the infusion of saline. This helped to convince Windhager & Giebisch (1976) of 'the unavoidable conclusion that most of the inhibition of absolute proximal reabsorption is mediated by the parallel decline in postglomerular capillary protein concentration'. However, de Wardener (1978), who cited some other observations, was more impressed by the importance of hydrostatic pressure, and stated that 'the overall conclusion from these investigations is that the plasma protein concentration in the peritubular capillaries has little effect on the reabsorption of fluid from the proximal tubule'. A little later he emphasized

LUMEN   PERITUBULAR CAPILLARY

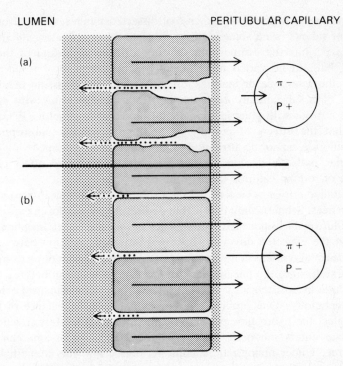

Fig. 7.3 The effect of 'physical factors'.
  (a) High pressure and low oncotic pressure in peritubular capillaries, resticted uptake of reabsorbed fluid, distended intercellular spaces, with increased back-flux reducing net rate of reabsorption.
  (b) Low pressure and high oncotic pressure in peritubular capillaries; narrow intercellular spaces, slower back-flux and faster net reabsorption.

that 'the doubt which surrounds the importance of the effect of the peritubular capillary oncotic pressure on proximal tubular sodium reabsorption does not extend to the effect of hydrostatic pressure'.

Giebisch (1978) admitted that not all observations supported the nice mechanistic hypothesis of GTB by Starling forces, and cited evidence that a faster flow of tubular fluid may promote its own reabsorption; in de Wardener's words, 'the stimulus for reabsorption is the filtrate itself'. This mechanism may be a major factor in maintaining GTB under normal hydropenic conditions (Häberle *et al.*, 1981). Individual tubules may show rates of reabsorption proportional to the rate of perfusion when they are perfused *in situ* with natural glomerular fluid, but not when they are perfused with isotonic saline solutions. The natural filtrate provides bicarbonate and organic solutes like glucose and amino acids whose co-transport enhances the active reabsorption of sodium, but unidentified stimulants of larger molecular weight may also be concerned (de Wardener, 1978).

Microperfusion of isolated segments of dissected tubules, mostly from the kidneys of rabbits, shed some light on these problems (Rector, 1983). This technique permits the compositions of the perfusing fluid and of the surrounding bath to be varied independently. One unequivocal result which indicates the relevance of Starling forces was that the omission of protein from the bath substantially impaired the absorption of water with sodium chloride, but not with glucose and sodium bicarbonate. Rector (1983) concluded that the effects of peritubular Starling forces on reabsorption of sodium chloride cannot be attributed to alterations in the permeability of the paracellular paths, and must be due to some unexplained effect on the transport of sodium chloride through the cells.

In a detailed critical review of the importance of the physical factors, with 276 references, Schnermann (1974) tabulated results of two dozen experimental procedures which indicated that changes in the rate of reabsorption were usually in the expected direction; but there was little relation between the magnitudes of alterations in the Starling forces and in the rates of reabsorption. He remarked; 'since the phenomenon resists lucid description because of the experimental inconsistencies it is not surprising that the mechanism behind it is quite nebulous'. One problem is that estimates of the balance of forces often neglect the hydrostatic pressure of the interstitial fluid from which the reabsorbate enters the peritubular capillaries, and also assume that it is protein-free. Under nondiuretic conditions, pressure in the interstitial fluid around the peritubular capillaries is of the order of 2 to 4 mmHg; its oncotic pressure varies around 5 mmHg. When uptake into the capillaries is inhibited following infusions of isotonic saline, the interstitial hydrostatic pressure can increase three- or four-fold, while the oncotic pressure is greatly reduced as the protein is diluted by fluid which the capillaries fail to take up (Wolgast et al., 1981). Alterations in proximal tubular reabsorption, however, are often small, and poorly correlated with these changes in pressure. More satisfactory correlations might be found with hydrostatic and oncotic pressures in the lateral intercellular spaces — if these were known.

Knox et al. (1983) suggested that intrarenal pressure might be a crucial variable affecting the excretion of sodium. They pointed out that in euvolaemic animals, renal vasodilatation with secretin increases hydrostatic pressure and reduces oncotic pressure in the peritubular capillaries without causing natriuresis. The same changes in blood flow, capillary hydrostatic pressure and oncotic pressure produced by acetylcholine are accompanied by a profuse natriuresis. The outstanding difference in the Starling forces is that acetylcholine increases the intrarenal pressure, while secretin does not. Bank & Aynedjian (1984) made micropuncture measurements on pairs of rats linked through cross-circulation. Despite changes of more than 10 mmHg in net intracapillary (oncotic−hydrostatic) pressure, there was no change in sodium excretion or in the absolute rate of proximal tubular reabsorption in recipient rats whose fluid volume was held constant while the donors were infused with plasma or saline; reducing peritubular oncotic pressure about 10 mmHg by plasmapheresis also failed to affect the rates of urinary excretion and of proximal tubular reabsorption of sodium. But when recipient rats were saline-expanded, their rates of excretion of sodium increased 50- to 90-fold, though there was still no change in the absolute rate of proximal reabsorption. Interstitial pressures measured through a subcapsular pipette were between 2 and 3 mmHg in the unexpanded and plasmapheresed rats, but between 9 and 11 mmHg in the saline-expanded recipients. Perhaps more importantly, the saline-expanded recipients also showed an increase of 40% in whole-kidney and 35% in single nephron filtration rate; consequently the unchanged absolute rate of proximal reabsorption implied a reduction in fractional reabsorption from 65% to 44% of the filtered load of sodium. Clearance data for the whole kidneys showed that the rate of natriuresis amounted to 10% of the extra filtered load, and that the rate of reabsorption beyond the proximal nephron was roughly doubled as 90% of the extra load was taken up there. Although the increased interstitial pressure may have helped to prevent the rates of proximal and more distal reabsorption from increasing enough to maintain GTB, the prime cause of the natriuresis appears to have been the large increase in filtration rate.

Third factors have been generally supposed to affect the large component of tubular reabsorption which occurs from the proximal tubules. The distal tubules, with their tight epithelia, should be less susceptible to the rate at which reabsorbed fluid is taken up into the peritubular capillaries, and distal reabsorption seems to be relatively unaffected by Starling forces while ECFV is normal. But there is convincing evidence that expansion of the ECF with saline inhibits reabsorption of sodium beyond the proximal tubules, and that this more distal inhibition is necessary for a maximal natriuretic response to loading with saline (Stein & Reineck, 1975). The loops of Henle and the distal convoluted tubules seem to reabsorb sodium in proportion to the load they receive, regardless of ECFV. But expansion of the ECFV seems to inhibit reabsorption from the collecting ducts, and their response probably accounts for the different effects of infusions of isotonic saline and of hyper-oncotic albumin. Both of these depress proximal tubular reabsorption of sodium to the same extent, but the saline infusions are followed by brisk natriuresis, and the albumin infusions are not. De Wardener (1978) regarded the collecting tubules as an important site controlling the urinary excretion of sodium, and Knox et al. (1983) considered that they might respond to variations in hydrostatic and oncotic pressures which would be unlikely to affect the distal convoluted tubules.

It is not yet possible to bring the discussion of the physical factors to a satisfactory conclusion. Although the Starling forces ought to control the rate of excretion of sodium, it is not certain how, or to what extent, they do so. There is the further difficulty of invoking phenomena that are only clearly demonstrable by rather drastic experimental procedures to explain what happens under normal physiological conditions.

7.4.4.4 ATRIAL NATRIURETIC FACTORS

The atrial natriuretic factors (ANFs) differ in several ways from what have been called third factors, and so deserve separate treatment; they resemble other natriuretic hormones in being humoral, but seem to act more on glomerular filtration than on tubular reabsorption. Marin-Grez *et al.* (1986) actually observed in rats treated with ANFs the widening of preglomerular and narrowing of postglomerular vessels inferred by Dunn *et al.* (1986).

Maack *et al.* (1985) traced the brief history of the atrial natriuretic factors since the description of what appeared to be secretory granules in atrial muscle cells in 1964, and the demonstration by DeBold *et al.* in 1981 that supernatants from homogenates of mammalian atria (but not of ventricles), injected intravenously into anaesthetized, nondiuretic rats, provoked within 1 or 2 minutes a brisk diuresis, lasting 10 to 20 minutes. The rate of excretion of sodium increased more than 30-fold, that of potassium doubled, with a 10-fold increase in the volume of urine. The responsible agent was also a vasodilator and relaxed intestinal as well as vascular smooth muscle; it was quickly purified, using these properties for biological assay, and within 3 years was characterized as a polypeptide and had its amino-acid sequence determined.

A number of names were used by different investigators for the products they studied, but ANFs or atrial natriuretic peptides (ANPs) are convenient comprehensive terms. Ballermann & Brenner (1985) referred to the active principle as 'atrin'. It appears that the substance first formed in the cells is a pre-pro-atrin which has 152 amino-acid residues in rats and 151 in human hearts. The first 26 residues (from the amino end) form a 'signal peptide' which appears to be necessary for intracellular transport but is not exported. The granules contain pro-atrin, with 126 residues. The active, circulating agent has 28 residues, numbers 123 to 150 of the original 152, pulled into a ring with two tails by a disulphide bridge which is essential for biological activity:

$$
\begin{array}{l}
\text{R}-\text{D}-\text{I}^*-\text{R}-\text{G}-\text{G}-\text{F}-\text{C}-\text{S}-\text{S}-\text{R}-\text{R}-\text{L}-\text{S} \quad \text{Amino end} \\
\qquad\qquad\qquad\qquad\qquad\quad | \\
\qquad\qquad\qquad\qquad\qquad\ \text{S} \\
\text{I} \\
\qquad\qquad\qquad\qquad\qquad\ \text{S} \\
\text{G}-\text{A}-\text{Q}-\text{S}-\text{G}-\text{L}-\text{G}-\text{C}-\text{N}-\text{S}-\text{F}-\text{R}-\text{Y} \qquad \text{Carboxy end}
\end{array}
$$

*Human atrin has methionine in place of this isoleucine residue. Synthetic peptides having 24 or more residues are also active (Needleman & Greenwald, 1986).

Synthetic ANPs were available in time for Maack and his colleagues to report the renal effects of a peptide containing 24 amino acids in anaesthetized dogs in 1984. While the peptide was being infused intravenously there was a sustained, but reversible, reduction in systemic arterial blood pressure of about 10% from 135 to 120 mmHg. Renal vascular resistance was not altered,

RBF was unchanged or reduced, but the GFR increased more than 20% and the FF increased from about 0.2 to 0.3. The volume flow of urine and the rate of excretion of sodium both increased about five times, and the rate of excretion of potassium was approximately doubled. At the same time plasma renin activity and the rate of release of renin fell to about a third of their control values, and the concentration of aldosterone in the plasma fell to half. Since the filtered load of sodium increased by up to 800 and the rate of excretion of sodium by up to 160 μmol/min, the natriuresis was never more than 10 to 20% of the increase in filtered load; the fraction of filtered sodium that was excreted increased from 1.2 to 4.3%.

These were striking effects, but the ANP could not be claimed as a hormone until Lang *et al.* (1985) reported that it was present in the plasma of rats. It had a very short half-life in the circulation. The rate at which it was released paralleled increases in right atrial pressure *in vivo*, following expansion of the plasma and ECF by saline infusions, or increases in the perfusion pressure of isolated, perfused hearts. The effects of intravenous infusions in anaesthetized dogs were confirmed in conscious dogs, except that the increased rate of excretion of potassium only occurred when the thoracic inferior vena cava was constricted — a manoeuvre which suppressed the increase in excretion of sodium, though ANF still greatly reduced the renin activity and the concentration of aldosterone in the plasma (Freeman *et al.*, 1985). Since in the 'caval' dogs the peptide produced the usual large increase in GFR without increasing their minimal rate of excretion of sodium, it cannot have depressed tubular reabsorption, which must have increased as much as the filtered load.

There is no evidence that ANPs inhibit the Na-K-ATPase like the natriuretic factors pursued by de Wardener and others. Binding sites for ^{125}I-labelled ANP occur predominantly in the glomeruli and renal vasculature (Healy & Fanestil, 1986) and also in the suprarenal cortex, especially the zona glomerulosa (Chai *et al.*, 1986). Although the increase in GFR is more than adequate to account for the extra sodium that is excreted after injections of ANFs, this may not be the only factor involved. Maack *et al.* (1985) suggested that a washing out of the medullary osmotic gradient in consequence of the vasodilator action of ANPs might reduce the reabsorption of sodium. Inhibition of the release of renin, together with the more direct inhibition of the secretion of aldosterone (acting on an early step and able to override many stimuli to increased production), cannot contribute to the acute natriuresis produced by these agents. Their extrarenal actions will, however, tend to maintain diuresis and natriuresis during prolonged exposure of the kidneys to ANP. Both the acute and the chronic effects therefore serve to reduce the sodium content of the body and the volumes of ECF and plasma.

The vasodilator actions of ANPs are most apparent where vascular tone is high — as in animals with genetically determined or experimentally induced hypertension; in the absence of high tone the lowering of blood pressure is due mainly to a reduced cardiac output. These agents seem well suited to spare the heart from the effects of overfilling of the circulation and from excessive work against high peripheral resistance. It is therefore appropriate that they are released into the circulation when the right atrium is distended, as by an excessive volume on the low-pressure side of the vascular system. Their possible importance is indicated by the large amounts which are produced. From 1 to 5% of all the messenger RNA in the atria seems to code for the synthesis of the atrial peptides, and the fraction varies in parallel with alterations in the intake of sodium (Ballermann & Brenner, 1985).

Finally, although there must be a vast amount still to be learned about the ANPs and their physiological actions, their short history, which includes the establishment of their source and precise composition, contrasts strongly with the long and relatively inconclusive history of the earlier postulated natriuretic hormones. The ANFs appear to be hormones which employ the kidneys to regulate sodium balance in the interests of stable ECFVs and the cardio-vascular system. Their concentrations in the plasma of conscious dogs reflect physiological alterations in the ECFV (Verburg *et al.*, 1986). Clinicians are beginning to explore their role in disease, and clinical pharmacologists see them and synthetic analogues as potential sources of valuable therapeutic agents.

7.4.4.5 THE RENAL NERVES

In 1956 Homer Smith was not convinced that the thoraco-lumbar sympathetic fibers could influence tubular reabsorption of sodium directly. Eighteen years later Pitts (1974) stated that 'because of the very significant vasomotor responses that result from excitation of the renal nerves and from renal denervation in anesthetized animals, direct tubular responses to nerve impulses have not been clearly demonstrated. Many believe them to be nonexistent — a view which the author shares'. Some later writers have been more optimistic. Gottschalk (1979) concluded that efferent renal nerve stimuli increase salt and water reabsorption, and added; 'any change in GFR that might occur concurrently will only magnify the effect'. This magnification may be physiologically desirable, but it must tend to mask the sought-after tubular effects. De Wardener's insistence (de Wardener & Clarkson, 1985) on the need to exclude all other factors in attempts to demonstrate the existence of natriuretic hormones applies equally to attempts to demonstrate direct effects of the renal nerves. Burg (1981) considered that the case for direct nervous effects was still marred by apparent inconsistencies in the experimental evidence.

Skorecki & Brenner (1981) accepted that 'stimulation of the renal nerves at a level below that which causes measurable changes in renal plasma flow or glomerular filtration rate results in diminished sodium excretion'. They added that 'proximal tubule reabsorption of salt and water has also been shown to decline following denervation of the kidney, again without measurable changes

in single nephron filtration rate'. Perhaps the greatest champion of the view
that the renal nerves directly control tubular reabsorption is Gerald DiBona.
His massive review (1982) presented evidence that the renal efferent sympathetic
nerves can increase proximal tubular reabsorption of sodium via α-adrenergic
receptors stimulated by transmitters released from nerve endings in contact
with the epithelial cells. This action is in addition to any haemodynamic
effects and consequent alterations in physical factors, independent of circulating hormones, and probably important in some oedematous states and
when the dietary intake of sodium is restricted.

DiBona (1985) expanded his earlier review with special reference to the
tubular reabsorption of sodium (and the secretion of renin). His Figure 1,
however, serves to emphasize the problem of separating tubular from haemodynamic and glomerular effects in data for the whole kidney. Stimulation
of the renal sympathetic nerves of hydropenic rats at a frequency of 0.9 Hz
reduced the average rate of excretion of sodium from 1.0 to 0.3 μmol/min.
There were no *detectable* changes in RBF, or in GFR measured as the
clearance of inulin. But the lengths of the error bars showed that the average
GFR was about 1.2 ml/min with a standard deviation of the order to 10%. If
the concentration of sodium in the plasma was 140 mM, the filtered load of
sodium would have averaged 168 μmol/min, which is more than 200 times
greater than the change in rate of excretion. Hence the change which was
attributed to an increased rate of tubular reabsorption could have been
caused by a reduction of 0.5% in the GFR — smaller by an order of
magnitude than the experimental error in the measurement. The data which
showed no *measurable* (i.e. statistically significant) change cannot exclude a
change which, though statistically insignificant, might have been at least
10 times larger than was required to account for the altered rate of excretion.
A later Figure (4), showing that denervated kidneys failed to protect against
a negative sodium balance when dietary intake was restricted, appears more
convincing; despite very long error bars the cumulative balances were clearly
different. But it is still possible that the denervated kidneys excreted more
sodium partly or wholly because they failed to reduce their filtration rate in
response to the deficiency. When arguments are based on changes in the rate
of excretion of sodium in the urine, the case for a direct tubular action
depends upon the proposal that stimulation of the nerves at low rates leads to
no vasomotor changes which might reduce the filtered load or influence
tubular reabsorption through physical factors depending upon renal hae-
modynamics. There must always be an element of uncertainty while GFRs
cannot be measured with much greater precision. Unfortunately the absence
of a measurable or detectable change does not prove that no change occurs;
indeed a non-zero standard deviation implies that changes are the rule rather
than the exception.

The problem of confusion from haemodynamic factors was circumvented
by perfusing the loop of Henle (DiBona, 1985); stimulation of the renal

nerves at low frequency apparently increased the rates of reabsorption of sodium and chloride from the loop by 7 to 10%. Another unambiguous approach is to measure the effects of neurotransmitters upon reabsorption from isolated segments of renal tubules, perfused *in vitro*. Bello-Reuss (1980) reported that 10^{-6}M noradrenaline added to the bath increased the average rate of uptake of fluid by segments of rabbits' proximal convoluted tubules from 1.19 to 1.71 nl/min per mm of tubule. No effect occurred with proximal straight tubules or when the noradrenaline was presented in the luminal fluid. Reabsorption of sodium was not measured directly and no more was claimed than that the results were consistent with a physiological role for the sympathetic nervous system in modulating proximal tubular transport. Such experiments demonstrate that the renal tubules are capable of responding to neurotransmitters *in vitro*. They make it likely, but cannot absolutely prove, that they respond in the same way to transmitters released from nerve endings in the intact kidney.

This all leads to the rather unsatisfying conclusion that a direct tubular influence of the renal nerves upon the reabsorption of sodium is not improbable, and may be physiologically important; but it is not proven. Until we can be quite certain that no haemodynamic changes are produced at the same time, the tubular actions of the renal efferent nerves must remain a matter of opinion, if not a matter of faith.

7.4.4.6 MISCELLANEOUS HORMONES, PROSTAGLANDINS AND KININS

A. Parathormone

Parathormone (PTH) is extrinsic to the kidney and is principally concerned with controlling the excretion of inorganic phosphate by inhibiting its tubular reabsorption; it also inhibits the reabsorption of sodium, especially from the proximal tubules (Aurbach & Heath, 1974; Goldberg *et al.*, 1976). This secondary action appears to be mediated by cAMP, but its mechanism is not clear. Phosphate is reabsorbed from the proximal tubule partly by co-transport as an anionic partner for sodium (Section 4.3.2C); and early work showed that parathyroid extracts increased the excretion of sodium and of bicarbonate as well as of phosphate. This might however have been because the crude extracts which were then available increased GFR substantially. Micropuncture techniques and the use of pure extracts revealed the inhibition of proximal tubular reabsorption, particularly of the fraction of sodium which is reabsorbed in association with bicarbonate. In the distal nephron, where little bicarbonate remains, phosphate and sodium are handled independently and most of the extra sodium delivered to the distal nephron when proximal reabsorption is inhibited by PTH is reabsorbed from the distal tubule, while much of the phosphate is excreted. Expansion of the ECFV increases the excretion of phosphate as well as of sodium and there is some evidence that the increased excretion of phosphate may be due to increased secretion of PTH from the parathyroid glands, for it is abolished by parathyroidectomy. But there is no compelling evidence that the inhibition of proximal tubular reabsorption of sodium by PTH is an important factor in the homeostatic control of the ECFV.

B. Oestrogens and progesterone

The well-known accumulation of water and salt which occurs during pregnancy and periodically during the menstrual cycle and its modification by oral contraceptives has led to a widespread belief that these steroids somewhat resemble the adrenal steroids in promoting the retention of salt and water in the body. So many other profound changes in the background of circulating hormones are going on at these times that it is difficult to disentangle their effects and discover just how oestrogens affect the kidney. Christy & Shaver (1974) reviewed this very difficult problem and concluded that there is evidence that oestrogens can promote the retention of sodium independently of associated increases in the secretion of adrenal salt-retaining steroids; they do not at the same time enhance the excretion of potassium. Alterations in the concentrations of circulating oestrogens are often accompanied by varying concentrations of progesterone, which was also once believed to promote the retention of sodium. It now appears more likely that, at least when the kidneys are under the influence of aldosterone with which it competes, progesterone exerts a natriuretic action (Katz & Lindheimer, 1977). These gonadal hormones should probably not be regarded as major factors controlling ECFV; their actions during the reproductive cycle lead rather to temporary disturbances than to homeostatic regulation.

C. Prostaglandins

The kidney produces several prostaglandins, chiefly PGI_2 in the cortex and PGE_2 in the medulla and papilla; these probably act near the cells that synthesize them and not as circulating hormones (Lote, 1982). The cortical PGs help to maintain the renal circulation and glomerular filtration by counteracting the actions of vasoconstrictors (Section 3.3.5.3); they may contribute to the control of sodium balance by mediating the release of renin, which is important as the initiator of a sequence leading to the secretion of aldosterone (Section 7.4.3C). The medullary PGs have been credited with direct tubular contributions to the homeostasis of the body fluids.

Prostaglandins can increase the excretion of water by antagonizing the hydro-osmotic action of ADH, by interfering with the cortico-medullary osmotic gradient, and possibly also by inhibiting reabsorption of salt from the thick ascending limb of the loop of Henle (Stokes, 1981). Inhibitors of PG synthesis can reduce the excretion of water and salt without detectably altering

GFR, and on-going synthesis of PGs seems necessary for the normal excretion of sodium loads in rats and dogs; inhibition can lead to the accumulation of excess fluid. But no dramatic effects have been consistently demonstrated, and the rate of synthesis of PGs does not respond to alterations in sodium status, though this may be partly because the rate of excretion of PGs has often been used as a measure of their synthesis. Kirschenbaum & Serros (1980) classified the references they reviewed into three groups, claiming that PGs are natriuretic, that they are antinatriuretic and that they do not affect sodium transport. The most consistent data in favour of a natriuretic action followed direct injections of depressor PGs into a renal artery, but other vasodilators are natriuretic when so administered, and this is not the natural route by which renal PGs reach cells upon which they are supposed to act. Prostaglandins undoubtedly *affect* the excretion of sodium, but cannot be claimed to regulate it (Lote, 1982). Discrepancies between published reports may be due to differences in experimental procedures, as well as in the physiological state of the experimental animals. Schlondorff & Ardaillou (1986) concluded that although there is convincing evidence that PGs affect renal RBF and glomerular filtration, the concentrating mechanism and the release of renin, there is no certainty about a tubular action on the excretion of sodium chloride. They suggested that renal PGs might 'maintain the internal milieu' of cells exposed to extreme changes in their environment, leaving the functions of the tubular cells to be controlled by other factors.

D. Kallikrein and kinins

The kallikreins are proteolytic enzymes, occurring in glandular organs and in plasma, which release vasodilator peptide kinins from circulating kininogens formed in the liver. The proximal tubule is so rich in kininases and other peptidases that plasma kallikrein and circulating kinins are unlikely to reach the renal cells. But the kidney has its own glandular kallikrein, produced by cells of the distal convoluted tubules in the cortex. Infusions of saline or glucose and vasodilators which increase the excretion of sodium, increase the excretion of kallikrein in the urine; adrenalectomy reduces it. The kininogens and kinins resemble the ANPs in having precisely known primary structures, but there is no precise knowledge about their functions in the kidney. Reviews which surveyed about 240 references revealed a complicated story, full of contradictions (Fuller & Funder, 1986; Scicli & Carretero, 1986).

Like the renal PGs, the kinins probably act only within the kidneys, and not as hormones controlling renal function from outside. The renal kallikrein occurs chiefly in the apical cell membranes, with the active site facing the lumen of the distal tubules, so that it can release kinins (kallidin, i.e. lysyl-bradykinin, later degraded to bradykinin) from kininogen in the tubular fluid. The distal convoluted tubules are probably the principal sites where kinins act, as well as the only sites where they are produced. Unlike kinins infused into the renal artery, kinins introduced into the distal tubules reach the urine, but it is not easy to deduce the concentrations normally present within the kidney because kininases destroy urinary kinins along the lower urinary tract and in the bladder.

Like other vasodilators, kinins infused into the renal artery increase RBF, urine volume and the rate of excretion of sodium. They also increase the synthesis of renal PGs, and these might mediate some of their actions if kinins naturally produced within the kidney also stimulate PG synthesis. Kinins produced in the distal tubules are unlikely to reach the glomerular vessels, and they are not known to affect glomerular filtration. Unlike other vasodilators the kinins do not increase the delivery of water and salt out of the proximal tubules, but act only in the distal nephron. Their production is reduced by sodium loading and stimulated by mineralocorticoids, restricted sodium intakes, and high intakes of potassium; all of which increase the secretion of aldosterone, so that their responses to altered sodium status might be secondary to altered rates of secretion of mineralocorticoids. Co-operative relations between the kallikrein−kinin and renin−angiotensin−aldosterone systems are still debatable. There is, however, a widespread belief that the kinins somehow affect transport in the distal nephron and so form part of an intrarenal hormone system controlling the homeostasis of water and electrolytes, but no detailed mechanism has been substantiated.

E. Angiotensin II

Besides stimulating the secretion of aldosterone, AT II may directly stimulate reabsorption of sodium from the proximal tubules. Hall (1986a) suggested that this immediate, proximal action might be more important for the day to day regulation of sodium balance than the delayed, long-term effect on the cortical collecting tubules mediated by aldosterone.

7.4.5 Integrated renal control of extracellular fluid volume

Since the kidneys are agents rather than initiators of regulatory action, the question of how they work to stabilize the volume of the ECFs becomes mainly a question of how they are driven. The facile notion put forward in the first 'Reflections on Renal Function' (Robinson, 1954) that two hypo-physial hormones, ADH from the neurohypophysis and ACTH from the adenohypophysis, were the two reins used to drive the kidneys, had to be abandoned when it was realized that renin rather than ACTH controls the secretion of aldosterone. Claims by Lockett & Roberts (1963) that something from the head, possibly GH, was needed to convert an inhibitory action of aldosterone to the familiar stimulant effect upon reabsorption of sodium seemed to offer an alternative adenohypophysial rein (Robinson, 1964), but this idea has not prospered.

Some of the evidence assembled by Robinson (1954) that renal function responds appropriately to alterations in the volume and distribution of circulating blood need not be repeated here. It is necessary, however, to consider how receptors in the cardiovascular system might monitor the total volume of ECF, most of which is outside the blood vessels. A litre of water added to the body of an adult person with 40 litres of TBW, and shared between the cells and the ECFs, would increase the volume of each by 2.5%. This would add about 100 ml to the volume of blood in the vessels but the water diuresis that would remove the excess water would be largely attributable to suppression of the secretion of ADH by the fall of 2.5% in osmolality. The addition of 140 mmol of sodium chloride to the extracellular compartment, followed by drinking to correct increased osmolality, would add 1 litre of isotonic saline to the ECF. Although the partition of excesses and deficits between the blood and the interstitial part of the ECF may vary under different conditions (Gauer & Henry, 1963), the intravascular and extravascular portions of the extracellular compartment normally have a similar compliance of about 300 ml/mmHg, so that the volume of blood should change about as much as that of the extravascular portion of the ECF (Gauer et al., 1970).

The interstitial fluid outside the vessels is not freely mobile. It does not flow down into the legs when we stand up, though there is a slow redistribution which makes shaving more effective after breakfast than immediately on rising from bed (Verel, 1955). Moreover the skin adheres closely to under lying structures as though pressed against them by atmospheric pressure, so that the muscles are well demarcated. The interstitial fluid is held in a mucopolysaccharide gel (Guyton et al., 1971). One gram of hyaluronic acid can hold up to 100 ml of fluid in a loose gel which offers no appreciable resistance to diffusion, but great resistance to flow under pressure. The gel is normally unsaturated; measurements made by means of wicks or in hollow perforated capsules placed under the skin indicate that its avidity for fluid keeps the interstitial pressure about 6 mmHg below atmospheric. The existence of this so-called 'negative pressure' is no longer controversial (Brace, 1981); it is maintained by low hydrostatic pressure in the capillaries, combined with lymphatic scavenging of protein which keeps the oncotic pressure low outside them.

If enough additional fluid is added to the interstitial space to saturate the gel, the interstitial pressure reaches atmospheric and the compliance of the extravascular compartment suddenly increases about 25-fold (Guyton et al., 1971). Instead of being evenly divided between the vascular and extravascular compartments, additional fluid now appears outside the vessels as oedema which shifts freely under gravitational forces. Since the normal close proportion between the volumes of blood and total ECF ceases to hold, receptors in the vascular system can no longer monitor volume outside the vessels, and physiological control of ECFV is both severely impaired and hard to regain.

Figure 7.4 shows how this breakdown might occur in a human subject. About 3.6 litres of additional ECF could be shared between the blood and the extravascular compartment, and would saturate the interstitial gel. Any further excess fluid would be extravascular, and not signalled by a proportionate increase in the volume of blood. This is in agreement with the common observation that it takes about 4 litres of excess ECF to produce clinically evident generalized oedema. Since the blood vessels normally contain less than 4 litres of plasma, such oedema cannot be produced merely by shifting fluid out of the vessels. Transfer of all the fluid out of the plasma into the tissue spaces would be fatal, but survival with oedema requires continual replenishment of fluid which leaves the vessels. It depends ultimately upon excessive reabsorption of sodium chloride by the kidneys, for oedema fluid can no more be made without salt than the biblical bricks without straw. The retained salt excites thirst and secretion of ADH, so that water is ingested and retained with the salt to make isotonic fluid. Hence the salt and water that accumulate as oedema, like excess food destined to be stored as fat, enter the body through the mouth.

The amount of circulating plasma protein should be an important factor determining the volume of the blood and the distribution of fluid between the vascular system and the interstitial compartment. Continuous production of plasma proteins by the liver makes up for metabolic and other losses, but

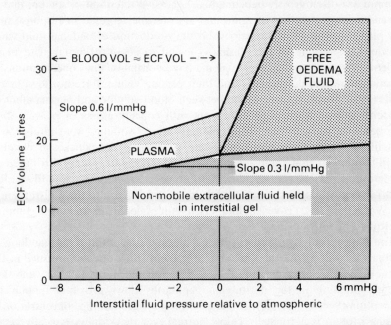

Fig. 7.4 The breakdown of the relation between plasma volume and total volume of ECF when interstitial gel becomes saturated. (Based on a figure by Guyton *et al.*, 1971, with figures modified to human orders of magnitude.)

little or nothing is known about how the rate of production and the total amount in the body are regulated. An adult man has about 500 g of plasma protein; 3 litres of plasma at 70 g/l hold 210 g; hence more than half the 'plasma' protein is actually outside the blood vessels, in the interstitial fluid, at a concentration of 20 to 30 g/l. About 10 g of albumin escapes from the capillaries every hour (Renkin, 1986), and a similar amount is returned by the lymphatic system, which carries new protein from the liver as well as protein scavenged from tissue spaces.

In so far as the oncotic pressure of the plasma proteins opposes the hydrostatic pressure of blood in the capillaries in the dynamic Starling equilibrium, and so keeps the water and low molecular solutes of the plasma inside the vessels, the volume of the plasma should be proportional to the amount of circulating protein. However, large alterations in the amount of protein can exist for long periods without the expected changes in plasma volume (Manning & Guyton, 1982). Moderate lowering of the oncotic pressure of the plasma leads to a temporary shift of fluid from the plasma into the interstitial space, which is later reversed by a comparable fall in the oncotic pressure of the interstitial fluid (Dorhout Mees *et al.*, 1984). Patients with nephrotic syndromes can lose so much albumin through their leaky glomerular membranes that the liver cannot supply enough to maintain a normal concentration in the plasma, and those with low concentrations of circulating albumin are often grossly oedematous. Excessive retention of sodium due to increased concentrations of renin and aldosterone secreted in response to a low plasma volume may contribute to the production of oedema fluid when the oncotic pressure of the plasma is less than about 10 mmHg. But many patients who are accumulating oedema have normal or low concentrations of plasma renin and aldosterone, and their plasma volumes are not low. Geers *et al.* (1984) found no correlation between blood volume and plasma albumin concentration in 60 nephrotic patients with concentrations of plasma albumin between 10 and 27 g/l. These patients' blood volumes were rarely lower and often higher than normal, despite substantial deficiencies in circulating albumin, so that their retention of sodium could not be attributed to depletion of plasma volume; they had, however, remarkably low FFs (13 to 15%) which would be consistent with some undefined intrarenal disturbance. De Wardener (1985) gave a helpful discussion of nephrotic and other common clinical forms of oedema.

The concentration of protein in the plasma affects the renal handling of sodium, as well as the total amount of protein. Low oncotic pressure in the glomerular capillaries favours faster filtration (Section 3.2.3.3), and low oncotic pressure in the peritubular capillaries slows proximal tubular reabsorption (Section 7.4.4.3). In the nephrotic syndrome, the concentration of plasma protein is chronically below normal, yet the kidneys typically retain too much sodium in the body. The circulating protein is also deficient in amount, however, and the kidneys are not normal. Temporary reductions in the concentration of plasma protein under otherwise normal circumstances do promote the excretion of sodium. O'Connor (1977) established that infusions of isotonic saline solutions into normal dogs were followed by increased rates of excretion of sodium which could be fully accounted for by increased rates of glomerular filtration associated with the reduced concentration of plasma proteins. He regarded the concentration of protein in the plasma as a very important factor controlling the excretion of sodium, and proposed that in the normal range of sodium intake, sodium excretion and plasma composition, the modulation of glomerular filtration by the oncotic pressure of the plasma would be sufficient to maintain sodium balance despite fluctuations in intake. Manning & Guyton (1982) pointed out that O'Connor's experiments lasting several hours did not allow time for alterations in oncotic pressure to extend to the interstitial fluid, so that the mechanism he proposed might be more suitable for correcting acute disturbances in the ECFV than for its long-term regulation.

7.4.5.1 PROTECTION OF BLOOD AND EXTRACELLULAR FLUID VOLUMES IN FACE OF LOSS OF WATER

Loss of water without solute increases osmolality and reduces the volumes of plasma, ECFs and ICFs approximately in proportion to their initial volumes. Thirst and the secretion of ADH are stimulated until enough water is replaced to correct the increase in osmolality; if no solutes have been lost or gained, this will restore the original volumes. If water is not replaced, haemoconcentration, with increasing oncotic pressure, tends immediately to reduce filtration and promote tubular reabsorption of sodium. Reduced discharge from cardiac receptors augments the release of ADH. The greater sympathetic discharge to the heart, blood vessels and kidney, that is required to maintain systemic arterial pressure with a smaller volume of blood, may immediately reduce filtration a little, and may also directly promote tubular reabsorption of sodium. It also increases the secretion of renin which, in physiological doses, may promote the proximal reabsorption of sodium immediately and directly (Schuster, 1986). More importantly, however, it stimulates the secretion of aldosterone (Section 7.4.3), which promotes a delayed increase in reabsorption of sodium downstream. Increasing reabsorption of sodium permits more complete reabsorption of water and augments the osmotic stimulation of thirst and release of ADH.

The traditional teaching that loss of water leads to avid retention of salt despite increasing osmolality and plasma sodium concentration (the 'dehydration reaction' which Peters (1950) attributed to activation of the adrenal cortex in response to the reduced volume of body fluid) needs some qualification. Rats, rabbits, sheep and dogs (even when depleted by diets poor in sodium) may greatly increase their urinary excretion of sodium when they are first deprived of water and so experience a smaller initial increase in osmolality (Merrill *et al.*, 1986). Circulating ADH and plasma renin increase appropriately, but there is an unexplained fall in secretion of aldosterone in spite of rising AT II, which may underlie the increased excretion of sodium because infusions of aldosterone can prevent the 'natriuresis of dehydration'. If water is supplied during this phase, therefore lowering the concentration of sodium in the plasma, the concentration of aldosterone increases and sodium is retained to repair the earlier loss (Ramsay, 1985). If access to water is still restricted, however, aldosterone is secreted as expected and the traditional dehydration reaction sets in after a day or two. Sodium is then avidly retained and potassium excreted; increasing osmolality maintains thirst and the secretion of ADH, while water leaves the cells to accompany retained sodium and sustain the volumes of the ECF and the circulating blood.

7.4.5.2 RESPONSE TO LOSS OF ISOTONIC FLUIDS INCLUDING BLOOD

These may be considered together, for there is no significant change in osmolality. Peters' (1952) statement that the kidneys are indifferent to the ECFV outside the blood vascular system is less pessimistic than it might appear. While the relationship between the volumes of the intravascular and extravascular portions of the ECF remains normal (Fig. 7.4), deficits of ECF reduce the volume of blood, and so can be monitored by receptors in the cardiovascular system.

The receptors in the central thoracic veins and the chambers of the heart are well placed to monitor changes in the volume of blood, and it would be convenient if their rates of discharge controlled the excretion of sodium. There is good evidence that they subserve reflex adjustments of the rate of secretion of ADH, which failed to occur in patients with allografted (and therefore denervated) hearts (Drieu *et al.*, 1986). But they do not seem to affect glomerular filtration, or the secretion of aldosterone which promotes the reabsorption of sodium (Linden & Kappagoda, 1982). In his last detailed examination of the problem, Homer Smith (1957) was convinced that reflexes from the left atrium control the output of ADH. But no receptor responding to volume and controlling the excretion of sodium could be defined; and, although retention of sodium gathers in water through the osmoregulatory mechanisms, retention of water does nothing to promote the conservation of sodium.

The other relevant receptors are the high-pressure arterial baroreceptors in the carotid sinus and the arch of the aorta. Small reductions in blood volume without a fall in blood pressure should not permanently reduce the discharge from these receptors; but the general increase in sympathetic tone to the heart and blood vessels that is needed to maintain blood pressure leads to increased efferent traffic in the renal sympathetic nerves. Even if moderately increased sympathetic activity has little effect on the GFR (Section 7.4.2), it may promote the reabsorption of sodium directly, as well as by stimulating the secretion of renin. Larger losses of blood call for greater sympathetic activity, which, with a falling perfusion pressure when blood pressure cannot be maintained, reduces GFR so that less sodium is filtered; and the arrival of less sodium at the macula densa augments the secretion of renin. Thus, retention of sodium might be related indirectly to the tightness of the vessels, which must be increased to maintain arterial pressure with a smaller volume of blood, rather than to the fullness of the circulation signalled by the cardiac receptors. The scheme presented by Gauer & Henry (1963) showed that larger losses of blood were needed to mobilize aldosterone than ADH.

Physical activity and changes of posture are departures from Homer Smith's (1956) ideal state of comfortably relaxed recumbent rest (Section 3.3.4.3A, 1 & 2), and are accompanied by temporary reductions in the rate of excretion of sodium and water. During exercise the flow of blood is diverted away from the kidneys to active muscles and the GFR is reduced. Renal sympathetic tone is also increased with changes from recumbency, and if a vertical posture is maintained without muscular activity, net efflux from capillaries in lower parts of the body reduces the volume of plasma and increases the concentration of the plasma proteins. The greater oncotic pressure may then reduce glomerular filtration further, and also enhance the tubular reabsorption of sodium (Section 7.4.4.3).

7.4.5.3 RESPONSES TO EXCESSES OF FLUID

Excess water dilutes and expands all the body fluids, and is corrected primarily by water diuresis through the osmoregulatory system (Section 7.2). Increased volumes of blood, alone or accompanying isotonic expansion of the ECF, lead to a natriuresis which removes ECF from the body. This saline diuresis results from the combined effects of dilution of plasma protein, increased peritubular capillary pressure, increased GFR, inhibition of sympathetic tone, and diminished secretion of renin. It may be augmented by third factors (Section 7.4.4) and by the release of ANPs from distended atria (Section 7.4.4.4), possibly also by a natriuretic hormone from an unknown source (Section 7.4.4.2). The effects of some of these factors were only demonstrable unequivocally with large, rapid increases in ECFV; but if smaller disturbances induce small changes in the same direction, these should work together to remove excess sodium and water from the body, and to restore normal volumes of body fluids.

7.4.5.4 'MINERALOCORTICOID ESCAPE'

It has been known for several decades that prolonged secretion or administration of large amounts of mineralocorticoids leads to a sustained loss of potassium in the urine, but only to a transient reduction in the rate of urinary excretion of sodium, which catches up with intake again after a few days. Primary aldosteronism from aldosterone-secreting tumours is marked by excessive urinary excretion of potassium and symptoms associated with a low concentration of potassium in the plasma; there is usually hypertension but not oedema (Williams *et al.*, 1977). The escape of renal retention of sodium after initial stimulation by salt-retaining steroids demonstrates that the mechanisms involved in volume homeostasis need not all work in the same direction. The escape seems to be confined to renal handling of sodium, for renal excretion of potassium is still enhanced and the concentration of sodium in the sweat is low. The initial retention of sodium increases the ECFV somewhat, and a small increase in the GFR could compensate for the increased tubular re-absorption without the aid of any other factor. 'Third factors' might also help the kidney to escape from the salt-retaining effects of aldosterone in patients with secreting tumours who do not develop oedema. But they fail to effect escape in secondary hyperaldosteronism, when cardiac failure or other conditions preclude an increase in GFR, and the patients are often oedematous.

Knox *et al.* (1980) reviewed many possible mechanisms of escape, and concluded that no single one of these could by itself provide a satisfactory explanation. Escape can occur without an increase in GFR, even when this is experimentally reduced. It cannot be attributed solely to changes in proximal tubular reabsorption or the amount delivered from the proximal tubules, to alterations in concentration of plasma protein, to other physical factors, to the renin–angiotensin system, to the renal PGs or to a natriuretic hormone. Atrial natriuretic peptides were naturally not considered, but it is doubtful whether they could be solely responsible. One problem is that experimental conditions which eliminate or exaggerate the contribution of one factor leave others free to compensate for the disturbance. Many patients with aldosteronism are hypertensive, and the increased arterial blood pressure, combined with renal vasodilatation, might increase the excretion of sodium. Romero *et al.* (1985) considered that reduced activity of the renal sympathetic nerves is itself an important factor. Mineralocorticoid escape remains an interesting but unexplained phenomenon and a reminder that multiple factors control the excretion of sodium.

7.4.5.5 THE QUESTION OF A SET POINT

After mineralocorticoid escape has been established, the body settles for a somewhat increased sodium content and a somewhat greater ECFV. The normal sodium content and ECFV which the homeostatic mechanisms are set to maintain appear to be determined in some way by habitual intake of sodium. Thus, a few days after the daily intake is abruptly increased by, say, 20 mmol, the urinary output increases by the same amount. The body then comes into balance again, with the somewhat larger sodium content and ECFV that are needed to achieve the greater rate of excretion — much as during mineralocorticoid escape. Similarly, if customary intake is reduced, it takes a few days for output to be correspondingly reduced and a new steady state established. Hollenberg (1980) was struck by the observation that a normal man who had lost 300 mmol of sodium in the course of attaining a state of balance on a low daily intake of 10 mmol rapidly excreted 30 mmol given inadvertently in an infusion — instead of avidly retaining it to repair his presumed deficit. This is not an isolated observation; Strauss *et al.* (1958) reported similar responses in a group of 10 normal subjects given 15 mmol of sodium when adapted to a daily intake of 5 mmol. The body thus preserved its lowered sodium status instead of guarding the original ECFV. However, if a further 100 mmol of sodium was removed by means of a diuretic, without time being allowed to adapt to the increased deficit, infused sodium up to a total of 100 mmol was retained until the augmented deficit was corrected.

One interpretation would be that the steady state reached on the low intake of sodium had become accepted as 'normal'; an unexpected bonus of 30 mmol was then treated as a surplus and promptly excreted, while a suddenly imposed further loss was treated as a deficit requiring correction. This would imply that the levels maintained by the homeostatic mechanisms were not fixed but were adapted to the habitual daily intake of sodium. The rate of excretion could be matched to a different current intake after a delay of a few days. Greater intakes would require greater rates of excretion, and the stimulus for these might be derived in some way from the increased body content and ECFV.

Hollenberg (1980) argued that there is a true, fixed set point — a sodium content and its corresponding ECFV below which the homeostatic mechanisms react to a true or absolute deficit. This set point is the amount of sodium in the body when balance has been achieved on a zero intake (which implies also zero extrarenal losses). Strauss *et al.* (1958) also considered that normal people who are excreting salt cannot strictly be said to be depleted. The fact that people normally operate considerably above the set point would readily explain why reducing the daily intake of sodium often fails to increase the secretion of aldosterone. The concept of a fixed set point was, however, challenged and debated but without agreement about what appear to be two alternative ways of describing what happens. Bonventre & Leaf (1982) preferred the notion of a number of interlocking mechanisms, each with its own set point, cooperating to permit a succession of steady states. On either view, the sodium content of the body and the ECFV are ultimately adjusted to make the rate of urinary excretion equal to the intake of sodium over periods of a day or more. Strauss *et al.* (1958) suggested that the stimulus required to increase the rate of excretion and regain metabolic balance with greater intakes comes from some function of the sodium content of the body and ECFV. An analysis of published results from a dozen studies of human subjects showed remarkably similar increases or decreases of about 13 mmol in body content for each 10 mmol step in daily sodium intake, and an average half-time of 21 hours for the change to a new steady state (Walser, 1985). Hence there is probably no rigidly fixed, 'normal' body content, and the actual amount of sodium in the body depends upon the customary intake.

7.4.5.6 SUMMARY OF SODIUM EXCRETION AND ITS CONTROL

The main points of what has become a lengthy and sometimes diffuse and inconclusive narrative can be illustrated conveniently by Fig. 7.5 (Bray *et al.*, 1986) which summarizes the principal glomerular and tubular mechanisms which have been discussed. More mechanisms than one are commonly employed to achieve any important physiological end, and the control of the urinary excretion of sodium is a typical example of Barcroft's (1934) notion that 'every adaptation is an integration'. The paramount importance of glomerular filtration is not generally recognized (Section 7.4.2), and no other single mechanism should be regarded as *the* mechanism which determines sodium balance. The round figures illustrating the contributions of different segments of the nephron are approximate and intended only to give an impression of orders of magnitude. Minor differences from corresponding figures in the text and elsewhere are not important — except as a reminder that the quantities they represent are, after all, variables.

Each day over 25 000 mmol of sodium is delivered to the renal tubules by glomerular filtration; this quantity can be reduced very quickly by reflex mechanisms involved in vasomotor homeostasis. About two thirds of the normal daily load of filtered sodium is reabsorbed by the proximal tubules; this quantity also can be quickly reduced, by so-called 'third factors' if the ECFV is suddenly expanded. Over 6000 mmol is reabsorbed each day from the loops of Henle, and most of what remains is reabsorbed from the distal tubules and the collecting system. This last component of reabsorption, especially that part of it which is located in the cortical collecting tubules, is subject to a slowly developing, long-term enhancement by aldosterone which is synthesized and released from the adrenal cortex after renin from the kidney has caused AT II to appear in the blood (Fig. 7.2). Only the small fraction of filtered sodium that escapes these phases of reabsorption remains to be excreted in the urine.

Figure 7.5 serves to emphasize the relatively large role of the autonomic nervous system in controlling the excretion of sodium, even if the renal nerves do not control tubular reabsorption directly. Both the neurogenic reduction in glomerular filtration and the release of renin which will increase the reabsorption of sodium downstream are subject to control by brisk reflexes arising from the cardiovascular system — though some distal adjustments are delayed by the slow action of aldosterone. In so far as homeostatic control of the ECFV serves to maintain the circulation of the blood, the regulation of sodium balance from monitors in the vascular tree is singularly

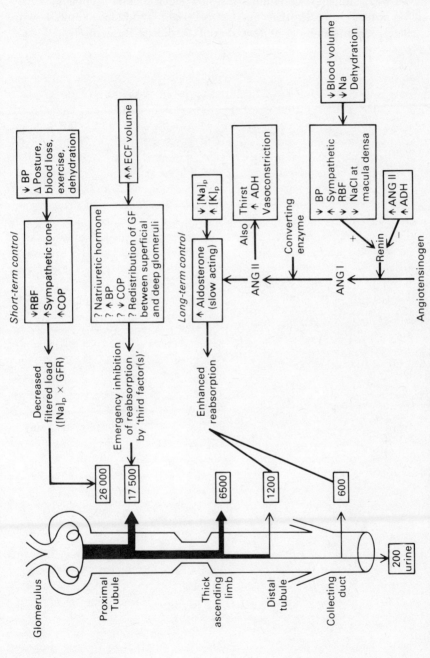

Fig. 7.5 A summary of the control of sodium handling by the kidneys in man. Quantities are in mmol per day.

appropriate. But many details still remain to be clarified and, until it is known what ultimately determines just how much sodium is enough, it may still be prudent to accept that 'one fact is certain. The kidney knows how to regulate sodium excretion, and we do not' (Orloff & Burg, 1971).

CHAPTER 8
Adaptation and regulation of renal function

8.1 INTRODUCTION

This chapter replaces the earlier Epilogue and an unsatisfying chapter on the regulation of renal function (Robinson, 1954). Since the kidneys process some 1800 litres of blood each day and control the quality and quantity of the plasma and of the ECFs in equilibrium with it, they might be expected to respond directly to alterations in the composition of the blood and indirectly to alterations in the quantities of blood and ECF. In fact, some important renal adjustments to altered composition of the blood are indirect, and renal functions also need to be modified to adapt to environmental influences as well as to respond to acute or chronic disturbances arising from physical activities.

Remote stimuli, external to the body, elicit alterations in renal functions by means of internal changes, and the final renal responses depend upon intrinsic determinants of renal function operating within the kidneys; these are the final common paths for regulating glomerular filtration and the functioning of segments of renal tubules. It will be convenient first to outline some of the principal stimuli that affect the kidneys, then to attempt to define the intrinsic determinants of renal function upon which extrinsic stimuli impinge to produce their integrated results and finally to examine some features of the ways in which the controls operate. The kidney's functional responses to remote and immediate stimuli may be categorized as: (1) inevitable; (2) automatic; and (3) indirectly controlled, or adjusted. Mechanisms which have been discussed in earlier chapters can be dismissed briefly with appropriate back-references.

Stimuli which modify renal function range from remote factors, wholly or partly external to the body, to internal factors including properties of the blood that flows into the kidneys. The most remote are environmental and climatic factors which affect the availability of particular nutrients. These may be bulk components of the diet like common foodstuffs and water; elements like calcium, iron, copper; or essential micronutrients like vitamins and trace elements — for one example, selenium, which appears to be handled more thriftily by the kidneys of New Zealanders who live off selenium-poor soils than by those of Americans whose environmental supplies, dietary intakes and body contents are several times greater (Robinson *et al.*, 1985). National customs, personal habits and patterns of physical activity affect the intakes of local foods, salt and water, as well as rates of loss by extrarenal channels, and leave the kidneys to make appropriate adjustments.

More immediate factors, internal to the body but still extrinsic to the kidney, are metabolic patterns dependent upon growth, ageing, physical activity, and current and recent absorption of foodstuffs, water, and foreign substances including drugs. These affect the rates of production of urea and other waste products and the concentrations of metabolic substrates and intermediates in the blood; these concentrations are also affected by diseases which disturb metabolism. Meanwhile posture, physical activity and the intake of food and water affect the volume, pressure and distribution of the blood and are accompanied by rapidly changing patterns of autonomic nervous activity which control the cardiovascular system and flow on to the kidney, though their effects upon the renal circulation are often surprisingly small (Section 2.2.8).

From the point of view of the kidney the immediate extrinsic factors are the blood pressure, what might be called the quality of the blood (its composition, including osmolality, oncotic pressure, pH, the partial pressures of respiratory gases), and circulating hormones; all of which can in principle act directly inside the kidneys. The volumes of blood and of ECF act indirectly through haemodynamic changes, hormones and the efferent renal nerves. The intrinsic renal factors through which all these operate are the determinants of glomerular and of renal tubular function (Sections 8.2, 8.3). Meanwhile the self-regulating mechanisms which link these two sets of determinants and underlie glomerulotubular balance and tubuloglomerular feedback help to maintain the kidneys' autonomy despite alterations in cardiovascular function. The extent to which the various determinants of glomerular and tubular function are involved together in adaptations to different circumstances emphasizes the great interdependence of the kidney's vascular and secretory organs (Section 1.3).

8.2 DETERMINANTS OF GLOMERULAR FUNCTION

Brenner and his group developed four 'determinants of glomerular filtration', linking extrinsic factors to the rate of filtration in each individual glomerulus (Section 3.3.5.2). These are (1) the filtration coefficient K_f; (2) the difference in pressure, P', between glomerular capillaries and Bowman's space; (3) the oncotic pressure, π_A; and, usually most important, (4) the rate of flow, Q_A, of afferent arteriolar plasma. Since K_f includes the area as well as the hydraulic conductivity of the glomerular filter, it is appropriate to add a further determinant of whole-kidney GFR: (5) the number of glomeruli; though this is more of pathological than of physiological relevance.

The most immediate extrinsic agents working through the intrinsic determinants which control glomerular filtration are the efferent renal nerves and the incoming blood. The nerves supply glomerular arterioles (affecting primarily determinants 4, 2, and possibly 1); they also stimulate the secretion of renin from the juxtaglomerular cells. The blood carries vasomotor hormones like catecholamines, AT, and ANFs, which may back up or modulate the actions of the autonomic nerves on the kidney's vessels; its oncotic pressure is important in its own right (determinant 3); its viscosity and haematocrit (PCV) may influence glomerular filtration through other determinants; and its pressure, transmitted to the afferent arterioles, may directly affect the release of renin as well as glomerular plasma flow (4) and filtration.

8.3 DETERMINANTS OF TUBULAR FUNCTION

Intrinsic determinants of tubular functions (reabsorptive, secretory and synthetic) are more complex than the relatively simple physical determinants of glomerular filtration because of the far greater heterogeneity of the tubules and their activities. The kidney is not only a collection of more or less similar nephrons; it is also an organized community of many kinds of cells. The most important functional components of the renal tubules are their epithelial cells, specialized for the transcellular transport of water and a variety of solutes, and arranged in parallel between the lumen and the interior of the body. The most obvious function of these cells is reabsorption; they are bathed on the luminal side by a filtrate containing substances to be reabsorbed, and supplied with oxygen from peritubular blood on the basal side where their major energy-requiring 'pumps' are located. The peritubular blood also takes up the reabsorbed fluid, and the rate of uptake affects the net rate of reabsorption through its effects upon physical forces and back-diffusion (Section 7.4.4.3). Besides reabsorption and the secretion of some substances into the urine, the tubular epithelial cells have important metabolic functions, including the synthesis of hormones and of some constituents of the blood and of the urine (Section 4.5).

Hence the determinants of tubular function include:

1 Properties and numbers of the epithelial cells. Differences between proximal tubules, loops of Henle, distal tubules, and collecting tubules, which are also epithelial, have been mentioned in earlier sections. Sophisticated histochemical techniques which can locate specific enzymes have filled in details of the component cells (Kinne & Schwartz, 1978; Guder & Ross, 1984), and Morel (1983) has applied micromethods for adenyl cyclase to indicate the sites of action of hormones which use cAMP as a messenger. Studies of isolated, cultured tubular epithelial cells may lead to greater understanding in the next decade. Such simplified systems reveal some of the things that renal cells can (or cannot) do under restricted experimental conditions, but may not fully account for their functioning in the intact kidney.

It is becoming increasingly recognized that some specialized functions are not performed by the tubular cells in general, but by special cells located in particular segments of the tubules. Moreover, the properties and distribution of these cells are not invariable. A few examples will illustrate how their capacities and numbers may vary during adaptation to chronic demands.

Potassium was, until fairly recently, supposed to be reabsorbed principally by the proximal tubules, and secreted by distal tubules. It now seems that at least four distinct cells are involved in handling potassium. Most of the filtered potassium is ordinarily reabsorbed by cells lining the proximal tubules, but the cells of the thick ascending limbs of the loops of Henle share in this activity and the notion of distal handling has been greatly refined. Secretion of potassium into the urine appears to be the function of two groups of cells — the principal cells of the connecting tubule and intercalated cells in the initial collecting tubule which develop a greater area of basolateral membrane in rats adapted to a high intake of potassium (Stanton *et al.*, 1981; Section 4.4.4). Depletion of potassium, however, led to a three-fold increase in the luminal membrane area, with an increased density of rod-shaped particles, presumably associated with transport, in some intercalated cells in the medullary collecting ducts of rats; these cells appear to be responsible for a late phase of active reabsorption mobilized when potassium is scarce (Stetson *et al.*, 1980; Section 4.3.4). Recirculation among currents and countercurrents may further complicate the handling of potassium (Jamison, 1987).

The carbonic anhydrase-rich cells capable of secreting protons and bicarbonate, described by Steinmetz (1986), were mentioned in Section 6.3. Diamond (1985) commented that the cortical collecting duct of the rabbit possesses a 'reversible epithelium' in the sense that it can secrete either bicarbonate or protons into the lumen during alkalosis or acidosis, as the population of carbonic anhydrase-rich cells alternates between the α-type and the β-type. This adaptation depends upon remarkably rapid changes in the numbers of cells, the area of the secreting membrane, and the density of its rod-shaped particles, in response to variations in carbon dioxide tension, bicarbonate, and pH (cf. Section 6.3.2). As with potassium, attainable rates of secretion probably depend more on numbers of pump sites than of cells.

Adaptive responses to varying demand also occur in the proximal convoluted tubules. A sustained increase in the GFR leads to an increased area of basolateral membrane in the proximal tubular cells, which may be the first stage in the development of tubular hypertrophy (Fine, 1986; Section 3.3.4.2).

Hence a number of distinct functions; routine reabsorption of sodium and potassium by cells of the proximal tubules and of the thick ascending limbs of the loops of Henle, emergency distal reabsorption of potassium, secretion of potassium, secretion of protons, and secretion of bicarbonate; are attributable to the proximal tubular cells and to several other distinct and morphologically recognizable types of cells. In the proximal tubule, with its leaky epithelium, active reabsorption of sodium provides the driving force for co-transport of many other solutes which are not handled independently (Sections 4.2, 4.3), as well as for the countertransport of protons against small electrochemical gradients which effects the 'reabsorption' of much of the filtered bicarbonate (Section 6.3.1). The lining of the proximal tubules is sufficiently permeable to water to permit the almost isotonic reabsorption of the bulk of the glomerular filtrate, and also sufficiently permeable to some solutes for anions to follow transported cations and for passive back-flux to affect net rates of transport (Giebisch, 1978; Rector, 1983). The more specialized cells that have been mentioned are confined to the tight epithelium of the distal nephron, where individual solutes are handled independently, and fine adjustments are made to the relatively small volume of tubular fluid left over after bulk reabsorption upstream.

To the extent that they share changes in other parts of the body, the composition and pH of the kidney's ICFs may be important determinants of renal responses to systemic disturbances. Some earlier doubts about the major importance of systemic acid–base status as a determinant of renal acid secretion during metabolic acidosis were resolved by Madias & Zelman (1986); and Al-Awqati (1985) emphasized the role of carbon dioxide and intracellular acidity as mediators of adaptive cellular changes in respiratory disturbances. The adaptive changes promoting secretion or reabsorption of potassium might depend upon the concentration of potassium in the renal cells (Stetson *et al.*, 1980). The simple idea (Section 6.4) that renal cells depleted of potassium are abnormally acid and secrete protons into the urine in preference to potassium must be abandoned if protons and potassium are secreted by different cells.

2   Energy supplies, including fuel and oxygen, may become limiting factors under unfavourable conditions, but are probably not important variables for physiological adjustment.

3   Supplies of substrates. These depend upon the circulation and the composition of the blood. They are rarely limiting factors because the blood supply of the kidneys is so much greater than their needs; but they are important determinants of metabolic activities of the kidney (Section 4.5).

4   Supplies of filtrate, more specifically, of filtered solutes. Under physiological conditions with normal kidneys, these depend upon the determinants of glomerular filtration and are more than adequate, like the RBF. The effect of chronically increased GFR upon the area of basolateral membrane in proximal tubular cells was mentioned under (1) above. The essential factor for this, as for more rapid responses to acute changes, is filtered load rather than GFR as such, and some solutes affect the reabsorption of others. For example, bicarbonate and co-transported glucose and amino acids promote the proximal tubular reabsorption of sodium. Hence the extra load of sodium due to an increase in GFR is better handled than an additional load due to a greater concentration of sodium chloride in the plasma (Langberg *et al.*, 1986). With a constant GFR, urea is excreted at a rate proportional to its concentration in the plasma; if GFR falls, the load and rate of excretion can be maintained by a greater concentration in the plasma (Section 4.2.1). Filtered loads set upper limits to possible rates of reabsorption. The filtered

load of glucose is less than the tubules can normally reabsorb, so that glucose does not appear in the urine; but it fails to be reabsorbed completely if the load is sufficiently increased (Section 4.2.2).

5 The rate of flow of tubular fluid. The rate at which a substance is secreted should be proportional to the concentration maintained by the secreting cells and to the rate at which the tubular fluid flows past them. Stimulation of the tubular secretion of potassium by the delivery of more sodium into the distal tubule is now attributed to the associated greater flow of tubular fluid rather than to the presence of more sodium to exchange (Field & Giebisch, 1985; Section 4.4.4C). The rate of excretion of ammonium generated in the kidney depends in part upon the partition between tubular urine and blood, which gives strongly acid urines an advantage to offset the far greater RBF (Section 4.4.4E). When this advantage was removed by making the urine slightly alkaline (pH 7.6 to 8.2) the rate of excretion of ammonium increased with the flow of urine up to more than 10 ml/min during water diuresis (Macknight *et al.*, 1962). The rate of excretion of ammonium was also proportional to minute volume during acidosis if the flow of urine was small enough (Richterich, 1962). Since substantial alterations in the flow of tubular fluid during water diuresis are confined to the collecting ducts, the increased rate of excretion of ammonium during water diuresis might be due in part to washing out ammonium from the medulla, similar to the washing out of urea discussed in Section 5.5.3. But even in steady states, more filtered urea is excreted when the final volume of urine (and hence the rate of flow through terminal portions of the nephrons) is greater (Section 4.2.2).

6 Physical factors. Factors including arterial blood pressure, the hydrostatic and oncotic pressures of plasma in peritubular capillaries, and renal interstitial pressure influence the uptake of reabsorbed fluid and probably affect net rates of proximal tubular reabsorption by altering the geometry and permeability of the paracellular pathways (Section 7.4.4.3). The phenomenon of pressure diuresis (faster excretion of water and salt when arterial perfusion pressure is increased) has been known for more than a century; it may help to control systemic arterial blood pressure. This diuresis cannot be explained solely by increased GFR and must depend partly upon a reduced rate of reabsorption, which is probably determined by physical factors (Hall, 1986b). Incompletely defined physical factors probably also contribute to the 'third factors' which can powerfully inhibit the proximal tubular reabsorption of sodium and water when the ECFV is expanded (Section 7.4.4).

7 Nerves. Although Homer Smith (1957) 'set aside as without adequate foundation the belief that the renal nerves play any role in the control of sodium excretion beyond those effects which may issue from changes in vasomotor activity', the possibility that stimulation of the renal sympathetic nerves promotes the proximal tubular reabsorption of sodium has not been abandoned (Section 7.4.4.5).

8 Hormones. Although some hormones discussed in earlier sections are primarily vasomotor and affect glomerular filtration, others, notably vasopressin (Section 5.5.3, 5.4), aldosterone (Section 7.3.3) and possible natriuretic hormones (Section 7.4.4.2) act on the tubular epithelium. Besides its major action in promoting the tubular reabsorption of calcium beyond the loop of Henle (Section 4.3.3), PTH has an important function in the proximal tubules, where it stimulates production of the biologically active, hormonal form of vitamin D_3 (Section 1.1).

9 Other constituents of the blood. These include: pH and partial pressure of carbon dioxide, bicarbonate and chloride, which affect the secretion of hydrogen ions; osmotic diuretics and other inhibitors of transport which interfere with the reabsorption of sodium; the concentration of potassium, which affects its secretion directly by affecting its uptake into the secreting cells, and may also mediate chronic changes in intracellular potassium which lead to adaptive changes in the special secreting and reabsorbing cells; concentrations of calcium and of inorganic phosphate — low concentrations stimulate production of the active form of vitamin D directly as well as indirectly by mobilizing PTH; the oncotic pressure of glomerular efferent blood in peritubular capillaries, which affects the uptake of reabsorbed fluid and may contribute to GTB and to the action of 'third factors'; and partial pressure of oxygen which affects the secretion of erythropoietin (Section 1.1).

These determinants of tubular function are not wholly independent. For example, supplies of filtrate (4), depend upon the composition of the blood (9) as well as upon the GFR set by the determinants of glomerular function. Concentrations of hormones might have been included among constituents of the blood; but they merit special listing as transmitters of stimuli rather than as major constituents whose concentrations are to be regulated. Supplies of substrates (3) could be regarded simply as products of GFR and their concentrations in the blood (9); the separate heading is a reminder that they are often products of other organs, such as the liver and muscles. Most of the nine determinants can be important for controlling tubular reabsorption; 1 to 3 and 5 to 9 seem most important for secretory, and 1, 8 and 9 for synthetic functions of the kidneys.

8.4 REGULATION OF RENAL FUNCTION

Besides mediating the control of the kidney by extrinsic factors, the determinants of glomerular and of tubular function contribute to two intrinsic mechanisms which link the magnitudes of glomerular filtration and bulk tubular reabsorption. These could not be wholly independent; reabsorption would be impossible without prior filtration; and glomerular filtration without reabsorption would be self-limiting, for all the ECF would be lost in a few hours and the pressure available for filtration would fall to zero. Glomerulo-tubular balance and TGFB help to keep the rates of filtration and bulk reabsorption well matched in each individual nephron (Sections 2.2.7; 3.3.5.3; 7.4.4). The most important determinant for GTB is probably the oncotic pressure of efferent glomerular plasma perfusing the peritubular capillaries; the loss of more filtrate leaves the plasma more concentrated and promotes the uptake of reabsorbed fluid. The flow of afferent arteriolar plasma and the rate of flow of tubular fluid into the distal tubule are probably most important for TGFB. Although there is still doubt about the most important solute, the 'data point to an influence of tubular flow rate at the macula densa on the vascular tone of the afferent arteriole' (Schnermann *et al.*, 1980). It is therefore important the ADH affects the rate of flow of tubular fluid only beyond the macula densa. Renal arterial pressure as such appears less important.

There are other links between glomerular and tubular activity which are not so direct or wholly internal to the kidney. When activity of the renal efferent nerves, circulating catecholamines, and alterations in tension in the walls of the glomerular afferent arterioles reduce the GFR, they also initiate a long, delayed loop by stimulating the secretion of renin from juxtaglomerular cells into the general circulation. The AT II thus generated stimulates the suprarenal glands to secrete aldosterone which enhances the reabsorption of sodium from the distal nephron — again beyond the macula densa (Section 7.4.3). The direct links operating within the kidney serve mainly to match filtered loads of water and solutes with routine bulk reabsorption from proximal nephrons, while the longer, indirect loop is involved in fine tuning and in defending the body's store of sodium.

Examples of renal responses to stimuli:

1 Inevitable responses. Some renal responses to external influences are inevitable results of constraints imposed by the structure and working of the kidneys. A trivial example is the anuria caused by a fall in arterial blood pressure that is large enough to abolish glomerular filtration. Another example is the impairment of water diuresis when insufficient sodium can be reabsorbed to generate solute-free water during Addison's disease (Section 5.4). Of greater importance is the fact that the greatest osmolar concentration that can be maintained in the inner medulla sets an upper limit to the concentration of the urine (Section 5.5.3). This limitation prevents ordinary urinary solutes from being concentrated so much that they precipitate out of solution and obstruct the tubules mechanically. But it limits the extent to which the volume of urine can be reduced, however great the need to conserve water may be. The faster flow of tubular fluid leads to dilution of the medullary osmolar gradient and depresses the maximal osmolarity of the urine; this constrains the volume of the urine to increase far more than in proportion to the amount of urinary solute excreted during osmotic diuresis. Osmotic diuresis removes water from the body in an approximately isotonic solution containing the osmotic diuretic and all other urinary solutes, so that the kidneys cannot correct hypertonicity of the plasma caused by the presence of an osmotic diuretic (Section 5.5.4).

2 Automatic responses. Some automatic responses to alterations in the composition of the blood are simple and direct; for example, the increase in the rate of secretion of protons with a rising partial pressure of carbon dioxide, and the greater filtered load of bicarbonate which accompanies an increase in its concentration in the plasma. These automatic responses help to stabilize the bicarbonate content and the pH of the ECFs; but the integrated renal response to disturbances of acid—base metabolism is a great deal more complicated because of interactions with metabolic and centrally controlled respiratory mechanisms (Section 6.4).

Not all the kidneys' responses are directed to keeping concentrations in the plasma constant. The concentration of glucose in the plasma may normally be increased by about 100% before the tubular reabsorbing mechanisms are saturated, and the concentration in the plasma is allowed to fluctuate widely; the kidneys do not primarily regulate it, though they may oppose large variations by excreting glucose rapidly or adding new glucose to the blood (Section 4.5). Peptide hormones which are destroyed by the proximal tubules are not excreted, but they are removed from the plasma at rates equal to their filtered loads, so that their concentrations in the plasma depend upon the rates at which they are released into the blood (Section 4.6).

The slow, automatic adjustments which match the excretion of urea to its rate of production actually depend upon variations in its concentration in the plasma. At ordinary rates of urine flow, the rate of excretion is proportional to the concentration of urea in the plasma, and so to the amount in the body. Temporary accumulation, during a reduction in GFR, an increase in the rate of production, or an increase in passive reabsorption when the minute volume of urine falls below 2 ml, increases the concentration of urea in the plasma and can maintain the filtered load. Elimination is therefore automatically matched to production; a rising concentration in the plasma which indicates the need for faster excretion is also the means of achieving it, but neither the amount in the body nor the concentration in the plasma need be constant. Foreign glomerular substances like inulin, and no-threshold substances (Section 4.6) like PAH and diodone which also have constant renal plasma clearances so long as their concentrations are below their saturation limits, are excreted at rates proportional to their concentrations in the plasma, so that these concentrations fall exponentially towards their normal value of zero.

3 Indirectly controlled, or adjusted responses. The rate of urinary excretion of water varies in parallel with its concentration in the plasma, but not automatically or in simple proportion. The kidney does not respond directly to the concentration of water in the blood; adding or subtracting water increases or decreases the amount in the body and the concentration of water

in all the body fluids. This is monitored by osmoreceptors in the brain, and they withhold or release AVP which promotes the reabsorption of water from the collecting tubules; hence small differences in concentration of water lead to disproportionately large alterations in its excretion, and the osmolarity of the body fluids is regulated quite precisely (Section 5.5.4).

The concentration in the plasma is not important for controlling the rate of excretion of sodium. The concentration of sodium in the plasma is regulated by controlling the excretion of water (through ADH), so that the addition or subtraction of sodium to the body affects principally the ECFV. The renal response is even more indirect than in the case of water. Substantial alterations in the ECFV with changes in the volume, oncotic pressure and hydrostatic pressure of the blood may affect determinants of glomerular as well as of tubular function. Hence a large number of factors conspire to adjust the rate of excretion of sodium for the homeostatic control of the ECFV (Section 7.4).

Thus the responses of the kidney range from simple reactions to changes in a single variable, through more complex but still automatic processes like those that control the excretion of urea, to alterations in the excretion of substances like water and sodium which are controlled indirectly by many extrinsic factors. The intrinsic determinants of glomerular filtration are subject to continuous control (or interference) by the autonomic nervous system, but the kidney's cells are not driven from minute to minute like muscle cells activated by motor or vasomotor nerves. Compared with cells in skeletal muscles and in intermittently secreting glands, they are spontaneously active all the time and relatively autonomous. It is hardly conceivable that each separate epithelial cell should be centrally controlled to suit remote events all over the body, and quite appropriate that the kidney's functioning should be largely automatic, based on routine reabsorption of most of what the glomeruli filter. The cells lining the proximal tubules reabsorb sodium along with co-transported solutes and water as these are presented to them. The gradients which drive the reabsorption of water and many solutes are set up by re-absorption of sodium and no further stimulus is required than the presence of suitable solutes in the filtrate. The elimination of waste products and foreign substances is also largely automatic. Small molecular solutes appear in the glomerular filtrate, and their excretion only requires that they not be re-absorbed; it is also the nature of cells in the proximal nephron to secrete compounds like PAH and diodone into the urine if they are present in the peritubular blood. Cells in the distal nephron are more discriminating, and subject to control by hormones like aldosterone; this part of the nephron, with its special segments, is able to excrete or retain important body constituents like water, salt and potassium, and to vary the acidity of the urine.

There are interesting analogies between the nephron and the gastro-intestinal tract. If the glomerulus corresponds to the stomach, the proximal and distal nephrons correspond the the small and large intestines. Once the contents of the small intestine have been broken down by digestive enzymes, most of the sodium, sugars and amino acids are taken up by the leaky epithelium of the proximal part of the jejunum. The absorbing cells have brush borders and the process resembles renal proximal tubular reabsorption in that the driving forces for transport of water and solutes across the epithelium are mainly derived from active transport of sodium. Glucose and amino acids enter by co-transport; their presence promotes the absorption of sodium, and corresponding defects of intestinal absorption accompany some genetically determined defects in renal tubular reabsorption that present as aminoacidurias.

The tight epithelium of the colon absorbs water and electrolytes in smaller quantities and more selectively. Sugars and amino acids have disappeared, as in the nephron. Sodium is absorbed in preference to potassium; indeed, potassium and protons may be secreted into the lumen, and these processes are stimulated by aldosterone (Bray *et al.*, 1986, Chapter 14). But unlike reabsorption from the distal nephron, intestinal absorption is everywhere approximately isosmolal. There is nothing corresponding to water diuresis, though the faeces may become inspissated as a result of avid uptake of sodium and water by the colon during dehydration. As in the renal tubule, unabsorbed solutes pre-empt water to keep the luminal fluid roughly isosmotic, and this may lead to diarrhoea, which is analgous to osmotic diuresis.

Both intestinal absorption and renal tubular reabsorption are directed from outside the body towards the blood; moreover, their maximal rates are comparable. The renal tubules can usually reabsorb glucose fast enough to avoid loss in the urine however rapidly the small intestine absorbs it. The small intestine can also absorb water as fast as the stomach delivers it, and when the absence of ADH suppresses facultative reabsorption, the kidneys can excrete water as fast as the gut absorbs it, and so prevent water intoxication. At the opposite extreme, when water and electrolytes are lacking, or are not absorbed from the intestinal tract, renal tubular reabsorption can be intensified, so that the deficient intake is matched by a low urinary output, and the body's stores are conserved.

Ordinarily, water and electrolytes are absorbed in excess of requirements, and then, as Homer Smith sagely remarked, the composition of the body depends not so much upon what the mouth takes in as upon what the kidney keeps. However, Smith's epigram need not imply that the kidney is the independent arbiter of what remains in the body. Its functions are executive rather than administrative and the foregoing account of renal function and its regulation might justify a final reflection that, in the long term, the composition of the body largely determines what the kidney excretes.

References

Abel FL & Murphy QR. 1962. Mesenteric, renal and iliac vascular resistance in dogs after hemorrhage. *American Journal of Physiology* **202**: 978–980. [2.2.6]

Agus ZS, Goldfarb S & Wasserstein A. 1981. Calcium transport in the kidney. *Reviews of Physiology, Biochemistry & Pharmacology* **90**: 155–169. [4.3.3]

Al-Awqati Q. 1978. H^+ transport in urinary epithelia (Editorial review). *American Journal of Physiology* **235**: F77–F88. [6.4]

Al-Awqati Q. 1985. The cellular renal response to respiratory acid–base disorders (Nephrology forum). *Kidney International* **28**: 845–855. [8.3]

Alexander EA, Churchill S & Bengele HH. 1980. Renal hemodynamics and volume homeostasis during pregnancy in the rat. *Kidney International* **18**: 173–178. [3.3.4.2]

Allen TH & Orahovats PD. 1951. Kinetics of reaction between T-1824 and liver slices in mixtures of plasma albumin. *American Journal of Physiology* **164**: 123–130. [2.3.2]

Allison MEM, Wilson CB & Gottschalk CW. 1974. Pathophysiology of experimental glomerulonephritis in rats. *Journal of Clinical Investigation* **53**: 1402–1423. [3.4.2, 3.4.3]

Anderson WP, Korner PI & Selig SE. 1981. Mechanisms involved in the renal responses to intravenous and renal artery infusions of noradrenaline in conscious dogs. *Journal of Physiology* **321**: 21–30. [2.2.5, 3.4.3]

Andersson B. 1978. Regulation of water intake. *Physiological Reviews* **58**: 582–603. [7.2]

Arendshorst WJ & Gottschalk CW. 1985. Glomerular ultrafiltration dynamics: an historical perspective (Editorial review). *American Journal of Physiology* **248**: F163–F174. [3.2.2]

Arndt JO & Gauer OH. 1965. Diuresis induced by water infusions into the carotid loop of unanaesthetized dogs. *Pflügers Archiv für gesamte Physiologie* **282**: 301–312. [5.3]

Aronson PS. 1983. Mechanisms of active H^+ secretion in the proximal tubule (Editorial review). *American Journal of Physiology* **245**: F547–F659. [6.3]

Atherton JC, Bulock D & Pirie SC. 1982. The effect of pseudopregnancy on glomerular filtration rate and salt and water reabsorption in the rat. *Journal of Physiology* **324**: 11–20. [3.3.4.2]

Atherton JC, Hai MA & Thomas S. 1969. Acute effects of lysine vasopressin injection (single and continuous) on urinary composition in the conscious water diuretic rat. *Pflügers Archiv für gesamte Physiologie* **310**: 281–296. [5.5.3]

Aukland K. 1976. Renal blood flow. In *Kidney and Urinary Tract Physiology II, Vol. II* (ed. Thurau K), pp. 25–79. Baltimore: University Park Press. [2.2.1, 2.3.3]

Aukland K. 1980a. Methods for measuring renal blood flow: total flow and regional distribution. *Annual Review of Physiology* **42**: 543–555. [2.3.2]

Aukland K. 1980b. 'Redistribution' of intrarenal blood flow: facts or methodological artifacts. In *Renal Pathophysiology* (eds. Leaf A, Giebisch G, Bolis L & Gorini G), pp. 145–154. New York: Raven Press. [2.3.2]

Aukland K & Berliner RW. 1964. Renal medullary countercurrent system studied with hydrogen gas. *Circulation Research* **15**: 430–442. [2.3.2]

Aukland K, Bower BF & Berliner RW. 1964. Measurement of local blood flows with hydrogen gas. *Circulation Research* **15**: 164–187. [2.3.2]

Aukland K. Tønder HK & Maes G. 1977. Capillary pressure in deep and superficial glomeruli of the rat kidney. *Acta Physiologica Scandinavica* **101**: 318–427. [3.2.2, 3.2.3]

Aurbach GD & Heath DA. 1974. Parathyroid hormone and calcitonin regulation of renal function. *Kidney International* **6**: 331–345. [7.4.4.6]

Baeyer H von. 1981. Transport of D-glucose in the mammalian kidney. In *Renal Transport of Organic Substances* (eds. Greger R, Lang F & Silbernagl S), pp. 154–177. Berlin, Heidelberg, New York: Springer-Verlag. [4.2.2]

Bagnasco S, Balaban R, Fales HM, Yang Yi-M & Burg M. 1986. Predominant osmotically active organic solutes in rat and rabbit renal medullas. *Journal of Biological Chemistry* **261**: 5872–5877. [7.3]

Balaban RS & Burg MB. 1987. Osmotically active organic solutes in the renal inner medulla. *Kidney International* **31**: 562–564. [5.5.1, 7.3]

Baldes EJ & Smirk FH. 1934. The effect of water drinking, mineral starvation, and salt administration on the total osmotic pressure of the blood in man, chiefly in relation to the problems of water absorption and water diuresis. *Journal of Physiology* **82**: 62–74. [5.3]

Baldwin D, Kahana EM & Clarke RW. 1950a. The renal excretion of sodium and potassium in the dog. *American Journal of Physiology* **162**: 655–664. [2.2.5]

Baldwin DS, Sirota JH & Villareal H. 1950b. Diurnal variations of renal function in congestive heart failure. *Proceedings of the Society for Experimental Biology and Medicine* **74**: 578–581. [3.3.4.2]

Bálint P. 1961. *Aktuelle Probleme der Nierenphysiologie*. Berlin: Verlag Volk and Gesundheit. [2.2.3, 2.2.5, 2.2.6, 3.3.1, 3.4.3]

Ballermann BJ & Brenner BM. 1985. Biologically active atrial peptides. *Journal of Clinical Investigation* **76**: 2041–2048. [7.4.4.4]

Bank N & Aynedjian HS. 1984. Failure of changes in intracapillary pressure to alter proximal fluid reabsorption. *Kidney International* **26**: 275–282. [7.4.4.3]

Barajas L. 1981. The juxtaglomerular apparatus; anatomical considerations in feedback control of glomerular filtration rate. *Federation Proceedings* **40**: 78–86. [2.2.7]

Barcroft H & Loughridge WM. 1938. On the accuracy of the thermostrohmuhr method for measuring blood flow. *Journal of Physiology* **93**: 382–400. [2.2.2]

Barcroft H & Swan HJC. 1953. *Sympathetic control of human blood vessels*. London: Edward Arnold & Co. [3.4.3]

Barcroft J. 1934. *Features in the Architecture of Physiological Function*. Cambridge: University Press. [7.4.5]

Barcroft J & Brodie TG. 1905. The gaseous metabolism of the kidney. *Journal of Physiology* **32**: 18–27. [2.2.2]

Barfuss DW & Schafer JA. 1981. Differences in active and passive glucose transport along the proximal nephron. *American Journal of Physiology* **241**: F322–F332. [4.2.2]

Barger AC, Berlin RD & Tukenko JF. 1958. Infusion of aldosterone, 9-α-fluorohydrocortisone and antidiuretic hormone into the renal artery of normal and adrenalectomized, unanesthetized dogs: effect on electrolyte and water excretion. *Endocrinology* **62**: 804–815. [7.4.3]

Barger AC & Herd JA. 1973. Renal vascular anatomy and distribution of blood flow. In *Handbook of Physiology: Renal Physiology* (eds. Orloff J & Berliner RW), pp. 249–313. Washington DC: American Physiological Society [2.3.2]

Bartter FC, Delea CS, Terakazu K & Gill JR, jr. 1974. The adrenal cortex and the kidney. *Kidney International* **6**: 272–280. [3.3.4.2]

Battle DC & Kurtzman NA. 1985. Renal regulation of acid–base homeostasis: integrated response. In *The Kidney: Physiology and Pathophysiology, Vol. 2* (eds. Seldin DW & Giebisch G), pp. 1539–1565. New York: Raven Press. [6.5]

Baumann K. 1981. Renal transport of proteins. In *Renal Transport of Organic Substances* (eds. Greger R, Lang F & Silbernagl S), pp. 118–133. Berlin, Heidelberg, New York: Springer-Verlag. [4.2.4]

Baylis C. 1981. Information on the determinants of glomerular utrafiltration derived from study of the Munich-Wistar rat. In *Proceedings of the 8th International Congress of Nephrology*, pp.95–101. Athens: Karger. [3.3.5.2]

Baylis C, Deen WM, Myers BD & Brenner BM. 1976. Effect of some vasodilator drugs on transcapillary exchange in the renal cortex. *American Journal of Physiology* **230**: 1148–1158. [3.3.4.2]

Baylis C, Rennke HR & Brenner BM. 1977. Mechanisms of the defect in glomerular ultrafiltration associated with gentamicin administration. *Kidney International* **12**: 344–353. [3.2.2, 3.2.3]

Bayliss LE. 1956. The process of secretion. In *Modern Views on the Secretion of the Urine* (ed. Winton FR), pp. 96–127. London: J & A Churchill. [4.3.1]

Bayliss LE & Lundsgaard E. 1932. The action of cyanide on the isolated mammalian kidney. *Journal of Physiology* **74**: 279–293. [3.2.4, 3.3.5.3, 4.3.1]

Bayliss WM. 1902. On the local reactions of the arterial wall to changes of internal pressure. *Journal of Physiology* **28**: 220–231. [2.2.7]

Bayliss WM. 1915. *Principles of General Physiology*. London: Longmans, Green & Co. [3.2.1]

Beeuwkes R. 1971. Efferent vascular patterns and early vascular–tubular relations in the dog kidney. *American Journal of Physiology* **221**: 1361–1374. [3.3.4]

Beeuwkes R & Bonventre JV. 1975. Tubular organization and vascular–tubular relations in the dog kidney. *American Journal of Physiology* **229**: 695–713. [3.3.4]

Bell PD. 1982. Luminal and cellular mechanisms for the mediation of tubuloglomerular feedback. *Kidney International* **22** (Suppl. 12): S97–S103. [2.2.7, 3.3.5.3]

Bell PD & Navar LG. 1982. Relationship between tubulo-glomerular feedback responses and perfusate hypotonicity. *Kidney International* **2**: 234–239. [2.2.7, 3.3.5.3]

Bell PD, Navar LG, Ploth DW & MacLean CB. 1980. Tubuloglomerular feedback response during perfusion with nonelectrolyte solutions in the rat. *Kidney International* **18**: 460–471. [2.2.7]

Bello-Reuss E. 1980. Effect of catecholamines on fluid reabsorption by the isolated proximal convoluted tubule. *American Journal of Physiology* **238**: 347–352. [7.4.4.5]

Bennett CM, Brenner BM & Berliner RW. 1968. Micropuncture study of nephron function in the rhesus monkey. *Journal of Clinical Investigation* **47**: 203–216. [5.2, 5.4, 5.5.1, 5.5.3]

Bennett CM, Clapp JR & Berliner RW. 1967. Micropuncture study of the proximal and distal tubule in the dog. *American Journal of Physiology* **213**: 1254–1262. [3.3.5.3, 5.2]

Bennett CM, Glasscock RJ, Chang RLS, Deen WM, Roberston CR & Brenner BM. 1976. Permselectivity of the glomerular capillary wall: studies of experimental glomerulonephritis in the rat using dextran sulfate. *Journal of Clinical Investigation* **57**: 1287–1294. [3.3.5]

Bennett T & Gardner SM. 1986 Influence of exogenous vasopressin on baroreflex mechanisms (Editorial review). *Clinical Science* **70**: 307–315. [7.2]

Berliner RW. 1961. Renal mechanisms of potassium excretion. *Harvey Lectures* **55**: 141–171. [4.4.3]

Berliner RW. 1976. The concentrating mechanism in the renal medulla. *Kidney International* **9**: 214–222. [5.5.2]

Berliner RW. 1982. Mechanisms of urine concentration. *Kidney International* **22**: 202–211. [5.5.2]

Berliner RW. 1985. Carbon dioxide tension of alkaline urine. In *The Kidney: Physiology and Pathophysiology*, *Vol. 2* (eds. Seldin DW & Giebisch G), pp. 1527–1537. New York: Raven Press. [6.4]

Berliner RW, Levinsky NG, Davidson DG & Eden M. 1958. Dilution and concentration of the urine and the action of antidiuretic hormone. *American Journal of Medicine* **24**: 730–744. [5.5.2]

Berliner RW & Orloff J. 1956. Carbonic anhydrase inhibitors. *Pharmacological Reviews* **8**: 137–174. [4.3.2, 6.4]

Bernanke D & Epstein FH. 1965. Metabolism of the renal medulla. *American Journal of Physiology* **208**: 541–545. [2.3.2, 4.2.5]

Bernard C. 1859. *Leçons sur les Propriétés Physiologiques et les Altérations Pathologiques des Liquides de l'Organisme.* Paris: Baillière. [2.1]

Berne RM & Levy MN. 1950. Effects of acute reduction of cardiac output on the renal circulation of the dog. *Journal of Clinical Investigation* **29**: 444–454. [2.2.6]

Berry CA. 1982. Heterogeneity of tubular transport processes in the nephron. *Annual Review of Physiology* **44**: 181–201. [4.2.1]

Berry CA. 1983. Water permeability pathways in the proximal tubule (Editorial review). *American Journal of Physiology* **245**: F279–F294. [5.2]

Bichara M, Paillard M, Leviel F, Prigent A & Gardin J-P. 1983. Na:H exchange and the primary H pump in the proximal tubule. *American Journal of Physiology* **244**: F165–F171. [6.3]

Bickford RG & Winton FR. 1937. The influence of temperature on the isolated kidney of the dog. *Journal of Physiology* **89**: 198–219. [3.2.4, 3.3.5.3, 4.3.1]

Bie P. 1980. Osmoreceptors, vasopressin, and control of renal water excretion. *Physiological Reviews* **60**: 961–1048. [5.3]

Bijvoet OLM. 1980. Indices for the measurement of the renal handling of phosphate. In *Renal Handling of Phosphate* (eds. Massry SG & Fleisch H), pp. 1–37. New York, London: Plenum Medical Book Co. [4.3.2]

Bishop JM, Wade OL & Donald KW. 1958. Changes in jugular and renal arterio-venous oxygen content difference during exercise in heart disease. *Clinical Science* **17**: 611–619. [2.2.5]

Bishop JVH & Green R. 1983. Glucose handling by distal portions of the nephron during pregnancy in the rat. *Journal of Physiology* **336**: 131–142. [4.2.2]

Bishop JVH, Green R & Thomas S. 1979. Free-flow reabsorption of glucose, sodium, osmoles and water in rat proximal tubule. *Journal of Physiology* **288**: 331–351. [5.2]

Black DAK, Davies HEF, Emery EW & Wade EG. 1956. Renal handling of radioactive potassium in man. *Clinical Science* **15**: 277–283. [4.4.3]

Blair-West JR, Coghlan JP, Denton DA, Goding JR, Wintour M & Wright RD. 1963. The control of aldosterone secretion. *Recent Progress in Hormone Research* **19**: 311–363. [7.4.3]

Blair-West JR, Coghlan JP, Denton DA, Hardy KJ, Scoggins BA & Wright RD. 1979. Effect of adrenal arterial infusion of P-113 on aldosterone secretion in Na-deficient sheep. *American Journal of Physiology* **236**: F333–F341. [7.4.3]

Blair-West JR, Gibson AP, Woods RL & Brook AH. 1985. Acute reduction of vasopressin levels by rehydration in sheep. *American Journal of Physiology* **248**: R68–R71. [7.2]

Blantz RC, Israelit AH, Rector FC, Jr & Seldin DW. 1972. Relation of distal tubular NaCl delivery and glomerular hydrostatic pressure. *Kidney International* **2**: 22–32. [3.2.2, 3.2.3]

Blantz RC & Pelayo JC. 1984. A functional role for the tubuloglomerular feedback mechanism. *Kidney International* **25**: 739–746. [3.3.5.3]

Blantz RC, Peterson OW, Gushna L & Tucker BJ. 1982. Effect of modest hyperglycemia on tubuloglomerular feedback activity. *Kidney International* **22** (Suppl. 12): S206–S212. [3.3.5.3]

Blantz RC, Rector FC, Jr & Seldin DW. 1974. Effect of hyperosmotic albumin expansion upon glomerular ultrafiltration in the rat. *Kidney International* **6**: 209–221. [3.2.3.3]

Bohle A, Christensen J, Meter DS, Laberke HG & Strauch M. 1982. Juxtaglomerular apparatus of the human kidney: correlation between structure and function. *Kidney International* **22** (Suppl. 12): S18–S23. [2.2.7]

Bohle A, Jahnecke J. Meyer D & Schubert GE. 1976. Morphology of acute renal failure: comparative data from biopsy and autopsy. *Kidney International* **10**: S9–S16. [3.3.4.3]

Bohrer MP, Baylis C, Humes HD, Glasscock RJ, Robertson CR & Brenner BM. 1978. Permselectivity of the glomerular capillary wall: facilitated filtration of circulating polycations. *Journal of Clinical Investigation* **61**: 72–78. [3.2.5]

Bohrer MP, Deen WM, Robertson CR & Brenner BM. 1977. Mechanism of angiotensin-II-induced proteinuria in the rat. *American Journal of Physiology* **233**: F13–F21. [3.2.5]

Bonjour JP & Fleisch H. 1980. Tubular adaptation to the supply and requirement of phosphate. In *Renal Handling of Phosphate* (eds. Massry SG & Fleisch H), pp. 243–264. New York, London: Plenum Medical Book Co. [4.3.2]

Bonventre JV & Leaf A. 1982. Sodium homeostasis without a set point. *Kidney International* **21**: 880–885. [7.4.5]

Borle AB. 1967. Membrane transfer of calcium. *Clinical Orthopedics* **52**: 267–291. [4.3.3]

Borst JGG. 1954. The characteristic renal excretion patterns associated with excessive or inadequate circulation. In *The Kidney* (eds. Lewis AAG & Wolstenholme GEW), pp. 255–284. London: J & A Churchill. [7.2]

Bounous G, Onnis M & Shumacker HB. 1960. The abolition of renal autoregulation by renal decapsulation. *Surgery Gynecology & Obstetrics* **111**: 682–690. [2.2.7]

Bowman W. 1842. On the structure and use of the Malpighian bodies of the kidney, with observations on the circulation through the gland. *Philosophical Transactions of the Royal Society, London* **132**: 57–80. [1.3, 3.2.1, 3.2.2]

Boylan JW. 1979. Introduction to a symposium on proteinuria and renal protein catabolism. *Kidney International* **16**: 247–250. [4.2.4]

Boylan JW & Asshauer A. 1962. Depletion and restoration of the medullary osmotic gradient in the dog kidney. *Pflügers Archiv für gesamte Physiologie* **276**: 99–116. [5.5.3]

Brace RA. 1981. Progress towards resolving the controversy of positive vs negative interstitial fluid pressure (Brief review). *Circulation Research* **49**: 281–297. [7.4.5]

Bradley SE. 1951. Kidney. *Annual Review of Physiology* **19**: 513–556. [2.2.6]

Bradley SE & Bradley GP. 1947. Renal function during chronic anaemia in man. *Blood* **2**: 192–202. [2.3.4.2]

Bradley SE, Chasis H, Goldring W & Smith HW. 1945. Hemodynamic alterations in normotensive and hypertensive subjects during the pyrogenic reaction. *Journal of Clinical Investigation* **24**: 749–758. [2.2.5, 2.2.6]

Bradley SE, Chien K-CH, Coelho JB & Mason RC. 1974a. Effect of uninephrectomy on glomerulotubular functional-structural balance in the dog. *Kidney International* **5**: 122–130. [3.3.4.2]

Bradley SE, Stephan F, Coelho JB & Réville P. 1974b. The thyroid and the kidney. *Kidney International* **6**: 346–365. [3.3.4.2, 3.3.4.3]

Bradley SE & Wheeler HO. 1958. On the diversities of structure, perfusion and function of the nephron population. *American Journal of Medicine* **24**: 692–708. [2.2.3.2]

Bray JJ, Cragg PA, Macknight ADC, Mills RG & Taylor DW. 1986. *Lecture notes on Human Physiology*. Oxford: Blackwell Scientific Publications. [7.4.5, 8.4]

Brenner BM, Baylis C & Deen WM. 1976a. Transport of molecules across renal glomerular capillaries. *Physiological Reviews* **56**: 502–534. [2.2.5, 3.2.7, 3.3.4.2, 3.3.5.2]

Brenner BM, Bennett CM & Berliner RW. 1968. Relationship between glomerular filtration rate and sodium reabsorption by proximal tubule of rat nephron. *Journal of Clinical Investigation* **47**: 1358–1374. [7.4.2]

Brenner BM & Berliner RW. 1969. Relationship between extracellular volume and fluid reabsorption *American Journal of Physiology* **217**: 6–12. [7.4.2]

Brenner BM, Bohrer MP, Bayliss C & Deen WM. 1977. Determinants of glomerular permselectivity: insights derived from observations *in vivo* (Editorial review). *Kidney International* **12**: 229–237. [3.2.5]

Brenner BM, Deen WM & Robertson CR. 1974. The physiological basis of glomerular ultrafiltration. In *Kidney and Urinary Tract Physiology* (ed. Thurau K), pp. 336–356. Baltimore: University Park Press. [3.2.2, 3.2.3, 3.3.4.2, 7.4.3]

Brenner BM, Deen WM & Robertson CR. 1976b. Determinants of glomerular filtration rate. *Annual Review of Physiology* **38**: 9–19. [3.2]

Brenner BM, Deen WM & Robertson CR. 1976c. Glomerular filtration. In *The Kidney*, *Vol. 1* (eds. Brenner BM & Rector FC), pp. 251–271. Philadelphia: W B Saunders Co. [3.2.4, 3.2.5, 3.3.5.2]

Brenner BM, Hostetter TH & Humes HD. 1978. Glomerular permselectivity: barrier function based on discrimination of molecular size and charge. *American Journal of Physiology* **234**: F455–F460. [3.2.5, 3.2.6]

Brenner BM, Troy JL & Daugharty TM. 1971a. The dynamics of glomerular ultrafiltration in the rat. *Journal of Clinical Investigation* **50**: 1776–1780. [3.2.2, 3.2.3]

Brenner BM, Troy JL & Daugharty TM. 1971b. On the mechanism of inhibition in fluid reabsorption by the proximal tubule of the volume-expanded rat. *Journal of Clinical Investigation* **50**: 1596–1602. [7.4.4.3]

Brenner BM, Troy JL, Daugharty TM, Deen WM & Robertson CR. 1972a. Dynamics of glomerular ultrafiltration in the rat. II. Plasma-flow dependence of GFR. *American Journal of Physiology* **223**: 1184–1190. [3.2.2, 3.2.3, 3.3.4.2, 3.3.4.3]

Brenner BM, Ueki IF & Daugharty TM. 1972b. On estimating colloid osmotic pressure in pre- and postglomerular plasma in the rat. *Kidney International* **2**: 51–53. [3.2.3.3]

Brewer DB. 1951. Renal clearance of dextran of varying molecular weights. *Proceedings of the Royal Society of Medicine* **44**: 561–563. [3.2.5]

Brezis M, Rosen S, Silva P & Epstein FH. 1984. Renal ischemia: a new perspective (Editorial review). *Kidney International* **26**: 375–383. [4.5.1]

Bricker NS. 1967. The control of sodium excretion with normal and reduced nephron populations. The pre-eminence of the third factor (Editorial). *American Journal of Medicine* **43**: 313–321. [7.4.4]

Bricker NS, Bourgoignie JJ & Weber H. 1976. The renal response to progressive renal loss. In *The Kidney*, *Vol. 1* (eds. Brenner BM & Rector FC), pp. 703–736. Philadelphia: W B Saunders Co. [3.3.4.2]

Bricker NS, Guild WR, Reardon JB & Merrrill JF. 1956. Studies on the functional capacity of a denervated homotransplanted kidney in an identical twin with parallel observations in the donor. *Journal of Clinical Investigation* **35**: 1364–1380. [2.2.5]

Briggs JP. 1981. The macula densa sensing mechanism for tubuloglomerular feedback. *Federation Proceedings* **40**: 99–103. [2.2.7]

Briggs JP. 1982. A simple steady-state model for feedback control of glomerular filtration rate. *Kidney International* **22** (Suppl. 12): S143–S150. [3.3.5.3]

Britton KE. 1979. Radionuclides in the investigation of renal disease. In *Renal Disease*, 4th edn (eds. Black DAK & Jones NF), pp. 270–304. Oxford: Blackwell Scientific Publications. [3.3.2]

Brøchner-Mortensen J & Ditzel J. 1982. Glomerular filtration rate and extracellular fluid volume in insulin-dependent patients with diabetes mellitus. *Kidney International* **21**: 696–698. [3.3.4.2]

Brøchner-Mortensen J, Rickers H & Balslev I. 1980. Renal function and body composition before and after intestinal bypass operation in obese patients. *Scandinavian Journal of Clinical and Laboratory Investigation* **40**: 695–702. [3.3.4.2]

Brod J & Fejfar Z. 1955. Die Pathogenese der Herzinsuffienz. *Schweizerische medizinische Wochenschrift* **85**: 84–92. [3.3.4.2]

Brod J & Sirota JH. 1949. Effects of emotional disturbance on water diuresis and renal blood flow in the rabbit. *American Journal of Physiology* **157**: 31–39. [3.3.4.2]

Brodie TG & Russell AE. 1905. On the determination of the rate of blood-flow through an organ. *Journal of Physiology* **32**: xlvii–xlix. [2.2.2]

Brun C, Crone C, Davidsen HG, Fabricius J, Tybjaerg A, Hansen NA & Munck O. 1955. Renal blood flow in anuric human subject determined by the use of radioactive krypton–85. *Proceedings of the Society for Experimental Biology & Medicine* **89**: 687–690. [2.2.5]

Brun C, Knudsen EDE & Raaschou F. 1945. The influence of posture on the kidney function. 1. The fall of diuresis in the erect posture. *Acta Medica Scandinavica* **122**: 315–331. [3.3.4.3]

Bucht H, Ek J, Eliasch H, Holmgren A, Josephson B & Werkö L. 1953. The effect of exercise in the recumbent position on the renal circulation and sodium excretion in normal individuals. *Acta Physiologica Scandinavica* **28**: 95–100. [2.2.5]

Bull GM. 1948. Postural proteinuria. *Clinical Science* **7**: 77–108. [3.3.4.3]

Bull GM & Metaxas P. 1962. The theory and applicability of clearance methods for determining renal blood and lymph flow. *Clinical Science* **23**: 515–523. [2.2.3]

Burg MB. 1976a. The renal handling of sodium chloride. In *The Kidney, Vol. 1* (eds. Brenner BM & Rector FC), pp. 272–298. Philadelphia: W B Saunders Co. [4.3.2]

Burg MB. 1976b. Mechanisms of action of diuretic drugs. In *The Kidney, Vol. 1* (eds. Brenner BM & Rector FC), pp. 737–762. Philadelphia: W B Saunders Co. [4.3.2]

Burg MB. 1981. Renal handling of sodium chloride, water, amino acids and glucose. In *The Kidney, Vol. 1*, 2nd edn (eds. Brenner BM & Rector FC), pp. 328–370. Philadelphia: W B Saunders Co. [7.4.4.5]

Burg MB. 1982a. Introduction: background and development of microperfusion technique. *Kidney International* **22**: 417–424. [4.1.1]

Burg MB. 1982b. Thick ascending limb of Henle's loop. *Kidney International* **22**: 454–464. [4.3.1]

Burger BM, Hopkins T, Tulloch A & Hollenberg NK. 1976. The role of angiotensin in the canine renal vascular response to barbiturate anesthesia. *Circulation Research* **38**: 196–202. [3.3.4.3]

Burton AC. 1965. *Physiology and Biophysics of the Circulation*. Chicago: Year Book Medical Publishers. [2.2.7]

Burton-Opitz R & Lucas DR. 1911. The blood supply of the kidney. V. The influence of the vagus nerve upon the vascularity of the left organ. *Journal of Experimental Medicine* **17**: 303–313. [2.2.7]

Carey RM & Sen S. 1986. Recent progress in the control of aldosterone secretion. *Recent Progress in Hormone Research* **42**: 251–296. [7.4.3]

Carone FA, Peterson DR, Oparil S & Pullman TN. 1979. Renal tubular transport and catabolism of proteins and peptides. *Kidney International* **16**: 271–278. [4.2.4]

Castenfors J. 1967a. Renal function during exercise. *Acta Physiologica Scandinavica* **70** (Suppl. 293): 1–44. [2.2.5, 3.3.5.3]

Castenfors J. 1967b. Renal clearances and urinary sodium and potassium excretion during supine exercise in normal subjects. *Acta Physiologica Scandinavica* **70**: 207–214. [2.2.5, 3.3.5.3]

Chai SY, Sexton PM, Allen AM, Figdor R & Mendelsohn FAO. 1986. *In vitro* autoradiographic localization of AVP receptors in rat kidney and adrenal gland. *American Journal of Physiology* **250**: F753–F757. [7.4.4.4]

Chang RLS, Deen WM, Robertson CR, Bennett CM, Glasscock RJ & Brenner BM. 1976. Permselectivity of the glomerular capillary wall: studies of experimental glomerulonephritis in the rat using neutral dextran. *Journal of Clinical Investigation* **5**: 1272–1286. [3.2.5]

Chang RLS, Deen WM, Robertson CR & Brenner BM. 1975a. Permeability of the glomerular capillary wall: restricted transport of polyanions. *Kidney International* **8**: 212–218. [3.2.5]

Chang RLS, Deen WM, Robertson CR & Brenner BM. 1975b. Permselectivity of the glomerular capillary wall to macromolecules. I. Theoretical considerations. *Biophysical Journal* **15**: 861–886. [3.2.5]

Chang RLS, Ueki IF, Deen WM, Robertson CR & Brenner BM. 1975c. Permselectivity of the glomerular capillary wall to macromolecules. II. Experimental studies in rats using neutral dextrans. *Biophysical Journal* **15**: 887–906. [3.2.5]

Chantler C. 1979. Renal failure in childhood. In *Renal Disease*, 4th edn (eds. Black DAK & Jones NF), pp. 825–868. Oxford: Blackwell Scientific Publications. [3.3.4.2]

Chasis H & Goldring W. (eds.) 1965. *Homer William Smith. His Scientific and Literary Achievements*. New York: University Press. [2.2.2]

Chasis H, Ranges HA, Goldring W & Smith HW. 1938. The control of renal blood flow and glomerular filtration in normal man. *Journal of Clinical Investigation* **17**: 683–697. [3.3.4.2, 5.3]

Chesley LC. 1972. Water, electrolyte, and acid base disorders in pregnancy. In *Clinical Disorders of Fluid and Electrolyte Metabolism*, 2nd edn (eds. Maxwell MH & Kleeman CR), pp. 995–1022. New York: McGraw Hill Book Co. [3.3.4.2]

Chinard FP. 1952. Derivation of an expression for the rate of formation of glomerular fluid (GFR). Applicability of certain physical and phyisco-chemical concepts. *American Journal of Physiology* **171**: 578–586. [3.2.8]

Christiansen JS, Gammelgaard J, Tronier B, Svensden PA & Parving HH. 1982. Kidney function and size in diabetes before and during initial insulin treatment. *Kidney International* **21**: 683–688. [3.3.4.2]

Christy NP & Shaver JC. 1974. Estrogens and the kidney. *Kidney International* **6**: 366–376. [7.4.4.6]

Clapp JR & Robinson RR. 1966. Osmolality of distal tubular fluid in the dog. *Journal of Clinical Investigation* **45**: 1847–1853. (5.4, 5.5.1, 5.5.5]

Clapp JR, Watson JF & Berliner RW. 1963. Osmolality, bicarbonate concentration, and water reabsorption in proximal tubules of the dog nephron. *American Journal of Physiology* **205**: 273–280. [5.2]

Clappison BH, Anderson WP & Johnston CI. 1981. Renal hemodynamics and renal kinins after angiotensin-converting enzyme inhibition. *Kidney International* **20**: 615–620. [3.3.5.3]

Coghlan JP, Blair-West JR, Denton DA, Scoggins BA & Wright RD. 1971. Perspectives in aldosterone and renin control. *Australia & New Zealand Journal of Medicine* **1**: 178–197. [7.4.3]

Cohen JJ. 1979. Is the function of the renal papilla coupled exclusively to an anaerobic pattern of metabolism? (Editorial review) *American Journal of Physiology* **236**: F423–F433. [2.3.3, 4.5]

Cohen JJ & Barac-Nieto M. 1973. Renal metabolism of substrates in relation to renal function. In *Handbook of Physiology. Section 8. Renal Physiology* (eds. Orloff J & Berliner RW), pp. 909–1002. Washington DC: American Physiological Society. [4.2.2, 4.5]

Cohen JJ & Kamm DE. 1976. Renal metabolism: relation to renal function. In *The Kidney*, Vol. 1 (eds. Brenner BM & Rector FC), pp. 126–214. Philadelphia: W B Saunders Co. [4.5]

Conn HL, Jr, Anderson W & Arena S. 1953. Gas diffusion technique for measurement of renal blood flow with special reference to the intact anuric subject. *Journal of Applied Physiology* **5**: 683–689. [2.2.3.3]

Conn HL, Jr, Wood JC & Schmidt CF. 1953. A comparison of renal blood flow results obtained in the intact animal by the nitrous oxide (derived Fick) method and by the para-aminohippurate (direct Fick) method. *Journal of Clinical Investigation* **32**: 1180–1183. [2.2.3]

Conway BE. 1981. *Ionic Hydration in Chemistry and Biophysics*. Amsterdam, Oxford, New York: Elsevier. [3.2.9]

Cook WF & Pickering GW. 1959. The location of renin in the rabbit kidney. *Journal of Physiology* **149**: 526–536. [1.3]

Corvilain J & Abramow M. 1962. Some effects of human growth hormone on renal hemodynamics and on tubular phosphate transport in man. *Journal of Clinical Investigation* **41**: 1230–1235. [3.3.4.2]

Cotter T, Gebruers EM, Hall WJ & O'Sullivan MF. 1986. Plasma expansion does not precipitate the fall in plasma vasopressin in humans drinking isotonic fluids. *Journal of Physiology* **376**: 429–438. [7.2]

Crabbe J. 1961. Stimulation of active sodium transport by the isolated toad bladder with aldosterone *in vitro*. *Journal of Clinical Investigation* **40**: 2103–2110. [7.4.3]

Crane RK. 1965. Na$^+$-dependent transport in the intestine and other animal tissues. *Federation Proceedings* **24**: 1000–1006. [4.2.2]

Crawford B & Ludemann H. 1951. The renal response to intravenous injection of sodium chloride solutions in man. *Journal of Clinical Investigation* **30**: 1456–1462. [3.3.4.2]

Cushny AR. 1917. *The Secretion of the Urine* London: Longmans, Green & Co. [3.2.1]

Cushny AR. 1926. *The Secretion of the Urine*, 2nd edn. London: Longmans, Green & Co. [2.2.2, 4.1, 4.6]

Daniel PM, Peabody CN & Prichard MML. 1951. Observations on the circulation through the cortex and the medulla of the kidney. *Quarterly Journal of Experimental Physiology* **36**: 199–203. [2.3.1]

Daniel PM, Peabody CN & Prichard MML. 1952. Cortical ischaemia of the kidney with maintained blood flow through the medulla. *Quarterly Journal of Experimental Physiology* **37**: 11–18. [2.3.1]

Dantzler WH. 1981. Comparative physiology of the renal transport of organic solutes. In *Renal Transport of Organic Substances* (eds. Greger R, Lang F & Silbernagl S), pp. 290–308. Berlin, Heidelberg, New York: Springer-Verlag. [4.4.3]

Dantzler WH. 1982. Reptilian glomerular and tubular functions and their control. *Federation Proceedings* **42**: 2371–2376. [3.3.4.3]

Darmady EM, Durant J, Matthews ER & Stranack F. 1960. Localization of ^{131}I-pitressin in the kidney by autoradiography. *Clinical Science* **19**: 229–241. [5.3]

Davies DF & Shock NW. 1950. Age changes in glomerular filtration rate, effective renal plasma flow and tubular excretory capacity in adult males. *Journal of Clinical Investigation* **29**: 496–507. [2.2.4, 3.4.4.3, 7.3]

Davis JO & Freeman RH. 1976. Mechanisms regulating renin release. *Physiological Reviews* **56**: 1–56. [3.3.5.3, 7.4.2]

Davison J & Cheyne GA. 1974. History of the measurement of glucose in urine: a cautionary tale. *Medical History* **18**: 194–197. [4.2.2]

Davison J & Dunlop W. 1980. Renal hemodynamics and tubular function in normal human pregnancy. *Kidney International* **18**: 152–161. [3.3.4.2, 4.2.2]

Davson H. 1954. Vertebrate physiology from the point of view of active transport. *Symposia of the Society for Experimental Biology* **8**: 16–26. [3.2.4]

Davson H. 1956. *Physiology of the Ocular and Cerebrospinal Fluids*. London: J & A Churchill. [3.2.4, 3.4.3]

DeBold AJ, Borenstein HB, Veress AT & Sonnenberg H. 1981. A rapid and potent natriuretic response to intravenous injection of atrial myocardial extract in rats. *Life Science* **28**: 89–94. [7.4.4.4]

Deen WM, Bohrer MP & Brenner BM. 1979. Macromolecule transport across glomerular capillaries: application of pore theory. *Kidney International* **16**: 353–365. [3.2.9]

Deen WM, Maddox DA, Robertson CR & Brenner BM. 1974. Dynamics of glomerular ultrafiltration in the rat. VII. Response to reduced renal mass. *American Journal of Physiology* **227**: 556–562. [3.3.4.2]

Deen WM, Robertson CR & Brenner BM. 1972. A model of glomerular ultrafiltration in the rat. *American Journal of Physiology* **223**: 1178–1183. [3.3.5.2]

Deen WM, Troy JL, Robertson CR & Brenner BM. 1973. Dynamics of glomerular ultra-filtration in the rat. IV. Determination of the ultrafiltration coefficient. *Journal of Clinical Investigation* **52**: 1500–1508. [3.2.3]

Deetjen P. 1970. Nierenphysiologie. In *Niere und Wasserhaushalt* (eds. Boylan JW, Deetjen P & Kramer K), pp. 1–97. München, Berlin, Wien: Urban & Schwarzenberg. [4.2.2, 4.2.3, 4.4.1]

Deetjen P. 1981. Introduction. In *Renal Transport of Organic Substrances* (eds. Gregor R. Lang F & Silbernagel S), pp. 1–5. Berlin, Heidelberg, New York: Springer-Verlag. [4.2.3]

Deetjen P, Brechtelsbauer H & Kramer K. 1964. Hämodynamik des Nierenmarks. III Mitteilung. Farbestoffpassagezeiten in aüßerer Markzone und V. renalis. Die Durchblutungsverteilung in der Niere. *Pflügers Archiv für gesamte Physiologie* **279**: 281–293. [2.3.1]

Denton DA, Goding JR & Wright RD. 1959. Control of adrenal secretion of electrolyteactive steroids. *British Medical Journal* **ii**: 447–456; 522–530. [7.4.3]

Depner TA & Gulyassi PF. 1979. Clinical renal failure. In *Strauss and Welt's Diseases of the Kidney*, 3rd edn (eds. Earley LE & Gottschalk CW), pp. 211–262. New York: Little, Brown & Co. [2.3.4]

Diamond JM. 1985. A reversible epithelium. *Nature* **318**: 311. [8.3]

Diamond JM & Bossert WH. 1967. Standing gradient osmotic flow. A mechanism for coupling of water and solute transport in epithelia. *Journal of General Physiology* **50**: 2061–2083. [5.2]

DiBona GF. 1982. The functions of the renal nerves. *Reviews of Physiology, Biochemistry & Pharmacology* **94**: 75–181. [3.3.5.4, 7.4.4.5]

DiBona GF. 1985. Neural regulation of renal tubular reabsorption and renin secretion. *Federation Proceedings* **44**: 2816–2822. [7.4.4.5]

Dicker SE. 1956. Standard renal clearances in mammals. In *Modern Views on the Secretion of Urine* (ed. Winton FR), pp. 5–33. London: J & A Churchill. [2.4.3, 3.3.4, 5.3]

Dicker SE, Greenbaum AL & Morris CA. 1977. Compensatory renal hypertrophy in hypophysectomized rats. *Journal of Physiology* **273**: 241–253. [3.3.4.2]

Dirks JH. 1983. The kidney and magnesium regulation. *Kidney International* **23**: 771–777. [4.3.3]

Dirks JH, Cirksena WJ & Berliner RW. 1965. The effect of saline infusion on sodium reabsorption by the proximal tubule of the dog. *Journal of Clinical Investigation* **44**: 1160–1170. [5.2, 7.4.4]

Dirks JH, Seely JF & Levy M. 1976. Control of extracellular fluid volume and the pathophysiology of edema formation. In *The Kidney*, Vol. *1* (eds. Brenner BM & Rector JC), pp. 495–552. Philadelphia: W B Saunders Co. [7.4.4]

Doolan PD, Alpen EL & GB. 1962. A clinical appraisal of the plasma concentration and endogenous clearance of creatinine. *American Journal of Medicine* **32**: 65–79. [3.3.2, 4.4.3]

Dorhout Mees EJ, Geers AB & Koomans HA. 1984. Blood volume and sodium retention in the nephrotic syndrome: a controversial pathophysiological concept (Editorial). *Nephron* **36**: 201–211. [7.4.5]

Dreser H. 1892. Ueber Diurese und ihrer Beeinflussung durch Pharmakologische Mittel. *Archiv für Experimentelle Pathologie und Pharmakologie* **29**: 303–319. [3.3.5.3, 5.5.3]

Drieu L, Rainfray M, Cabrol G & Ardaillou R. 1986. Vasopressin, aldosterone and renin responses to volume depletion in heart-transplanted recipients. *Clinical Science* **70**: 233–241. [7.4.5]

Du Bose TD, Jr. 1983. Application of the disequilibrium pH method to investigate the mechanism of urinary acidification (Editorial review). *American Journal of Physiology* **245**: F535–F544. [6.3]

Dunn BR, Ichikawa I, Pfeffer JM, Troy JL & Brenner BM. 1986. Renal and systemic effects of synthetic atrial natriuretic peptide in the anesthetized rat. *Circulation Research* **59**: 237–246. [7.4.4.4]

Durbin RP. 1960. Osmotic flow of water across permeable cellulose membranes. *Journal of General Physiology* **44**: 315–326. [3.2.9]

Dworkin LD, Ichikawa I & Brenner BM. 1983. Hormonal modulation of glomerular function (Editorial) *American Journal of Physiology* **244**: F95–F104. [3.3.5.2]

Earle DP, Jr, Taggart JV & Shannon JA. 1944. Glomerulonephritis. A survey of the functional organization of the kidney in various stages of diffuse glomerulonephritis. *Journal of Clinical Investigation* **23**: 119–137. [3.4.4.3]

Earley LE & Daugharty TM. 1969. Sodium metabolism. *New England Journal of Medicine* **281**: 72–86. [7.4.2, 7.4.4]

Edelman IS & Leibman J. 1959. Anatomy of body water and electrolytes. *American Journal of Medicine* **27**: 256–277. [3.3.2, 7.4.1]

Eggleton MG & Habib YA. 1951. The mode of excretion of creatinine and inulin by the kidney of the cat. *Journal of Physiology* **112**: 191–200. [3.3.2]

Eisenbach GM, Van Liew JB & Boylan JW. 1975. Effect of angiotensin on the filtration of protein in the rat kidney: a micropuncture study. *Kidney International* **8**: 80–87. [3.2.3]

Ekehorn G. 1931. On the principles of renal function. *Acta Medica Scandinavica* Suppl. **36**: 1–716. [3.3.2]

Elias H. 1956. The renal glomerulus by light and electron microscopy. *Research in the Service of Medicine* (GD Searle & Co) **46**: 1–29. [3.2.6]

Elkinton JR. 1956. Hyponatremia: clinical state or biochemical sign. *Circulation* **14**: 1027–1034. [7.3]

Elkinton JR. 1960. Regulation of water and electrolytes. *Circulation* **21**: 1184–1192. [7.1]

Elkinton JR & Danowski TS. 1955. *The Body Fluids. Basic Physiology and Practical Therapeutics*. Baltimore: Williams & Wilkins. [7.4]

Ellis KJ, Vaswani A, Zanzi I & Cohn SH. 1976. Total body sodium and chlorine in normal adults. *Metabolism* **25**: 645–654. [7.4.1]

Emerson K, Jr & Dole VP. 1943. Diodrast and inulin clearances in nephrotic children with supernormal urea clearances. *Journal of Clinical Investigation* **22**: 447–450. [3.3.4.2]

Epstein FH, Goodyer AVN, Lawrason FD & Relman AS. 1951. Studies of the antidiuresis of quiet standing: the importance of changes in plasma volume and glomerular filtration rate. *Journal of Clinical Investigation* **30**: 63–72. [3.3.4.3]

Epstein FH, Kleeman CR, Lamdin E & Rubini ME. 1956. Studies of the antidiuresis of quiet standing: observations of electrolyte and acid–base excretion during sulfate diuresis. *Journal of Clinical Investigation* **35**: 308–313. [3.3.4.3]

Epstein M. 1978. Renal effects of head-out water immersion in man: implications for an understanding of volume homeostasis. *Physiological Reviews* **58**: 529–581. [2.2.6, 3.3.4.2]

Falchuk KH & Berliner RW. 1971. Hydrostatic pressures in peritubular capillaries and tubules in the rat kidney. *American Journal of Physiology* **220**: 1422–1426. [3.2.3]

Falkheden T & Sjøgren B. 1964. Extracellular fluid volume and renal function in pituitary insufficiency and acromegaly. *Acte Endocrinologica (Copenhagen)* **46**: 80–86. [3.3.4.3]

Farquhar MG. 1975. The primary glomerular filtration barrier — basement membrane or epithelial slits? (Editorial review). *Kidney International* **8**: 197–211. [3.2.6]

Field MJ & Giebisch GJ. 1985. Hormonal control of renal potassium excretion (Editorial review). *Kidney International* **27**: 379–387. [8.2]

Filehne W & Biberfeld H. 1902. Beiträge Zur Diurese. I. Einleitende Versuche. *Pflügers Archiv für gesamte Physiologie* **91**: 569–593. [5.5.1]

Fine L. 1986. The biology of renal hypertrophy (Editorial review). *Kidney International* **29**: 619–634. [3.3.4.2, 8.3]

Fizsimons JT. 1976. The physiological basis of thirst. *Kidney International* **10**: 3–11. [7.2]

Forbes GB. 1962. Sodium. In *Mineral Metabolism, Vol. 2, Part B* (eds. Comar CJ & Bronner F), pp. 1–72. New York, London: Academic Press. [7.4.1]

Foreman H, Vier M & Magee M. 1953. The metabolism of C^{14}-labelled ethylenediamine-tetraacetic acid in the rat. *Journal of Biological Chemistry* **203**: 1045–1053. [4.4.1]

Forster RP. 1947. An examination of some factors which alter glomerular activity in the rabbit kidney. *American Journal of Physiology* **150**: 523–533. [3.3.4.2]

Forster RP. 1952. Stability of glomerular filtration rates with uncomplicated water diuresis in rabbits. *American Journal of Physiology* **168**: 666–673. [3.3.4.2]

Forster RP & Maes JP. 1947. Effect of experimental neurogenic hypertension on renal blood flow and glomerular filtration rates in denervated kidney of unanesthetized rabbits with adrenal glands demedullated. *American Journal of Physiology* **150**: 534–540. [2.2.7]

Fourman JF & Moffatt DB. 1971. *The Blood Vessels of the Kidney*. Oxford: Blackwell Scientific Publications. [1.2, 3.2.2]

Franklin KJ, McGee LE & Ullman E. 1951. Effects of severe asphyxia on the kidney and urine flow. *Journal of Physiology* 112: 43–53. [2.2.5]

Franklin SS & Merrill JP. 1960. The kidney in health; the nephron in disease (Editorial). *American Journal of Medicine* 28: 1–7. [3.3.4.2]

Fraser R, Brown JJ, Lever AF, Mason M & Robertson JIS. 1979. Control of aldosterone secretion (Editorial review) *Clinical Science* 56: 389–399. [7.4.3]

Freeman RH, Davis JO & Vari RC. 1985. Renal response to atrial natriuretic factors in dogs with caval constriction. *American Journal of Physiology* 248: R495–R500. [7.4.4.4]

Frega NS, Davalos M & Leaf A. 1980a Effect of endogenous angiotensin on the efferent glomerular arteriole of rat kidney. *Kidney International* 18: 323–327. [2.2.7]

Frega NS, Di Bona DR & Leaf A. 1980b. Enhancement of recovery from experimental ischemic acute renal failure. In *Renal Pathophysiology* (ed. Leaf A), pp. 203–212. New York: Raven Press. [2.2.5]

Frömter E. 1979. Solute transport across epithelia: what can we learn from micropuncture studies on kidney tubules? *Journal of Physiology* 288: 1–31. [4.2.2]

Frömter E. 1981. Electrical aspects of tubular transport of organic substances. In *Renal Transport of Organic Substances* (eds. Greger R, Lang F & Silbernagl S), pp. 30–44. Berlin, Heidelberg, New York: Springer-Verlag. [4.2.2, 4.2.3]

Frömter E. 1984. Homer Smith Award Lecture: viewing the kidney through microelectrodes. *American Journal of Physiology* 247: F695–F705. [4.1.1]

Frömter E, Rumrich G & Ullrich KJ. 1973. Phenomenologic description Na^+, Cl^- and HCO_3^- absorption from proximal tubules of the rat kidney. *Pflügers Archiv für gesamte Physiologie* 343: 189–220. [4.3.1]

Fuller PJ & Funder JW. 1986. The cellular physiology of glandular kallikrein (Editorial review). *Kidney International* 29: 953–964. [7.4.4.6]

Fulton JF. 1966. *Selected Readings in the History of Physiology*, 2nd edn. Springfield, Illinois: Thomas. [1.3]

Funder JW, Blair-West JR, Coghlan JP, Denton DA, Scoggins BA & Wright RD. 1969. Effect of plasma $[K^+]$ on the secretion of aldosterone. *Endocrinology* 85: 381–384. [7.4.3]

Gaizutis M, Pesce AJ & Lewy JE. 1972. Determination of nanogram amounts of albumin by radioimmunoassay. *Microchemical Journal* 17: 327–337. [3.2.3]

Garby L. 1955. On the mechanism of the formation of the glomerular fluid. *Acta Physiologica Scandinavica* 35: 88–92. [3.2.8]

Gauer OH & Henry JP. 1963. Circulatory basis of fluid volume control. *Physiological Reviews* 43: 424–481. [2.2.6, 3.3.4.3, 7.2, 7.4.5]

Gauer OH, Henry JP & Behn C. 1970. The regulation of extracellular fluid volume. *Annual Review of Physiology* 32: 547–595. [7.4.5]

Gauer OH & Tata PS. 1968. Vasopressin studies in the rat. IV. The vasopressin-water equivalent and vasopressin clearance by the kidney. *Pflügers Archiv für gesamte Physiologie* 298: 241–257. [5.5.4]

Gebruers EM, Hall WJ, O'Brien NIH, O'Leary D & Plant WD. 1985. Signals from the oropharynx may contribute to the diuresis which occurs in man to drinking isotonic fluids. *Journal of Physiology* 363: 21–33. [7.2]

Geers AB, Koomans HA, Roos JC, Boer P & Dorhout Mees EJ. 1984. Functional relationships in the nephrotic syndrome. *Kidney International* 26: 324–330. [7.4.5]

Gekle D, Bruchhausen FV & Fuchs G. 1966. Über die Größe der Porenäquivalenten in isolierten Basalmembranen der Rattennierenrinde. *Pflügers Archiv für gesamte Physiologie* 289: 180–190. [3.2.5]

Gerber JG, Olson RD & Nies AS. 1981. Interrelationship between prostaglandins and renin release. *Kidney International* 19: 816–821. [7.4.3]

Gertz KH & Boylan JW. 1973. Glomerular-tubular balance. In *Handbook of Physiology. Section 8. Renal Physiology* (eds. Orloff J & Berliner RW), pp. 763–790. Washington DC: American Physiological Society. [7.4]

Gertz KH, Mangos JA, Braun G & Pagel HD. 1966. Pressure in the glomerular capillaries of the rat kidney and its relation to arterial blood pressure. *Pflügers Archiv für gesamte Physiologie* **288**: 369. [3.2.2]

Gibbons GH, Dzau VJ, Farhi ER & Barger AC. 1984. Interaction of signals influencing renin release. *Annual Review of Physiology* **46**: 291–308. [2.2.7, 7.4.3]

Giebisch G. 1975. Some reflections on the mechanism of renal tubular potassium transport. *Yale Journal of Biology & Medicine* **48**: 318–336. [4.3.3]

Giebisch G. 1976. Effects of diuretics on renal transport of potassium. In *Methods in Pharmacology* (ed. Martinez-Moldonado M), pp. 121–164. New York: Plenum Publishing Co. [4.3.3]

Giebisch G. 1978. The proximal nephron. In *Physiology of Membrane Disorders* (eds. Andreoli TE, Hoffman JF & Fanestil DD), pp. 629–660. New York: Plenum Publishing Co. [4.2.2, 4.3.1, 7.4.4.3, 8.3]

Giebisch G, Klose RM, Malnic G, Sullivan WJ & Windhager EE. 1964. Sodium movement across single perfused proximal tubules of rat kidneys. *Journal of General Physiology* **47**: 1175–1194. [4.3.1]

Giebisch G, Lauson HD & Pitts RF. 1954. Renal excretion and volume of distribution of various dextrans. *American Journal of Physiology* **178**: 168–176. [3.2.5]

Giebisch G & Malnic G. 1976. Studies on the mechanism of tubular acidification. *The Physiologist* **19**: 511–524. [6.3.1]

Giebisch G & Windhager EE. 1964. Renal tubular transport of sodium, chloride and potassium. *American Journal of Medicine* **36**: 643–669. [4.4.3]

Gilmore JP. 1964. Influence of tissue pressure on renal blood flow autoregulation. *American Journal of Physiology* **206**: 707–713. [2.2.7]

Gmaj P & Murer H. 1986. Cellular mechanisms of inorganic phosphate transport in kidney. *Physiological Reviews* **66**: 36–70. [4.3.2]

Goetz KL, Bond GC & Bloxham DD. 1975. Atrial receptors and renal function. *Physiological Reviews* **55**: 157–205. [7.2]

Goldberg M, Agus ZS & Goldfarb S. 1976. Renal handling of phosphate, calcium and magnesium. In *The Kidney, Vol. 1* (eds. Brenner BM & Rector FC) pp. 344–390. Philadelphia: W B Saunders Co. [7.4.4.6]

Goldring W, Chasis H, Ranges HA & Smith HW. 1941. Effective renal blood flow in patients with essential hypertension. *Journal of Clinical Investigation* **20**: 637–653. [3.3.4.3]

Good DW & Knepper MA. 1985. Ammonia transport in the mammalian Kidney. *American Journal of Physiology* **248**: F459–F471. [6.3]

Goodyer AV, Peterson ER & Relman AS. 1949. Some effects of albumin infusions on renal function and electrolyte excretion in normal man. *Journal of Applied Physiology* **1**: 671–682. [3.3.4.2]

Goormaghtigh N. 1937. L'appareil neuro-myo-arterial juxta-glomerulaire du rein: ses réactions en pathologie et ses rapports avec le tube urinifère. *Compte rendus des séances de l'Académie des Sciences* **124**: 293–296. [2.2.7]

Gottschalk CW. 1961. Fifth Bowditch Lecture: micropuncture studies of tubular function in the mammalian kidney. *The Physiologist* **4**: 35–55. [5.4]

Gottschalk CW. 1962–63. Renal tubular function: lessons from micropuncture. *Harvey Lectures* **58**: 99–124. [5.2]

Gottschalk CW. 1979. Renal nerves and sodium excretion. *Annual Review of Physiology* **41**: 229–240. [7.4.4.5]

Gottschalk CW Mylle M. 1959. Micropuncture study of the mammalian urinary concentrating mechanism: evidence for the countercurrent hypothesis. *American Journal of Physiology* **196**: 927–936. [5.5.1]

Graber ML, Bengele HH & Alexander EA. 1982. Elevated urinary P_{CO_2} in the rat: an intrarenal event. *Kidney International* **21**: 795–799. [6.4]

Granath KA & Kvist BE. 1967. Molecular weight distribution analysis by gel chromatography on sephadex. *Journal of Chromatography* **28**: 69–81. [3.2.5]

Grantham JJ. 1976. Fluid secretion in the nephron: relation to renal failure. *Physiological Reviews* **56**: 248–258. [4.4.1]

Green G & Giebisch G. 1984. Luminal hypotonicity: a driving force for fluid absorption from the proximal tubule. *American Journal of Physiology* **246**: F167–F174. [5.2]

Green R, Windhager EE & Giebisch G. 1974. Protein oncotic pressure effects on proximal tubular fluid movement in the rat. *American Journal of Physiology* **262**: 265–276. [7.4.4.3]

Greger R. 1981. Renal transport of oxalate. In *Renal Transport of Organic Substances* (eds. Greger R, Lang F & Silbernagl S), pp. 224–233. Berlin, Heidelberg, New York: Springer-Verlag. [4.4.3]

Grimby G. 1965. Renal clearance during prolonged supine exercise at different loads. *Journal of Applied Physiology* **20**: 1294–1298. [3.3.4.3]

Grimellec CL, Poujeol P & Rouffignac C de. 1975. ^{3}H-inulin and electrolyte concentrations in Bowman's capsule in rat kidney: comparison with artificial ultrafiltration. *Pflügers Archiv für gesamte Physiologie* **354**: 117–131. [3.2.4]

Gross R, Hackenberg HM, Hackenthal E & Kirchheim H. 1981. Interaction between perfusion pressure and sympathetic nerves in renin release by carotid baroreflex in conscious dogs. *Journal of Physiology* **313**: 237–250. [2.2.8]

Gross R & Kirchheim H. 1980. Effects of carotid occlusion and auditory stimulation on renal blood flow and sympathetic nerve activity in the conscious dog. *Pflügers Archiv für gesamte Physiologie* **283**: 233–239. [2.2.5, 2.2.8]

Guder WG & Ross BD. 1984. Enzyme distribution along the nephron (Editorial review). *Kidney International* **26**: 101–111. [1.1, 4.5, 8.3]

Guder WG & Wirthensohn G 1981. Renal turnover of substrates. In *Renal Transport of Organic Substances* (eds. Greger R, Lang F & Silbernagl S), pp. 66–77. Berlin, Heidelberg, New York: Springer-Verlag. [4.5, 4.6]

Gunther RA & Rabinowitz L. 1980. Urea and renal concentrating ability in the rabbit. *Kidney International* **17**: 205–222. [5.5.2]

Guyton AC. 1963. Theory for autoregulation of glomerular filtration rate and blood flow in each nephron by the juxtaglomerular apparatus (Abstract). Physiologist **6**: 194. [2.2.7]

Guyton AC, Granger HJ & Taylor AE. 1971. Interstitial fluid pressure. *Physiological Reviews* **51**: 527–563. [7.4.5]

Haas LF, Holdaway IM & Robinson JR. 1965. Transient alterations in excretion of urea with diuresis in man. *Australasian Annals of Medicine* **14**: 40–48. [4.2.1, 5.5.3]

Häberle DA. 1981. Characteristics of *p*-aminohippurate transport in the mammalian kidney. In *Renal Transport of Organic Substances* (eds. Greger R, Lang F & Silbernagl S), pp. 189–209. Berlin, Heidelberg, New York: Springer-Verlag. [4.4.1]

Häberle DA & Davis JM. 1982. Interrelationship between proximal tubular hydrodynamics and tubuloglomerular feedback in the rat kidney. *Kidney International* **22** (Suppl. 12): S193–S197. [3.3.5.3]

Häberle DA, Shigai TT, Maier G. Schiffl H & Davis JM. 1981. Dependency of proximal tubular fluid transport on the load of glomerular filtrate. *Kidney International* **20**: 18–28. [7.4.4.3]

Hai NA & Thomas S. 1969. The time-course of changes in renal tissue composition during lysine vasopressin infusions in the rat. *Pflügers Archiv für gesamte Physiologie* **310**: 297–319. [5.5.3]

Hall CL & Hardwicke J. 1979. Low molecular weight proteinuria. *Annual Review of Medicine* **30**: 199–211. [3.2.5]

Hall JE. 1986a. Control of sodium excretion by angiotensin II: intrarenal mechanisms and blood pressure regulation (Invited review). *American Journal of Physiology* **250**: R960–R972. [7.4.5]

Hall JE. 1986b. Symposium: Arterial pressure and body fluid homeostasis. Introductory comments. *Federation Proceedings* **45**: 2862–2863. [8.3]

Hall PW & Selkurt EE. 1951. Effects of graded venous occlusion on electrolyte clearance by the dog kidney. *American Journal of Physiology* **164**: 143–154. [3.3.4.3]

Halperin ML & Jungas RL. 1983. Metabolic production and renal disposal of hydrogen ions (Editorial review). *Kidney International* **24**: 709–713. [6.2, 6.3]

Hammerman M, 1986. Phosphate transport across renal proximal tubular cell membranes (Editorial review). *American Journal of Physiology* **251**: F385–F398. [4.3.2]

Handler JS. 1986. Studies of kidney cells in culture. *Kidney International* **30**: 208–215. [4.1]

Hansen AaP & Mogensen CE. 1972. Growth hormone secretion and kidney function during normalization of the metabolic state in newly diagnosed juvenile diabetics. *Hormone & Metabolic Research* **4**: 11–15. [3.3.4.2]

Hargitay B & Kuhn W. 1951. Das Multiplikationsprinzip als Grundlage der Harnkonzentrierung in der Niere. *Zeitschrift für Elektrochemie* **55**: 539–558. [5.5.2]

Hargitay B, Kuhn W & Wirz H. 1951. Ein mikrocryoskopische Methode für sehr kleine Lösungsmengen (0.1–1 gamma). *Experientia* **7**: 276–278. [5.5.1]

Harris CA, Baer PG, Chirito E & Dirks JH. 1974. Composition of mammalian glomerular filtrate. *American Journal of Physiology* **227**: 972–976. [3.2.2]

Harris RM & Gill JM. 1981. Changes in glomerular filtration rate during complete ureteral obstruction in rats. *Kidney International* **19**: 603–608. [3.3.2]

Hartmann H. Ørskov SL & Rein H. 1937. Die Gefäßreaktion der Niere im Verlaufe allgemeiner Kreislauf-Regulationsvorgänge. *Pflügers Archiv für gesamte Physiologie* **238**: 239–250. [2.2.6, 2.2.7]

Harvey AM & Malvin RL. 1966. The effect of androgenic hormones on creatinine secretion in the rat. *Journal of Physiology* **184**: 883–888. [3.3.2]

Hayman JM, Jr. 1927. Estimations of afferent arteriole and glomerular capillary pressures in the frog kidney. *American Journal of Physiology* **79**: 389–409. [3.2.2]

Hays RM. 1983. Alteration of luminal membrane structure by antidiuretic hormone (Editorial review). *American Journal of Physiology* **245**: C289–C296. [5.5.3]

Hays RM, Franki N & Ding G. 1987 Effect of antidiuretic hormone on the collecting ducts. *Kidney International* **31**: 530–537. [5.5.3]

Hayslett JP. 1979. Functional adaptation to reduction in renal mass. *Physiological Reviews* **59**: 137–164. [7.3.4.2]

Hayslett JP, Kashgarian M & Epstein FH. 1968. Functional correlates of compensatory renal hypertrophy. *Journal of Clinical Investigation* **47**: 774–782. [7.3]

Healy DP & Fanestil DD. 1986. Localization of atrial natriuretic peptide binding sites within the rat kidney. *American Journal of Physiology* **250**: F573–F578. [7.4.4.4]

Hebert SC & Andreoli TE. 1984. Control of NaCl transport in the thick ascending limb. *American Journal of Physiology* **246**: F745–F756. [5.5.3]

Hebert SC, Schafer JA & Andreoli TE. 1981. The effects of antidiuretic hormone (ADH) on solute and water transport in the mammalian nephron. *Journal of membrane Biology* **58**: 1–19. [5.3, 5.4, 5.5.3]

Heidenhain R. 1883. Die Harnabsonderung. In *Handbuch der Physiologie, Vol. V* (ed. Hermann L), pp. 279–373. Leipzig: Vogel. [3.3.3]

Heinrich WL. 1981. Role of prostaglandins on renin secretion. *Kidney International* **19**: 822–830. [7.4.3]

Heinrich WL, Walker BR, Handelman WA, Erickson AL, Arnold PE & Schrier RW. 1986. Effects of angiotensin II on plasma antidiuretic hormone and water excretion. *Kidney International* **30**: 503–508. [7.4.3]

Hervey GR, McCance RA & Tayler RQC. 1946. Forced diuresis during hydropenia. *Nature (London)* **157**: 338. [5.5.3]

Heymans C. Bouckaert JJ & Regniers P. 1933. *Le Sinus Carotidien et la Zone Homologue Cardioaortique.* Paris: Doin. [2.2.6]

Heymans C & Neil E. 1958. *Reflexogenic areas of the cardiovscular system*. London: J & A Churchill. [2.2.6]

Hiatt EP. 1942. The effect of denervation on the filtration rate and blood flow in dog kidneys rendered hyperemic by administration of pyrogen. *American Journal of Physiology* **136**: 38−41. [2.2.5, 3.3.4.2]

Hiatt EP & Hiatt RB. 1942. The effect of food on the filtration rate and renal blood flow of the harbor seal (*Phoca vitulina* L.). *Journal of Cellular & Comparative Physiology* **19**: 221−227. [3.3.4.2]

Hierholzer K, Tsiakiras D, Schöneshöfer M, Siebe H & Weskamp P. 1981. Renal handling of hormones. In *Renal Transport of Organic Substances* (eds. Greger R, Land F & Silbernagi S), pp. 278−289. Berlin, Heidelberg, New York: Springer-Verlag. [4.2.4]

Hierholtzer K & Ullrich KJ. 1969. Grundzüge der Nierenphysiologie. In *Handbuch der experimentelle Pharmakologie* , pp. 1−61. Berlin, Heidelberg, New York: Springer-Verlag. [3.3.3]

Hilger HH, Klümper JD & Ullrich KJ. 1958. Wasserrückresorption und Ionentransport durch die Sammelrohrzellen der Saugetierniere. *Pflügers Archiv für gesamte Physiologie* **267**: 218−237. [5.4]

Hill AV. 1931. *Adventures in Biophysics*. London: Humphrey Milford, Oxford University Press. [5.3]

Hitchcock DI. 1945. Some properties of aqueous solutions. In *Physical Chemistry of Cells and Tissues* (ed. Höber R), pp. 75−91. Philadelphia: Blakiston. [3.2.3]

Hogg RJ & Kokko JH. 1979. Renal countercurrent multiplication system. *Reivews of Physiology, Biochemistry & Pharmacology* **86**: 95−135. [5.5.2]

Hollenberg NK. 1979. The physiology of the renal circulation. In *Renal Disease*, 4th edn (eds. Black DAK & Jones NF), pp. 30−63. Oxford: Blackwell Scientific Publications. [3.3.4.3]

Hollenberg NK. 1980. Set point for sodium homeostasis: surfiet, deficit, and their implications (Editorial review). *Kidney International* **17**: 423−429. [7.4.5]

Hoppe F. 1859. Ueber die Bildung des Harns. *Virchows Archiv für pathologische Anatomie und Physiologie* **16**: 412−413. [1.3, 5.2]

Hostetter TH. 1986. Human renal response to a meat meal. *American Journal of Physiology* **250**: F613−F618. [3.3.4.2]

Hostetter TH, Olson JL, Rennke HG, Venkatachalam MA & Brenner BM. 1981a. Hyperfiltration in remnant nephrons: a potentially adverse response to renal ablation. *American Journal of Physiology* **241**: F85−F93. [3.3.4.2]

Hostetter TH, Troy JL & Brenner BM. 1981b. Glomerular hemodynamics in experimental diabetes mellitus. *Kidney International* **19**: 410−415. [3.3.4.2]

House CR. 1974. *Water Transport in Cells and Tissues*. London: Edward Arnold. [5.2]

Hulter HN. 1985. Effects of interrelationships of PTH, Ca^{2+}, vitamin D, and Pi on acid−base homeostasis (Editorial review). *American Journal of Physiology* **248**: F739−F752. [6.4]

Hunsicker LG, Shearer TP & Shaffer SJ. 1981. Acute reversible proteinuria induced by infusion of the polycation hexadimethrine. *Kidney International* **20**: 7−17. [3.2.6]

Huth EJ, Squires RD & Elkinton JR. 1959. Experimental potassium depletion in normal human subjects II. Renal and hormonal factors in the development of extracellular alkalosis during depletion. *Journal of Clinical Investigation* **38**: 1149−1165. [6.4]

Ichikawa I. 1982. Hemodynamic influence of altered distal salt delivery on glomerular microcirculation. *Kidney International* **22** (Suppl. 12): S109−S113. [3.3.5.3]

Ikkos D, Ljunggren H & Luft R. 1956. Glomerular filtration rate and renal plasma flow in acromegaly. *Acta Endocrinologica (Copenhagen)* **21**: 226−236. [3.3.4.2]

Ishikawa T, Koizumi K & Brooks C McC. 1966. Electrical activity recorded from the pituitary stalk of the cat. *American Journal of Physiology* **210**: 417−431. [5.3]

Israelit AH, Long DL, White MG & Hull AR. 1973. Measurement of glomerular filtration rate utilizing a single subcutaneous injection of ^{125}I-iothalamate. *Kidney International* **4**: 346−349. [3.3.2]

Jackson B & Oken DE. 1982. Internephron heterogeneity of filtration fraction and disparity between protein- and hematocrit-derived values. *Kidney International* **21**: 309–315. [3.3.5.2]

Jackson EK, Branch RA, Margolius HS & Oates JA. 1985. Physiological function of the renal prostaglandin, renin and kallikrein systems. In *The kidney: Physiology and Pathophysiology* (eds. Seldin DW & Giebisch G), pp. 613–644. New York: Raven Press. [7.4.3]

Jacobs MH. 1935. Diffusion processes. *Ergebnisse der Biologie* **12**: 1–160. [3.4.4.3]

Jacobson HR. 1981. Functional segmentation of the mammalian nephron. *American Journal of Physiology* **241**: F203–F218. [4.2.1, 4.3.1]

Jacobson HR & Kokko JP. (eds.) 1982. Symposium: Isolated perfused tubule. *Kidney International* **22**: 415–570. [4.1, 4.1.1]

Jamison RL. 1974. Countercurrent systems. In *Kidney and Urinary Tract Physiology* (ed. Thurau K), pp. 199–245. Baltimore, Maryland: University Park Press. [5.5.2]

Jamison RL. 1976. Urinary concentration and dilution. The role of antidiuretic hormone and the role of urea. In *The Kidney* (eds. Brenner BM & Rector FC), pp. 391–441. Philadelphia: W B Saunders Co. [5.5.2]

Jamison RL. 1987. Potassium recycling (Editorial review). *Kidney International* **31**: 695–703. [8.3]

Jamison RL, Bennett CM & Berliner RW. 1967. Countercurrent multiplication by the loops of Henle. *American Journal of Physiology* **212**: 357–366. [5.5.2]

Jamison RL & Maffly RH. 1976. The urinary countercurrent mechanism. *New England Journal of Medicine* **292**: 1059–1067. [5.5.2]

Jamison RL & Robertson CR. 1979. Recent formulations of the urinary concentrating mechanism: a status report. *Kidney International* **16**: 537–545. [5.5.2]

Jelkman W. 1986. Renal erythropoietin: properties and production. *Reviews of Physiology, Biochemistry & Pharmacology* **104**: 139–215. [1.1, 8.3]

Jewell PA & Verney EB. 1957. An experimental attempt to determine the site of the neurohypophysial osmoreceptors in the dog. *Philosophical Transactions of the Royal Society of London* **240**: 197–324. [5.3]

Johnston CI & Davies JO. 1966. Evidence from cross circulation studies for a humoral mechanism in the natriuresis of saline loading. *Proceedings of the Society for Experimental Biology & Medicine* **121**: 1058–1063. [7.4.4]

Jones NF. 1972. Renal aspects of electrolyte disorders. In *Renal Disease*, 3rd edn (ed. Black DAK), pp. 615–653. Oxford: Blackwell Scientific Publications. [3.3.4.3]

Jungermann K. 1985. Metabolische Zonierung des Leberparenchyms. Bedeutung für die Regulation des Glucostaten Leber. *Naturwissenschaften* **72**: 76–84. [4.6]

Källskog O, Lindbom LO, Ulfendahl HR & Wolgast M. 1975. Kinetics of the glomerular ultrafiltration in the rat kidney: an experimental study. *Acta Physiologica Scandinavica* **95**: 293–300. [3.2.2, 3.3]

Kanwar YS & Farquhar MG. 1979. Presence of heparan sulfate in the glomerular basement membrane. *Proceedings of the National Academy of Sciences, Washington* **76**: 1301–1307. [3.2.6]

Karim F, Poucher SM & Summerill RA. 1984. The reflex effects of changes in carotid sinus pressure upon renal function in dogs. *Journal of Physiology* **355**: 557–566. [7.4.2]

Karlmark B, Jaeger P & Geibisch G. 1983. Luminal buffer transfer in rat cortical tubule: relationship to potassium metabolism. *American Journal of Physiology* **245**: F584–F592. [6.3]

Karnovsky MJ & Ainsworth SK. 1972. The structural basis of glomerular filtration. *Advances in Nephrology* **2**: 35–60. [3.2.6]

Kassirer JP & Gennari FJ. 1979. Laboratory evaluation of renal function. In *Strauss and Welt's Diseases of the Kidney, Vol. 1*, 3rd edn (eds. Earley LE & Gottschalk CW), pp. 41–91. Boston: Little, Brown & Co. [3.3.2]

Katz AI & Lindheimer MD. 1977. Action of hormones on the kidney. *Annual Review of Physiology* **39**: 97–134. [7.4.4.6]

Kerr DNS. 1979. Acute renal failure. In *Renal Disease*, 4th edn (eds. Black DAK & Jones NF), pp. 437–493. Oxford: Blackwell Scientific Publications. [3.3.4.3]

Keyl MJ, Scott BJ, Dabney JM, Haddy PJ, Harvey RB, Bell RD & Ginn HE. 1965. Composition of canine renal hilar lymph. *American Journal of Physiology* **209**: 1031–1033. [2.2.3]

Khuri RN, Wiederholt M, Strieder N & Giebisch G. 1975. Effects of flow rate and potassium intake on distal tubular potassium transfer. *American Journal of Physiology* **228**: 1249–1261. [4.4.3]

Kinne RN & Schwartz IL. 1978. Isolated membrane vesicles in the evaluation of the nature, localization and regulation of renal transport processes. *Kidney International* **14**: 547–556. [4.1.1, 8.3]

Kirchheim HR. 1976. Systemic arterial baroreceptor reflexes. *Physiological Reviews* **56**: 100–176. [2.2.8, 2.2.8.1]

Kirschenbaum MA & Serros ER. 1980. Are prostaglandins natriuretic? (Editorial). *Mineral & Electrolyte Metabolism* **3**: 113–121. [7.4.4.6]

Klahr S & Slatopolsky E. 1973. Renal regulation of sodium excretion. *Archives of Internal Medicine* **131**: 780–791. [7.4.2]

Kleeman CR. 1972. Water metabolism. In *Clinical Disorders of Fluid and Electrolyte Metabolism*, 2nd edn (eds. Maxwell MH & Kleeman CR), pp. 215–295. New York: McGraw-Hill Book Co. [5.5.4]

Kleinman LI. 1982. Developmental renal physiology. *The Physiologist* **25**: 104–110. [3.3.4.2]

Klisiecki A, Pickford M, Rothschild P & Verney EB. 1933. The absorption and excretion of water by the mammal. Part I. The relation between absorption of water and its excretion by the innervated and denervated kidney. *Proceedings of the Royal Society of London* **B112**: 496–521. [5.3]

Knepper M & Burg M. 1983. Organization of nephron function. *American Journal of Physiology* **244**: F579–F589. [4.1]

Knox FG. 1982. Comparative physiology of the control of renal function. *Federation Proceedings* **41**: 2382–2384. [3.3.4.3]

Knox FG, Burnett JC, Jr, Kohan DE, Spielman WS & Strand JC. 1980. Escape from the sodium-retaining effects of mineralocorticoids (Editorial review). *Kidney International* **17**: 263–276. [7.4.5]

Knox FG & Haas JA. 1982. Factors influencing renal sodium reabsorption in volume expansion. *Reviews of Physiology, Biochemistry & Pharmacology* **92**: 75–113. [7.4.2]

Knox FG, Mertz JI, Burnett JC, Jr & Haramati A. 1983. Role of hydrostatic and oncotic pressures in renal sodium reabsorption. *Circulation Research* **52**: 491–500. [7.4.4.3]

Knox FG, Schneider EG, Willis LR, Strandhoy JW & Ott CE. 1973. Site and control of phosphate reabsorption by the kidney. *Kidney International* **3**: 347–353. [4.3.2]

Knox FG & Spielman WS. 1983. Renal circulation. In *Handbook of Physiology, Section 2. The Cardiovascular System, Vol. III, Peripheral Circulation, Part 1* (eds. Shepherd JT & Abboud FM), pp. 183–217. Bethesda, Maryland: American Physiological Society. [2.2.7, 7.4.4.3]

Kokko JP. 1985. Nephrology forum. Primary acquired hypoaldosteronism. *Kidney International* **27**: 690–702. [7.4.2]

Kokko JP & Rector FC, Jr. 1972. Countercurrent multiplication system without active transport in inner medulla. *Kidney International* **2**: 214–223. [5.5.2]

Kokko JP & Tisher CC. 1976. Water movement across nephron segments involved with the countercurrent multiplication system. *Kidney International* **10**: 64–81. [5.4]

Kon I & Ichikawa I. 1983. Renal nerve control of cortical microcirculation. *American Journal of Physiology* **245**: F535–F553. [3.3.5.3]

Korner PI. 1963. Effects of low oxygen and of carbon monoxide on the renal circulation in unanaesthetized rabbits. *Circulation Research* **12**: 361–374. [2.2.6, 2.2.8, 3.3.4.3]

Korner PI. 1967. Control of the renal circulation by the autonomic nervous system. *Bulletin of the Post-graduate Committee in Medicine, University of Sydney* **23**: 162–180. [2.2.6, 3.3.4.3]

Korner PI. 1971. Integrative cardiovascular control. *Physiological Reviews* **51**: 312–367. [2.2.5, 2.2.6, 2.2.8, 2.2.8.1, 2.3.3]

Korner PI. 1974. Control of blood flow to special vascular areas: brain, kidney, muscle, skin, liver and intestine. In *MTP International Review of Science, Physiology Series 1, Vol. 1, Cardiovascular Physiology* (eds. Guyton AC & Jones CE), pp. 123–162. Baltimore: University Park Press. [2.2.8, 2.2.8.1, 3.3.5.2]

Kramer K & Deetjen P. 1960. Beziehungen des O_2-Verbrauchs der Niere zur Durchblutung und Glomerulusfiltrat bei Änderung des arteriellen Druckes. *Pflügers Archiv für gesamte physiologie* **271**: 782–796. [2.2.4]

Kramer K, Lochner W & Wetterer E. 1963. Methods of measuring blood flow. In *Handbook of Physiology, Section 2, Circulation, Vol. II* (eds. Hamilton WF & Dow P), pp. 1277–1324. Washington, DC: American Physiological Society. [2.2.2]

Kramer K, Thurau K & Deetjen P. 1960. Hämodynamik des Nierenmarks. I Capilläre Passagezeit, Blutvolumen, Durchblutung, Gewebshämatokrit und O_2-Verbrauch des Nierenmarks *in situ*. *Pflügers Archiv für gesamte Physiologie* **270**: 251–269. [2.3.2]

Kramp RA & Lorenz WB. 1982. Glucose transport in chronically altered nephrons. *American Journal of Physiology* **243**: F393–F403. [4.2.2]

Kramp RA, MacDowell M, Gottschalk CW & Oliver JR. 1974. A study by microdissection and micropuncture of the structure and function of the kidneys and the nephrons of rats with chronic renal damage. *Kidney International* **5**: 147–176. [3.3.4.3]

Krebs HA. 1950. Body size and tissue respiration. *Biochimica et Biophysica Acta* **4**: 249–269. [2.2.1]

Kregenow FM. 1977. Cell volume control. In *Water relations in membrane transport in plants and animals* (eds. Jungreis AM, Hodges TK, Kleinzeller A & Schultz SG), pp. 291–302. New York, San Francisco, London: Academic Press. [7.3]

Kriz W. 1981. Structural organization of the renal medulla: comparative and functional aspects. *American Journal of Physiology* **241**: R3–R16. [5.5.1, 5.5.2]

Krohn AG, Ogden DA & Holmes JH. 1966. Renal function before and after nephrectomy. *Journal of the American Medical Association* **196**: 322–324. [2.2.4, 3.3.4]

Kruhøffer P. 1960. Handling of alkali metal ions by the kidney. In *The Alkali Metal Ions in Biology* (eds. Ussing HH, Kruhøffer P. Thaysen JH & Thorn NA), pp. 233–423. Berlin, Göttingen, Heidelberg: Springer-Verlag. [3.3.4.2, 3.3.5.3]

Kumar R. 1986. The metabolism and mechanism of action of 1,25-dihydroxyvitamin D_3 (Editorial review). *Kidney International* **30**: 793–803. [1.1]

Kuhn W & Ramel A. 1959. Aktiver Satztransport als möglicher (und wahrscheinlicher) Einzeleffekt bei der Harnkonzentrierung in der Niere. *Helvetica Chimica Acta* **42**: 628–660. [5.5.2]

Ladd M. 1951. Effect of prehydration on the renal excretion of sodium in man. *Journal of Applied Physiology* **3**: 603–609. [3.3.4.2]

Ladd M & Raisz LG. 1949. Response of the normal dog to dietary sodium chloride. *American Journal of Physiology* **159**: 149–152. [3.3.4.2]

Ladd M, Raisz LG, Crowder CH & Page LB. 1951. Filtration rate and water diuresis in the seal *Phoca vitulina*. *Journal of Cellular and Comparative Physiology* **38**: 157–164. [3.3.4.2]

Lameire MI, Lifschitz MD & Stein JH. 1977. Heterogeneity of renal function. *Annual Review of Physiology* **39**: 159–184. [1.2]

Landergren E & Tigerstedt R. 1893. Die Blutzufuhr zu der Niere. *Skandinavisches Archiv für Physiologie* **4**: 241–280. [2.2.2]

Landis EM & Pappenheimer JR. 1963. Exchange of substances through the capillary walls, in *Handbook of Physiology, Section 2, Circulation, Vol. II* (eds. Hamilton WF & Dow P), pp. 961–1034. Washington, DC: American Physiological Society. [3.2.3]

Landwehr, DM, Klose RM & Giebisch G. 1967. Renal tubular sodium and water reabsorption in the isotonic sodium chloride-loaded rat. *American Journal of Physiology* **216**: 1327–1333. [3.3.4.2]

Lang F. 1981. Renal handling of urate. In *Renal Transport of Organic Substances* (eds. Greger R, Lang F & Silbernagl S), pp. 234–261. Berlin, Heidelberg, New York: Springer-Verlag. [4.3.2]

Lang RE, Thölken H, Ganten E, Luft FC, Ruskoaho H & Unger Th. 1985. Atrial natriuretic factor — a circulating hormone stimulated by volume loading. *Nature* **314**: 264–266. [7.4.4.4]

Langberg H, Hartmann A, Østensen M & Kiil F. 1986. Hypernatremia inhibits NaHCO$_3$ reabsorption and associated NaCl reabsorption in dogs. *Kidney International* **29**: 820–828. [8.3]

Lassen NA, Munck O & Thaysen JH. 1961. Oxygen consumption and sodium reabsorption in the kidney. *Acta Physiologica Scandinavica* **51**: 371–384. [4.3.1]

Lassiter WE. 1970. Urea transport in the mammalian nephron. In *Urea and the Kidney* (ed. Schmidt-Nielsen B), pp. 206–213. Amsterdam: Excerpta Medica Foundation. [4.2.1]

Latta H. 1973. Ultrastructure of the glomerulus and juxtaglomerular apparatus. In *Handbook of Physiology, Section 8, Renal Physiology* (eds. Orloff J & Berliner RW), pp. 1–29. Washington DC: American Physiological Society. [3.2.6]

Lauson HD, Bradley SE & Cournand A. 1944. The renal circulation in shock. *Journal of Clinical Investigation* **23**: 381–402. [2.2.6, 3.3.4.2, 3.3.4.3]

Leaf A. 1970. Regulation of intracellular fluid volume and disease (Editorial). *American Journal of Medicine* **49**: 291–295. [2.2.5]

Leaf A. 1982. From toad bladder to kidney (Homer Smith Award Lecture). *American Journal of Physiology* **242**: F103–F111. [4.6]

Leaf A & Cotran RS. 1976. *Renal pathophysiology*. New York: Oxford University Press. [2.3.2, 3.3.4.3]

Leaf A & Sharp GWG. 1971. The stimulation of sodium transport by aldosterone. *Philosophical Transactions of the Royal Society of London* **B.262**: 323–332. [7.4.3]

Lee MR. 1982. Dopamine and the kidney. *Clinical Science and Molecular Medicine* **62**: 439–448. [3.3.5.3]

Levens NR, Peach MJ & Carey RM. 1981. Role of the intrarenal renin–angiotensin system in the control of renal function. *Circulation Research* **48**: 157–167. [2.2.7]

Levine DZ & Jacobson HR. 1986. The regulation of renal acid secretion: new observations from studies of distal nephron segments (Editorial review). *Kidney International* **29**: 1099–1109. [6.3]

Levinsky NG & Levy M. 1973. Clearance techniques. In *Handbook of Physiology, Section 8, Renal Physiology* (eds. Orloff J & Berliner RW), pp. 103–117. Washington, DC: American Physiological Society. [3.3.2]

Levy MN & Sauceda G. 1959. Diffusion of oxygen from arterial to venous segments of renal capillaries. *American Journal of Physiology* **196**: 1336–1339. [2.3.2]

Leyssac PP. 1963. Dependence of glomerular filtration rate on proximal tubular reabsorption of salt. *Acta Physiologica Scandinavica* **58**: 236–242. [3.3.5.3]

Lifshitz MD. 1981. Prostaglandins and renal blood flow: *in vivo* studies. *Kidney International* **19**: 781–785. [3.3.5.3]

Lilien DM & Phillips H. 1966. Photographic micropuncture and the countercurrent system. *Journal of Urology* **95**: 90–98. [5.5.1]

Linden RJ & Kappagoda CT. 1982. *Atrial Receptors*. Cambridge: University Press. [3.3.5.3, 7.4.2, 7.4.5]

Liu FY, Cogan MG & Rector FC, Jr. 1984. Axial heterogeneity in the rat proximal convoluted tubule. II. Osmolality and osmotic water permeability. *American Journal of Physiology* **247**: F822−F826. [5.2]

Ljungberg E. 1947. On the reabsorption of chloride in the kidney of the rabbit. *Acta Medica Scandinavica Supplement* **186**: 1−189. [5.5.1]

Lockett MF & Roberts CN. 1963. Some actions of growth hormone in the perfused cat kidney. *Journal of Physiology* **169**: 879−888. [7.4.5]

London GM, Safar ME, Levenson JA, Simon AC & Temmar MA. 1981. Renal filtration fraction, effective vascular compliance, and partition of fluid volumes in sustained essential hypertension. *Kidney International* **20**: 97−103. [3.3.4.3]

Longuet-Higgins HC & Austin G. 1966. The kinetics of osmotic transport through pores of molecular dimensions. *Biophysical Journal* **6**: 271−224. [3.2.8]

Lönnerholm G, Wistrand PJ. 1984. Carbonic anhydrase in the human kidney: a histo-chemical and immunocytochemical study. *Kidney International* **25**: 886−898. [6.3]

Lote CJ. 1982. Renal prostaglandins and sodium excretion. *Quarterly Journal of Experimental Physiology* **67**: 377−385. [3.3.5.3, 7.4.4.6]

Lotspeich WD. 1959. *Metabolic Aspects of Renal Function*. Springfield, Illinois: Charles C Thomas. [4.5]

Ludwig C. 1844. Nieren und Harnbereitung. In *Handwörterbuch der Physiologie* (ed. Wagner R), pp. 628−640. Braunschweig: Vieweg. [1.3, 3.2.1, 4.3.1, 5.2, 7.4.4.3]

McCance RA. 1936. Medical problems in mineral metabolism (Goulstonian Lectures). III. Experimental human salt deficiency. *Lancet* **i**: 823−830. [3.3.4.3]

McCance RA. 1937. The changes in the plasma and cells during experimental human salt deficiency. *Biochemical Journal* **31**: 1278−1284. [7.4.3]

McCance RA. 1945. The excretion of urea, salts and water during periods of hydropenia in man. *Journal of Physiology* **104**: 196−209. [5.5.3]

McCance RA. 1948. Renal function in early life. *Physiological Reviews* **28**: 331−348. [2.2.4]

McCance RA. 1950. Renal function in infancy. *American Journal of Medicine* **9**: 229−241. [2.2.4]

McCance RA & Widdowson EM. 1952. The correct physiological basis on which to compare infant and adult renal function. *Lancet* **ii**: 860−862. [3.3.3]

McDonald MS & Emery JL. 1959. The late intra-uterine and postnatnal development of human renal glomeruli. *Journal of Anatomy* **93**: 331−340. [3.3.4.2]

McKay A, Eadie AS, Cumming AMM, Graham AG, Adams FG & Horton PW. 1981. Assessment of total and divided renal plasma flow by ^{123}I-hippuran renography. *Kidney International* **19**: 49−57. [2.2.3.3]

McKinley MJ, Denton DA & Weisinger RS. 1978. Sensors for antidiuresis and thirst — osmoreceptors or csf sodium detectors? *Brain Research* **141**: 89−103. [7.2]

Macknight ADC, DiBona DR & Leaf A. 1980. Sodium transport across toad urinary bladder: a model 'tight' epithelium. *Physiological Reviews* **60**: 615−715. [4.6, 5.5.3]

Macknight ADC & Leaf A. 1977. Regulation of cellular volume. *Physiological Reviews* **57**: 510−573. [7.3]

Macknight ADC, Macknight JM & Robinson JR. 1962. The effect of urinary output upon the excretion of 'ammonia' in man. *Journal of Physiology* **163**: 314−323. [8.3]

McLachlan MSF. 1978. The ageing kidney. *Lancet* **ii**: 143−146. [3.3.4.2, 3.3.4.3]

McManus JFM. 1966. *General Pathology*. Chicago: Year Book Medical Publishers. [3.3.3]

McNay JL, Rosello S & Dayton PG. 1976. Effects of azotemia on renal extraction and clearance of PAH and TEA. *American Journal of Physiology* **230**: 901−906. [4.4.2]

Maack T, Camargo MJF, Kleinert HD, Laragh JH & Atlas SA. 1985. Atrial natriuretic factor: Structure and functional properties (Editorial review). *Kidney International* **27**: 607−615. [7.4.4.4]

Maack T, Johnson V,-Kau ST, Figueiredo J & Sigulem D. 1979. Renal filtration, transport, and metabolism of low-molecular-weight proteins: a review. *Kidney International* **16**: 251−270. [4.2.4]

Maddox DA, Deen WM & Brenner BM. 1974. Dynamics of glomerular filtration. VI. Studies on the primate. *Kidney International* **5**: 271–278. [3.2.2, 3.2.3]

Madias NE & Zelman SJ. 1986. The renal response to chronic mineral acid feeding: a re-examination of the role of systemic pH. *Kidney International* **29**: 667–674. [8.3]

Malnic G. 1974. Tubular handling of H. In *Kidney and Urinary Tract Physiology* (ed. Thurau K), pp. 107–127. London: Butterworths. [6.3, 6.4]

Malnic G. 1980. CO_2 equilibria in renal tissue. *American Journal of Physiology* **239**: F307–F318. [6.4]

Malnic G, Klose RM & Giebisch G. 1964. Micropuncture study of renal potassium excretion in the rat. *American Journal of Physiology* **206**: 674–686. [4.3.3, 4.4.3]

Malnic G, Klose RM & Giebisch G. 1966. Micropuncture study of distal tubular potassium and sodium transport in rat nephron. *American Journal of Physiology* **211**: 529–547. [5.2]

Malvin RL & Wilde WS. 1959. Washout of renal countercurrent Na gradient by osmotic diuresis. *American Journal of Physiology* **197**: 177–180. [5.5.3]

Malvin RL, Wilde WS & Sullivan LP. 1958. Localization of nephron transport by stop flow analysis. *American Journal of Physiology* **194**: 135–142. [4.1.1, 4.2.3]

Manning RD, Jr & Guyton AC. 1982. Control of blood volume. *Reviews of Physiology, Biochemistry and Pharmacology* **93**: 70–114. [7.4.5]

Marchand GR. 1978. Direct recording of glomerular capillary hydrostatic pressure in the dog (Abstract). *Kidney International* **14**: 768. [3.2.2, 3.2.3]

Maren TH 1978. Carbon dioxide equilibria in the kidney: the problems of elevated carbon dioxide tension, delayed dehydration, and disequilibrium pH. *Kidney International* **14**: 395–405. [6.4]

Marin-Grez M, Fleming JT & Steinhausen M. 1986. Atrial natriuretic peptide causes pre-glomerular vasodilatation and post-glomerular vasoconstriction in rat kidney. *Nature* **324**: 473–476. [7.4.4.4]

Markley K, Bocanegra M, Morales G & Chiappori M. 1957. Oral sodium loading in normal individuals. *Journal of Clinical Investigation* **36**: 303–308. [3.3.4.2]

Marriott HL. 1950. *Water and Salt Depletion*. Springfield, Illinois: Charles C Thomas. [3.3.4.3]

Marsh DJ. 1982. Frequency response of autoregulation. *Kidney International* **22**: (Suppl. 12): S165–S172. [3.3.5.3]

Marshall EK, Jr & Crane MM. 1924. The secretory function of the renal tubules. *American Journal of Physiology* **70**: 465–488. [4.4.1]

Marshall EK, Jr & Vickers JL. 1923. The mechanism of the elimination of phenolsulpho-nephthalein by the kidney — a proof of secretion by the convoluted tubules. *Bulletin of the Johns Hopkins Hospital* **34**: 1–7. [4.4]

Martinez-Maldonado M. 1980. Inappropriate antidiuretic hormone secretion of unknown origin. *Kidney International* **17**: 554–567. [7.3]

Mason J & Moore LC. 1982. A new way of investigating tubuloglomerular feedback: the closed-loop mode. *Kidney International* **22** (Suppl. 12): S151–S156. [3.3.5.3]

Massry SG. 1979. Effects of electrolyte disorders on the kidney. In *Strauss and Welt's Diseases of the Kidney*, 3rd edn (eds. Earley LE & Gottschalk CW), pp. 1403–1430. Boston: Little, Brown & Co. [3.3.4.3]

Massry SG & Fleisch H. 1980. *Renal Handling of Phosphate*. New York, London: Plenum Medical Book Company. [4.3.2]

Mayerson HS. 1963. The lymphatic system with particular reference to the kidney (1962 Baxter Lecture). *Surgery Gynecology & Obstetrics* **116**: 259–272. [2.2.3]

Menninger RP. 1985. Current concepts of volume receptor regulation of vasopressin release. *Federation Proceedings* **44**: 55–58. [7.2]

Merrill AJ. 1946. Edema and decreased renal blood flow in patients with chronic congestive heart failure: evidence of 'forward failure' as the primary cause of edema. *Journal of Clinical Investigation* **25**: 389–400. [2.2.5]

Merrill AJ & Cargill WH. 1948. The effect of exercise on the renal plasma flow and filtration rate of normal and cardiac patients. *Journal of Clinical Investigation* **27**: 272–282. [2.2.5, 3.3.4.3]

Merrill DS, Skelton MM & Cowley AW, Jr. 1986. Humoral control of water and electrolyte excretion during water restriction. *Kidney International* **29**: 1152–1161. [7.4.5]

Michel CC. 1980. Filtration coefficients and osmotic reflexion coefficients of the walls of single frog mesenteric capillaries. *Journal of Physiology* **309**: 341–355. [3.2.9]

Mills IH. 1982. The renal kallikrein–kinin system and sodium excretion. *Quarterly Journal of Experimental Physiology* **67**: 393–399. [3.3.5.3]

Mills JN. 1966. Human circadian rhythms. *Physiological Reviews* **46**: 128–171. [3.3.3.2, 4.3.2]

Mitchell GAG. 1950. The nerve supply to the kidney. *Acta Anatomica* **10**: 1–37. [2.2.5]

Moffatt DB. 1979. The anatomy of the renal circulation. In *Renal Disease*, 4th edn (eds. Black DAK & Jones NF), pp. 3–29. Oxford: Blackwell Scientific Publications. [3.3.4]

Mogensen CE. 1968. The glomerular permeability determined by dextran clearance using Sephadex gel filtration. *Scandinavian Journal of Clinical and Laboratory Investigation* **21**: 77–82. [3.2.5]

Mogensen CE. 1971. Glomerular filtration rate and renal plasma flow in short-term and long-term juvenile diabetes mellitus. *Scandinavian Journal of Clinical and Laboratory Investigation* **28**: 91–100. [3.3.4.2]

Mogensen CE. 1973. Elevated glomerular filtration rates in insulin-treated short-term diabetes. *Acta Medica Scandinavica* **194**: 559–561. [3.3.4.2]

Möllendorff W von. 1930. Der Exkretionsapparat. *Handbuch der mikroskopisches Anatomie* **VII/I**: 1–328. Berlin: Springer, 1930. [4.2]

Möller E, McIntosh JF & van Slyke DD. 1929. Studies of urea excretion. II. Relationship between urine volume and the rate of urea excretion by normal adults. *Journal of Clinical Investigation* **6**: 427–465. [2.2.3.1]

Moore LC. 1982. Interaction of tubuloglomerular feedback and proximal nephron re-absorption in autoregulation. *Kidney International* **22** (Suppl. 12): S173–S178. [3.3.5.3]

Morel F. 1983. Regulation of kidney functions by hormones: a new approach. *Recent Progress in Hormone Research* **39**: 271–302. [8.3]

Morris GCR. 1976. Growth of rats' kidneys after unilateral uretero-caval anastomosis. *Journal of Physiology* **258**: 755–767. [3.3.3]

Morrison RBI. 1979. Urinalysis and assessment of renal function. In *Renal Disease*, 4th edn (eds. Black DAK & Jones NF), pp. 305–327. Oxford: Blackwell Scientific Publications. [3.3.2]

Mountcastle VB. 1974. Sleep, wakefulness and the conscious state. In *Medical Physiology*, 13th edn (ed. Mountcastle VB), pp. 254–281. St Louis: C V Mosby Co. [3.3.4.2]

Mudge GH, Berndt WD & Valtin H. 1973. Tubular transport of urea, glucose, phosphate, uric acid, sulfate and thiosulfate. In *Handbook of Physiology*, Section 8, *Renal Physiology* (eds. Orloff J, Berliner RW), pp. 587–652. Washington, DC: American Physiological Society. [4.4.3]

Muehrke RC & Pirani CL. 1972. Renal biopsy: an adjunct in the study of kidney disease, in *Renal Disease* 3rd edn (ed. Black DAK), pp. 111–153. Oxford: Blackwell Scientific Publications. [3.232]

Müller-Suur R, Persson AEG & Ulfendahl HR. 1982. Tubuloglomerular feedback in juxtamedullary nephrons. *Kidney International* **22** (Suppl. 12): S104–S108. [2.2.7, 3.3.5.3]

Murdaugh HV, Jr, Schmidt-Nielsen B, Doyle EM & O'Dell R. 1958. Renal tubular regulation of urea excretion in man. *Journal of Applied Physiology* **13**: 263–268. [3.3.4.2]

Murdaugh HV, Sieker HO & Manfredi F. 1959. Effect of altered intrathoracic pressure on renal hemodynamics, electrolyte excretion and water clearance. *Journal of Clinical Investigation* **38**: 834–842. [3.3.4.3]

Murer H, Barac-Nieto M, Ullrich KJ & Kinne R. 1981. Renal transport of lactate. In *Renal Transport ot Organic Substances* (eds. Greger R, Lang F & Silbernagl S), pp. 210–223. Berlin: Heidelberg, New York: Springer-Verlag. [4.3.2]

Musajo L & Benassi CA. 1964. Aspects of disorders of the kynurenine pathway of tryptophan metabolism in man. *Advances in Clinical Chemistry* 7: 63–135. [4.4]

Navar LG. 1978a. Renal autoregulation: perspectives from whole kidney and single nephron studies (Editorial review). *American Journal of Physiology* 234: F357–F370. [2.2.7]

Navar LG. 1978b. The regulation of glomerular filtration rate in mammalian kidneys. In *Physiology of Membrane Disorders* (eds. Andreoli TE, Hoffman JF & Fanestil DD), pp. 593–627. New York, London: Plenum Medical Book Company. [3.2.3]

Navar LG, Bell PD & Burke TJ. 1982. Role of a macula densa feedback mechanism as a mediator of renal autoregulation. *Kidney International* 22 (Suppl. 12): S157–S164. [2.2.7, 3.3.5.3]

Navar LG, Bell PD, White RW, Watts RL & Williams RH. 1977. Evaluation of the single nephron glomerular filtration coefficient in the dog. *Kidney International* 12: 137–149. [3.2.2, 3.2.3]

Navar LG & Rosivall L 1984. Contributions of the renin-angiotensin system to the control of intrarenal hemodynamics (Editorial review). *Kidney International* 25: 857–868. [2.2.7]

Needleman P & Greenwald JP. 1986. Atriopeptin: a cardiac hormone intimately involved in fluid, electrolyte, and blood pressure homeostasis. *New England Journal of Medicine* 314: 828–834. [7.4.3, 7.4.4]

Nevins TE & Michael AF. 1981. Isolation of anionic sialoproteins from the rat glomerulus. *Kidney International* 19: 553–563. [3.2.6]

Nichols G, Jr, Nichols N, Weil WB & Wallace WM. 1953. The direct measurement of the extracellular phase of tissues. *Journal of Clinical Investigation* 32: 1299–1308. [3.3.2]

Nicholson TF. 1949. Renal function as affected by experimental unilateral kidney lesions 2. The effect of cyanide. *Biochemical Journal* 45: 112–115. [3.2.4]

Nowinsky WW & Goss RJ. (eds.) 1969. *Compensatory Renal Hypertrophy*. New York: Academic Press. [3.3.4.2]

Nussbaum M. 1878. Fortgesetzte Untersuchungen über die Sekretion der Niere. *Pflügers Archiv für gesamte Physiologie* 17: 580 [3.1]

Nutbourne DM. 1968. The effect of small hydrostatic pressure gradients on the rate of active sodium transport across isolated living frog-skin membranes. *Journal of Physiology* 195: 1–18. [4.3.1]

Ochwadt B. 1963. On the measurement of intrarenal blood flow distribution by wash-out technique. *Proceedings of 2nd International Congress of Nephrology*, pp. 62–64. Prague: Karger. [2.3.2]

Ochwadt BK & Pitts RF. 1956. Effects of intravenous infusion of carbonic anhydrase on carbon dioxide tension of alkaline urine. *American Journal of Physiology* 185: 426–429. [6.4]

O'Connell JMB, Romeo JA & Mudge GH. 1962. Renal tubular secretion of creatinine in the dog. *American Journal of Physiology* 203: 985–990. [3.3.2]

O'Connor WJ. 1962. *Renal Function*. London: Edward Arnold. [3.3.4.2, 3.3.5.2, 7.4.3]

O'Connor WJ. 1977. Normal sodium balance in dogs and in man. *Cardiovascular Research* 11: 375–408. [3.3.4.2, 7.4.2, 7.4.5]

O'Connor WJ & Summerill RA. 1976a. The effect of a meal of meat on glomerular filtration rate in dogs at normal urine flows. *Journal of Physiology* 256: 81–91. [3.3.4.2]

O'Connor WJ & Summerill RA. 1976b. The excretion of urea by dogs following a meat meal. *Journal of Physiology* 256: 93–102. [3.3.4.2]

O'Connor WJ & Summerill RA. 1979. Sodium excretion in normal conscious dogs. *Cardiovascular Research* 13: 22–30. [3.3.5.2, 7.4.2]

Oken DE & Choi SC. 1981. Filtration pressure equilibrium: a statistical analysis. *American Journal of Physiology* 242: F196–F200. [3.3.5.2]

Oken DE & Flamenbaum W. 1971. Micropuncture studies of proximal tubular albumin concentrations in normal and nephrotic rats. *Journal of Clinical Investigation* **50**: 1498–1505. [3.2.3.1]

Oliver J. 1939. Urinary system. In *Problems of Ageing* (ed. Cowdrey EV), pp. 257–277. Baltimore: Williams & Wilkins. [2.2.4]

Oliver J. 1950. When is the kidney not a kidney? *Journal of Urology* **63**: 373–402. [3.3.4.2, 3.3.4.3]

Oliver J. 1968. *Nephrons and Kidneys. A quantitative study of developmental and evolutionary mammalian renal architecture.* New York: Harper & Row, Hoeber Medical Division. [1.2]

Opitz E & Smyth DH 1937. Nierendurchblutung bei Reizung des Carotis-Sinus. *Pflügers Archiv für gesamte Physiologie* **238**: 633–637. [2.2.6]

Orloff J & Burg M. 1971. Kidney. *Annual Review of Physiology* **33**: 83–130. [7.4.5]

Osgood RW, Reineck HJ & Stein JH. 1982. Methodologic considerations in the study of glomerular ultrafiltration (Editorial review). *American Journal of Physiology* **242**: F1–F7. [3.2.7, 3.3.5.2]

Ott CE, Marchand GR, Diaz-Buxo JA & Knox FG. 1976. Determinants of glomerular filtration rate in the dog. *American Journal of Physiology* **231**: 235–239. [3.2.2, 3.2.3]

Pabico RC, McKenna BA & Freeman RB. 1975. Renal function before and after unilateral nephrectomy in renal donors. *Kidney International* **8**: 166–175. [3.3.4.2]

Pang PKT, Uchiyama M & Sawyer WH. 1982. Endocrine and neural control of amphibian renal function. *Federation Proceedings* **41**: 2365–2370. [3.3.4.3]

Pappenheimer JR. 1953. Passage of molecules through capillary walls. *Physiological Reviews* **23**: 387–423. [3.2.7, 3.2.8]

Pappenheimer JR. 1960. Central control of renal circulation. *Physiological Reviews* **40**: (suppl.) 35–37. [2.2.8]

Pappenheimer JR & Kinter WB. 1956. Hematocrít ratio of blood within mammalian kidney and its significance for renal hemodynamics. *American Journal of Physiology* **185**: 379–390. [2.2.7]

Parsons V & Watkins PJ. 1979. Diabetes and the kidney, 4th edn. In *Renal Disease* (eds. Black DAK, Jones NF), pp. 687–712. Oxford: Blackwell Scientific Publications. [3.3.4.2]

Peart WS. 1978. Renin 1978. *Johns Hopkins Medical Journal* **143**: 193–206. [2.2.7, 7.4.3]

Pelletier M, Ludens JH & Fanestil DD. 1972. The role of aldosterone in active sodium transport. *Archives of Internal Medicine* **129**: 248–257. [7.4.3]

Persson AEG, Roberg U, Hahne B, Müller-Suur R, Norlen B-J & Selén G. 1982. Interstitial pressure as a modulator of tubuloglomerular feedback control. *Kidney International* **22** (Suppl. 12): S122–S128. [3.3.5.3]

Peter K. 1909. *Untersuchungen über Bau und Entwicklung der Niere.* Jena: Gustav Fischer. [5.5]

Peters JP. 1944. Water exchange. *Physiological Reviews* **24**: 491–531. [5.4]

Peters JP. 1950. Sodium, water and edema. *Journal of the Mount Sinai Hospital* **17**: 159–175. [7.4.5]

Peters JP. 1952. The problem of cardiac edema. *American Journal of Medicine* **12**: 66–76. [7.4.5]

Petersdorf RG & Welt LG. 1953. The effect of an infusion of hyperoncotic albumin on the excretion of water and solutes. *Journal of Clinical Investigation* **32**: 283–291. [3.3.4.3]

Pitts RF. 1933. The excretion of urine in the dog. VII. Inorganic phosphate in relation to plasma phosphate level. *American Journal of Physiology* **106**: 1–8. [4.3.2]

Pitts RF. 1959. *The Physiological Basis of Diuretic Therapy.* Springfield, Illinois: Charles C Thomas. [3.3.4.2, 6.3]

Pitts RF. 1974. *Physiology of the Kidney and Body Fluids*, 3rd edn. Chicago: Year Book Medical Publishers Inc. [1.2, 3.2.5, 4.2.2, 7.4.4.5]

Pitts RF, Ayer JL & Schiess WA. 1949. The renal regulation of acid base balance in man. III. The reabsorption and excretion of bicarbonate. *Journal of Clinical Investigation* **28**: 35–44. [6.4]

Pitts RF & Lotspeich WD. 1946. Bicarbonate and the renal regulation of acid base balance. *American Journal of Physiology* **147**: 138–159. [4.3.2, 6.4]

Pitts RF, Sullivan WJ & Dorman PJ. 1954. Regulation of the content of bicarbonate bound base in body fluids. In *The Kidney* (eds. Lewis AAG & Wolstenholme GEW), pp. 125–144. London: J & A Churchill. [6.1, 6.4]

Platt R. 1951 Renal Failure. *Lancet* **i**: 1239–1242. [4.2]

Platt R. 1952. Structural and functional adaptation in renal failure. *British Medical Journal* **i**: 1313–1317; 1372. [3.3.4.3]

Ploth DW & Roy RN. 1982. Renin–angiotensin influences on tubuloglomerular feedback activity in the rat. *Kidney International* **22** (Suppl. 12): S114–S121. [3.3.5.3]

Pollock AS, & Arieff AI. 1980. Abnormalities of cell volume and their functional consequences (Editorial review). *American Journal of Physiology* **239**: F195–F205. [7.3]

Provoost AP & Molenaar JC. 1980. Changes in the glomerular filtration rate after unilateral nephrectomy in rats. *Pflügers Archiv für die gesamte Physiologie* **385**: 161–165. [3.3.4.2]

Pullman TN, Alving SA & Landowne M. 1949. Effect of protein in the diet upon certain aspects of renal function (Abstract). *Federation Proceedings* **8**: 129. [3.3.4.2]

Radigan LR & Robinson S. 1949. Effects of environmental heat stress on renal blood flow and filtration rate. *American Journal of Physiology* **159**: 585–586. [3.3.4.3]

Ramsay DJ. 1985. Osmoreceptors subserving vasopressin secretion and drinking — an overview. In *Vasopressin* (ed. Schrier RW), pp. 291–298. New York: Raven Press. [7.4.5]

Ramsay DJ & Coxon RV. 1967. The effect of intravenously infused saline on the renal clearances of inulin and para-aminohippurate in dogs. *Quarterly Journal of Experimental Physiology* **52**: 145–149. [3.3.4.2]

Ranson SW, Fisher C & Ingram WR. 1938. The hypohalamic-hypophysial mechanism in diabetes insipidus. *Research Publications of the Association for Nervous and Mental Diseases.* **17**: 410–432. [5.3]

Rapoport S, Brodsky WA, West CD & Mackler B. 1949. Urinary flow and excretion of solutes during osmotic diuresis in hydropenic man. *American Journal of Physiology* **156**: 433–442. [5.5.3]

Rascher W. 1985. Kardiovaskuläre Wirkung des antidiuretischen Hormons Arginin-Vasopressin. *Klinische Wochenschrift* **19**: 989–999. [7.2]

Rector FC, Jr. 1973. Acidification of the urine. In *Handbook of Physiology, Section 8, Renal Physiology* (eds. Orloff J & Berliner RW), pp. 431–454. Washington, DC: American Physiological Society. [6.3]

Rector FC, Jr. 1977. Renal concentrating mechanisms. In *Disturbances of Body Fluid Osmolality* (eds. Andreoli TE, Grantham J & Rector FC, Jr), pp. 179–196. Bethesda, Maryland: American Physiological Society. [5.5.2]

Rector FC, Jr. 1983. Sodium, bicarbonate, and chloride reabsorption by the proximal tubule (Homer Smith Award Lecture). *American Journal of Physiology* **244**: F461–F471. [5.2, 6.2, 6.4, 7.4.4.3, 8.3]

Rehberg PB. 1926. Studies on kidney function. 1. The rate of filtration and reabsorption in the human kidney. 2. The excretion of urea and chlorine analysed according to a modified filtration–reabsorption theory. *Biochemical Journal* **20**: 447–460; 461–482. [3.3.2]

Reif MC, Troutman SL & Schafer JA. 1984. Sustained response to vasopressin in isolated rat cortical collecting tubules. *Kidney International* **26**: 725–732. [5.3, 5.3.3]

Rein H. 1929. Die Thermo-Stromuhr. II. Mitteilung. Arbeitsbedingungen und Arbeitsmöglichkeiten in Tierversuch. *Zeitschrift für Biologie* **89**: 195–201. [2.2.2]

Reiter RJ. 1969. The endocrines and compensatory renal enlargement, in *Compensatory Renal Hypertrophy* (eds. Nowinsky WW & Goss RJ), pp. 183–204. New York: Academic Press. [3.3.4.2]

Renkin EM. 1970. Permeability and molecular size in 'peripheral' and glomerular capillaries. In *Capillary Permeability (Alfred Benzon Symposium II)* (eds. Crone C & Lassen NA), pp. 544–547. Copenhagen: Munksgaard. [3.2.5, 3.2.9]

Renkin EM. 1986. Some consequences of capillary permeability to macromolecules: Starling's hypothesis reconsidered. *American Journal of Physiology* **250**: H706–H710. [7.4.5]

Renkin EM & Gilmore JP. 1973. Glomerular filtration. In *Handbook of Physiology. Renal Physiology* (eds. Orloff J & Berliner, RW), pp. 185–248. Washington DC: American Physiological Society. [3.2.2, 3.2.4]

Rennick BR. 1981. Renal tubular transport of organic cations. *American Journal of Physiology* **240**: F83–F89. [4.4.2]

Rennick BR, Moe GK, Lyons RM, Hoobler SW & Neligh R. 1947. Absorption and renal excretion of the tetraethylammonium ion. *Journal of Pharmacology and Experimental Therapeutics* **91**: 210–217. [4.4.2]

Rennie DW, Reeves RB & Pappenheimer JR. 1958. Oxygen pressure in urine and its relation to intrarenal blood flow. *American Journal of Physiology* **195**: 120–132. [2.3.2]

Rennke HG, Cotran RS & Venkatachalam MA. 1975. Role of molecular charge in glomerular permeability. Tracer studies with cationized ferritin. *Journal of Cellular Biology* **67**: 638–646. [3.2.5]

Rennke HG, Patel Y & Venkatachalam MA. 1978. Glomerular filtration of proteins: Clearance of anionic, neutral and cationic horseradish peroxidase in the rat. *Kidney International* **13**: 278–288. [3.2.5]

Reubi FC & Vorburger C. 1976. Renal hemodynamics in acute renal failure after shock in man. *Kidney International* **10**: S137–S143. [3.3.4.3]

Rhodin JAG. 1962. The diaphragm of capillary endothelial fenestrations. *Journal of Ultrastructure Research* **6**: 171–185. [3.2.6]

Richards AN. 1922. Kidney function. *American Journal of the Medical Sciences* **158**: 1–19. [3.2.1, 3.3.4]

Richards AN. 1938. Processes of urine formation (The Croonian Lecture). *Proceedings of the Royal Society, London* **B126**: 398–432. [3.2.3, 3.2.4]

Richards AN & Plant OH. 1922. Urine formation in the perfused kidney. The influence of adrenaline on the volume of the perfused kidney. *American Journal of Physiology* **59**: 184–190. [3.3.4.3]

Richterich R. 1962. Physico-chemical factors determining ammonia excretion. *Helvetica Physiologica et Pharmacologica Acta* **20**: 326–345. [8.3]

Rioch DMcK. 1930. Water diuresis. *Journal of Physiology.* **70**: 45–52. [5.3]

Robertson GL. 1984. Abnormalities of thirst regulation. *Kidney International* **25**: 460–469. [7.2]

Robertson GL, Athar S & Shelton RL. 1977. Osmotic control of vasopressin function. In *Disturbances of Body Fluid Osmolality* (eds. Andreoli TE, Grantham JJ & Rector FC, Jr) pp. 125–148. Bethesda, Maryland: American Physiological Society. [5.5.4]

Robertson GL, Shelton RL & Athar S. 1976. The osmoregulation of vasopressin. *Kidney International* **10**: 25–37. [5.3, 5.5.4, 7.2]

Robertson JA & Gray CH. 1953. Mechanism of lowered renal threshold for glucose in diabetes. *Lancet* **ii**: 12–15. [3.3.4.2]

Robinson JR. 1954. *Reflections on Renal Function.* Oxford: Blackwell Scientific Publications. [Passim]

Robinson JR. 1960. Metabolism of intracellular water. *Physiological Reviews* **40**: 112–149. [2.2.5]

Robinson JR. 1964. Renal handling of salt and water. *Australasian Annals of Medicine* **13**: 183–191. [7.4.4]

Robinson JR. 1975a. Colloid osmotic pressure as a cause of pathological swelling of cells. In *Pathophysiology of cell membranes* (eds. Trump BF & Arstilla AU), pp. 173–189. New York: Academic Press. [2.2.5]

Robinson JR. 1975b. *A Prelude to Physiology.* Oxford: Blackwell Scientific Publications. [3.2.3, 4.1, 4.3.1, 4.3.2, 6.2]

Robinson JR. 1975c. *Fundamentals of Acid Base Regulation* 5th edn. Oxford: Blackwell Scientific Publications. [4.3.2, 6.1]

Robinson JR. 1978. Claude Bernard's internal environment revisited. In *Studies in Neurophysiology presented to AK McIntyre* (ed. Porter R), pp. 413–427. Cambridge: University Press. [5.5.4, 6.5]

Robinson JR, Robinson MF, Levander OA & Thomson CD. 1985. Urinary excretion of selenium by New Zealand and North American human subjects on differing intakes. *American Journal of Clinical Nutrition* **41**: 1023–1031. [8.1]

Robinson, RR. 1980. Nephrology forum: isolated proteinuria in asymptomatic patients. *Kidney International* **18**: 395–406. [3.3.4.3, 4.2.4]

Robson JS. 1972. The nephrotic syndrome. In *Renal Disease* 3rd edn. (ed. Black DAK), pp. 331–366. Oxford: Blackwell Scientific Publications. [3.3.4.2]

Rocha A, Marcondes M & Malnic G. 1973. Micropuncture study in rats with experimental glomerulonephritis. *Kidney International* **3**: 14–23. [3.3.4.3]

Roch-Ramel F & Peters G. 1981. Renal transport of urea. In *Renal Transport of Organic Substances* (eds. Greger R, Lang F & Silbernagl S), pp. 134–153. Berlin, Heidelberg, New York: Springer-Verlag. [4.2.1]

Roddie IC & Shepherd JT. 1958. Receptors in the high-pressure and low-pressure vascular systems. Their role in the reflex control of the human circulation. *Lancet* **i**: 493–496. [2.2.6]

Rodewald R & Karnovsky MJ. 1974. Porous substructure of the glomerular slit diaphragm in the rat and mouse. *Journal of Cellular Biology* **60**: 423–435. [3.2.6]

Romero JC, Knox FG, Opgenorth TJ, Granger JP & Keiser JA. 1985. Contribution of sympathetic neural reflexes to mineralocorticoid escape. *Federation Proceedings* **44**: 2382–2397. [7.4]

Rosenbaum RW, Hruska KA, Anderson C, Robson AM, Slatopolsky E & Klahr S. 1979. Inulin: an inadequate marker of glomerular filtration rate in kidney donors and transplant recipients? *Kidney International* **16**: 179–186 [3.3.2]

Ross BD. 1978. The isolated perfused rat kidney (Editorial review). *Clinical Science and Molecular Medicine.* **55**: 513–521. [2.2.7]

Ross B & Lowry M. 1981. Recent developments in renal handling of glutamine and ammonia. In *Renal Tubular Transport of Organic Substances* (eds. Greger R, Lang F & Silbernagl S), pp. 78–92. Berlin, Heidelberg, New York: Springer-Verlag. [4.5]

Rouffignac C de & Bonvalet JP. 1974. Heterogeneity of nephron population. In *MTP International Review of Science, Series 1, Vol. 6. Kidney and Urinary Tract Physiology* (ed. Thurau K), pp. 391–409. Baltimore: University Park Press. [3.3.2]

Rouffignac C de & Jamison RL. (eds.) 1987. Symposium on the urinary concentrating mechanism. *Kidney International* **31**: 501–672. [5.5.2]

Rowell LB. 1974. Human cardiovascular adjustments to exercise and thermal stress. *Physiological Reviews* **54**: 75–159. [2.2.5]

Ryan GB. 1981. The glomerular seive and the mechanisms of proteinuria. *Australia and New Zealand Journal of Medicine* **11**: 197–206. [3.2.6]

Ryan GB & Karnovsky MJ. 1976. Distribution of endogenous albumin in the rat glomerulus: Role of hemodynamic factors in glomerular barrier functions. *Kidney International* **9**: 36–45. [3.2.6]

Sabatini S & Kurtzman NA. 1984. The maintenance of metabolic alkalosis: Factors which decrease bicarbonate excretion (Editorial review). *Kidney International* **24**: 357–361. [3.3.4.3, 6.4]

Sadowski J & Wocial B. 1977. Renin release and autoregulation of blood flow in a nonfiltering, nontransporting kidney. *Journal of Physiology* **266**: 219–233. [3.3.5.3]

Sarre H. 1938. Untersuchungen über die Sauerstoff- und Kohlensaüre-spannung im Harn und ihre Beziehung zum Nierengewebe und zur Nierenfunktion. *Pflügers Archiv für gesamte Physiologie* **239**: 377–399. [2.3.2]

Savin VJ, Lindsley HB, Nagle RB & Cachia R. 1982. Ultrafiltration coefficient and glomerular capillary resistance in a model of immune complex glomerulonephritis. *Kidney International* **21**: 28–35. [3.2.7]

Sawyer WH, Munsick RA & Van Dyke HB. 1960. Antidiuretic hormones. *Circulation* **21**: 1027–1037. [5.3]

Scatchard G. 1956. General introduction to a discussion on membrane phenomena. *Faraday Society Discussions* **21**: 27–30. [3.2.9]

Schafer JA. 1979. Response of the collecting duct to the demands of homeostasis. *The Physiologist* **22**: 44–53. [5.5.3]

Schafer JA. 1982. Salt and water absorption in the proximal tubule. *The Physiologist* **25**: 95–103. [7.4.4.3]

Schafer JA. 1984. Mechanisms coupling the absorption of solute and water in the proximal nephron (Robert F Pitts Memorial Lecture). *Kidney International* **25**: 708–716. [4.3.2, 5.2]

Schlondorff D & Ardaillou R. 1986. Prostaglandins and other arachidonic acid metabolites in the kidney. *Kidney International* **29**: 108–119. [7.4.3, 7.4.4.6]

Schmidt-Nielsen B. 1958. Urea excretion in mammals. *Physiological Reviews* **38**: 139–168. [4.2.1]

Schmidt-Nielsen B. 1987. The renal pelvis. *Kidney International* **31**: 621–628. [5.5.2]

Schmidt-Nielsen B & O'Dell R. 1961. Structure and concentrating mechanism in the mammalian kidney. *American Journal of Physiology* **200**: 1119–1124. [5.5]

Schmidt-Nielsen K. 1975. *Animal Physiology: Adaptation to Environment*. Cambridge: University Press. [2.2.5, 2.2.8]

Schnermann J. 1974. Physical forces and transtubular movement of solutes and water. In *MTP International Review of Science. Physiology Series One. Kidney and Urinary Tract Physiology, Vol. 6* (ed. Thurau K), pp. 157–198. London: Butterworths. Baltimore: University Park Press. [7.4.4.3]

Schnermann J & Briggs JP. 1981. Participation of renal cortical prostaglandins in the regulation of glomerular filtration rate. *Kidney International* **19**: 802–815. [3.3.4.2, 3.3.5.3]

Schnermann J & Briggs JP. 1982. Concentration-dependent sodium chloride transport as the signal in feedback control of glomerular filtration rate. *Kidney International* **22** (Suppl. 12): S82–S89. [2.2.7, 3.3.5.3]

Schnermann J & Briggs J. 1986. Role of the renin–angiotensin system in tubuloglomerular feedback. *Federation Proceedings* **45**: 1426–1430. [3.3.5.3]

Schnermann J, Briggs J, Kriz W, Moore L & Wright FS. 1980. Control of glomerular vascular resistance by the tubuloglomerular feedback mechanism. In *Renal Pathophysiology* (eds. Leaf A, Bolis L, Giebisch G & Gorini S), pp. 165–182. New York: Raven Press. [8.4]

Schnermann J, Briggs J & Schubert G. 1982. *In situ* studies of the distal convoluted tubule in the rat: evidence for NaCl secretion. *American Journal of Physiology* **243**: F160–F166. [3.3.5.3]

Schnermann J, Briggs JP & Weber PC. 1984. Tubuloglomerular feedback, prostaglandins, and angiotensin in the autoregulation of glomerular filtration rate. *Kidney International* **25**: 53–64. [3.3.5.3]

Scholander PF. 1954. Secretion of gases against high pressures in the swimbladder of deep sea fishes. II. The rete mirabile. *Biological Bulletin. Marine Biological Laboratory, Woods Hole Mass* **107**: 260–277. [5.5.1]

Schor N, Ichikawa I & Brenner BM. 1981. Mechanisms of action of various hormones and vasoactive substances on glomerular ultrafiltration in the rat. *Kidney International* **20**: 442–451. [3.3.5.2]

Schrier RW, Berl T & Anderson RJ. 1979. Osmotic and nonosmotic control of vasopressin release (Editorial review). *American Journal of Physiology* **236**: F321–F332. [5.5.4, 7.2]

Schultze RG & Berger H. 1973. The influences of GFR and saline expansion on Tm_G of the dog kidney. *Kidney International* **3**: 291–297. [4.2.2]

Schuster VL. 1986. Effects of angiotensin on proximal tubular reabsorption. *Federation Proceedings* **45**: 1444–1447. [7.4.5]

Schwartz WB & Relman AS. 1953. Metabolic and renal studies in chronic potassium depletion resulting from overuse of laxatives. *Journal of Clinical Investigation* **32**: 258–271. [3.3.4.3]

Scicli AG & Carretero OA. 1986. Renal kallikrein–kinin system. *Kidney International* **29**: 120–130. [7.4]

Scriver CR, Chesney RW & McInnes RR. 1976. Genetic aspects of renal tubular transport: diversity and topology of carriers. *Kidney International* **9**: 149–171. [4.2.2, 4.2.3]

Seely JF & Dirks JH. 1969. Micropuncture study of hypertonic mannitol diuresis in proximal and distal tubules of the dog kidney. *Journal of Clinical Investigation* **48**: 2330–2340. [5.5.3]

Seely JF & Dirks JH. 1977. Site of action of diuretic drugs. *Kidney International* **11**: 1–8. [3.3.4.2]

Seldin DW & Rector FC, Jr. 1972. The generation and maintenance of metabolic alkalosis. *Kidney International* **1**: 306–321. [6.4]

Selkurt EE. 1946. Comparison of renal clearances with direct renal blood flow under control conditions and following renal ischemia. *American Journal of Physiology* **145**: 376–386. [2.2.3.3]

Selkurt EE. 1963. The renal circulation. In *Handbook of Physiology*, Section 2, Circulation, Vol. 2 (eds. Hamilton WF & Dow P), pp. 1457–1516. Washington, DC: American Physiological Society. [2.2.3.3, 2.2.5, 2.3.1, 4.3.1]

Selkurt EE, Brandfonbrener M & Geller HM. 1952. Effects of ureteral pressure increase on renal hemodynamics and the handling of electrolytes and water. *American Journal of Physiology* **170**: 61–71. [3.3.4.3]

Selkurt, EE, Deetjen P & Brechtelsbauer H. 1965. Tubular pressure gradients and filtration dynamics during urinary stop flow in the rat. *Pflügers Archiv für gesamte Physiologie* **286**: 19–35. [3.3.5.3]

Sellwood RV & Verney EB. 1955. The effect of water and of isotonic saline administration on the renal plasma and glomerular filtrate flows in the dog, with incidental observations on the effects on these flows of compression of the carotid and renal arteries. *Philosophical Transactions of the Royal Society, London* **B238**: 361–396. [2.2.7, 3.3.4.2, 5.3]

Severinghaus JW, Mitchell RA, Richardson BW & Singer MM. 1963. Respiratory control at high altitude suggesting active transport regulation of CSF pH. *Journal of Applied Physiology* **18**: 1155–1166. [6.4]

Shannon JA. 1936. Glomerular filtration and urea excretion in relation to urine flow in the dog. *American Journal of Physiology* **117**: 206–225. [3.3.4.3, 4.2.1]

Shannon JA. 1938a. Urea excretion in the normal dog during forced diuresis. *American Journal of Physiology* **122**: 782–787. [3.3.4.2]

Shannon JA. 1938b. The renal reabsorption and excretion of urea under conditions of extreme diuresis. *American Journal of Physiology* **123**: 182–183. [4.2.1, 5.2]

Shannon JA, Jolliffe N & Smith HW. 1932. The excretion of urine in the dog. IV. The effect of maintenance diet feeding etc upon the quantity of glomerular filtrate. *American Journal of Physiology* **101**: 625–646. [3.3.4.2]

Sheehan HL. 1936. The renal elimination of phenol red in the dog. *Journal of Physiology* **87**: 237–253. [4.4]

Sieker HO, Gauer OH & Henry JP. 1954. The effect of continuous negative pressure breathing on water and electrolyte excretion by the human kidney. *Journal of Clinical Investigation* **33**: 572–577. [3.3.4.3]

Silbernagl S. 1981. Renal transport of amino acids and oligopeptides. In *Renal Transport of Organic Substances* (eds. Greger R, Lang F & Silbernagl S), pp. 93–117. Berlin, Heidelberg, New York: Springer-Verlag. [4.2.3]

Silverman M, Vinay P, Shinobu L, Gougoux A & Lemieux G. 1981. Luminal and antiluminal transport of glutamine in dog kidney: effect of metabolic acidosis. *Kidney International* **20**: 359–365. [4.5]

Simpson DP. 1983. Citrate excretion: a window on renal metabolism. *American Journal of Physiology* **244**: F223–F234. [4.5]

Simpson SA, Tait JF, Wettstein A, Neher R, Euw JV & Reichstein TS. 1953. Isolierung eines neues kristallisierten Hormons aus Nebennieren mit besonders hoher Wirksamkeit auf den Mineralstoffwechsel. *Experientia* **9**: 333–335. [7.4.3]

Sirota H, Baldwin DS & Villarreal H. 1950. Diurnal variations of renal function in man *Journal of Clinical Investigation* **29**: 187–192. [3.3.4.2]

Skorecki KL & Brenner BM. 1981. Body fluid homeostasis in man. A contemporary overview. *American Journal of Medicine* **70**: 77–88. [7.4.2, 7.4.4, 7.4.4.5]

Smith HW. 1937. *The Physiology of the Kidney*. London: Oxford University Press. [3.3.2, 4.4, 5.3, 5.5.3, 7.4]

Smith HW. 1939–40. The physiology of the renal circulation. *Harvey Lectures* **35**: 166–222. [2.2.5, 3.3.4.3]

Smith HW. 1943. *Lectures on the Kidney*. Lawrence, Kansas: Kansas University Press. [3.3.2, 4.4.1]

Smith HW. 1951. *The Kidney. Structure and Function in Health and Disease*. New York: Oxford University press. [Passim]

Smith HW. 1956. *Principles of renal physiology*. New York: Oxford University Press, 1956. [Passim]

Smith HW. 1957. Salt and water volume receptors: an exercise in physiological apologetics. *American Journal of Medicine* **23**: 623–652. [7.4.2, 7.4.4, 8.3]

Smith HW. 1959. The fate of sodium and water in the renal tubules. *Bulletin of the New York Academy of Medicine* **35**: 293–316. [5.5]

Smith HW. 1964. Renal physiology. In *Circulation of the Blood, Men and Ideas* (eds. Fishman AP & Richards DW), pp. 545–606. New York: Oxford University Press. [3.2.1]

Solomon S. 1957. Transtubular potential differences of rat kidney. *Journal of Cellular and Comparative Physiology* **49**: 351–365. [3.3.4.2, 4.3.1]

Sperber I. 1947. The mechanism of renal excretion of some detoxication products in the chicken. *Proceedings of the 17th International Congress of Physiology*. Oxford. pp. 217–218. [4.4.2, 4.4.3]

Spitzer A & Edelman CM, Jr. 1971. Maturational changes in pressure gradient for glomerular filtration. *American Journal of Physiology* **221**: 1431–1435. [3.3.4.2]

Squires RD & Huth EJ. 1959. Experimental potassium depletion in normal human subjects. Relation of ionic intakes to the renal conservation of potassium. *Journal of Clinical Investigation* **38**: 1134–1148. [4.3.3]

Stanton BA, Biemesderfer D, Wade JB & Giebisch G. 1981. Structural and functional study of the rat distal nephron: effects of potassium adaptation and potassium depletion. *Kidney International* **19**: 36–48. [4.4.3, 8.3]

Starling EH. 1898. The mechanism of the secretion of urine. In *A Textbook of Physiology, Vol I* (ed. Schäfer EA), pp. 639–661. Edinburgh, London: Young J Pentland. [2.2.2]

Starling EH. 1899. The glomerular functions of the kidney. *Journal of Physiology* **24**: 317–330. [3.2.3, 5.2]

Starling EH. 1909. *The Fluids of the Body*. London: Constable. [3.3.5.3, 5.5.3]

Stein JH. 1976. The renal circulation. In *The Kidney* (eds. Brenner BM & Rector FC, Jr), pp. 215–250. Philadelphia: W B Saunders Co. [2.2.5, 2.3.2]

Stein JH & Reineck HJ. 1975. Effect of alterations in extracellular fluid volume on segmental sodium transport. *Physiological Reviews* **55**: 127–141. [7.4.4.3]

Steinhausen M, Loreth A & Olson S. 1965. Messungen des tubulären Harnstromes, sein beziehungen zum blutdruck und zur inulin-clearance. *Pflügers Archiv für gesamte Physiologie* **286**: 118–141. [3.4.4]

Steinhausen M, Zimmerhackl B, Thederan H, Dussel R, Parekh N, Eblinger HU, von Hasens G, Komitowski D & Dallenbach FD. 1981. Intraglomerular microcirculation: measurements of single glomerular loop flow in rats. *Kidney International* **20**: 230–239. [3.2.9]

Steinmetz PR. 1974. Cellular mechanisms of urinary acidification. *Physiological Reviews* **54**: 890–956. [6.3]

Steinmetz PR. 1986. Cellular organization of urinary acidification (Homer Smith Award Lecture). *American Journal of Physiology* **251**: F173–F187. [8.3]

Stephenson JL. 1966. Concentration in renal countercurrent systems. *Biophysical Journal* **6**: 539–551. [5.5.2]

Stephenson JL. 1972. Concentration of urine in a central core model of the renal countercurrent system. *Kidney International* **2**: 85–94. [5.5.2]

Stephenson JL. 1987. Models of the urinary concentrating mechanism. *Kidney International* **31**: 648–661. [5.5.2]

Stern L. Backman KA & Hayslett JP 1985. Effect of cortical-medullary gradient for ammonia on urinary excretion of ammonia. *Kidney International* **27**: 652–661. [6.3]

Stetson DL, Wade JB & Giebisch G. 1980. Morphological alterations in the rat medullary collecting duct following potassium depletion. *Kidney International* **17**: 45–56. [4.3.3, 8.3]

Stokes JB. 1981. Integrated actions of renal medullary prostaglandins in the control of water excretion. *American Journal of Physiology* **240**: F471–F480. [7.4.4.6]

Strauss MB, Davis RK, Rosenbaum JO & Rossmeisl EC. 1951. 'Water diuresis' produced during recumbency by the intravenous infusion of isotonic saline solution. *Journal of Clinical Investigation* **30**: 862–868. [7.2]

Strauss HW, Kirchner PT & Wagner HN. 1979. Nuclear medicine in the evaluation of renal disease. In *Strauss and Welt's Diseases of the Kidney*, 3rd edn (eds. Earley LE & Gottschalk CW), pp. 149–164. New York: Little, Brown & Co. [2.3.2, 3.2.3.4]

Strauss MB, Lamdin E, Smith WP & Bleifer SJ. 1958. Surfiet and deficit of sodium. *Archives of Internal Medicine* **102**: 527–536. [7.4.5]

Summerill RA. 1982. The effect of increased amounts of meat on glomerular filtration and urea production in the conscious dog. *Journal of Physiology* **322**: 29P. [3.3.4.2]

Surtshin A, White HL. 1956. Postural effects on renal tubular activity. *Journal of Clinical Investigation* **35**: 267–271. [3.3.4.3]

Sutton RAL. 1983. Disorders of renal calcium excretion. *Kidney International* **23**: 665–673. [4.3.3]

Swanson RE & Hakim AA. 1962. Stop-flow analysis of creatinine excretion in the dog. *American Journal of Physiology*. **203**: 980–984. [3.3.2]

Takabatake T. 1982. Feedback regulation of glomerular filtration rate in the denervated kidney. *Kidney International* **22** (Suppl. 12): S129–S135. [3.3.5.3]

Tamman G. 1896. Die Thätigkeit der Niere im Lichte der Theorie des osmotischen Drucks. *Zeitschrift der Physikalischen Chemie* **20**: 180–197. [4.3.1, 5.2]

Tannen RL. 1978. Ammonia metabolism. *American Journal of Physiology* **235**: F265–F277. [4.5.2, 6.3]

Taylor MG & Ullman E. 1961. Glomerular filtration after obstruction of the ureter. *Journal of Physiology* **157**: 38–63. [3.3.5.3, 4.1.1]

Thomas CE, Bell PD & Navar LG. 1979. Glomerular filtration dynamics in the dog during elevated plasma colloid osmotic pressure. *Kidney International* **15**: 502–519. [3.2.2, 3.2.3, 3.2.5.2]

Thorburn GD, Kopald HH, Herd AJ, Hollenberg M, O'Morchoe DCC & Barger, AC, 1963. Intrarenal distribution of nutrient blood flow determined with krypton[85] in the unanesthetized dog. *Circulation Research* **13**: 290–307. [2.3.2]

Thompson CJ, Bland J, Burd J & Baylis PH. 1986. The osmotic thresholds for thirst and vasopressin release are similar in healthy man. *Clinical Science* **71**: 651–556. [7.2]

Thurau K. 1963. Fundamentals of the renal circulation. *Proceedings of the 2nd International Congress of Nephrology*. pp. 51–61. Prague: Karger. [2.2.7, 3.3.5.3]

Thurau K. 1964. Renal hemodynamics. *American Journal of Medicine* **36**: 698–719. [2.2.5, 2.2.7, 2.3.1, 2.3.3, 3.2.2, 4.5.1]

Thurau K. 1966. Nature of autoregulation of renal blood flow. *Proceedings of the 3rd*

International Congress of Nephrology, *Vol. 1*, pp. 162–173. Washington, DC, Basel, New York: Karger. [2.2.7]

Thurau K. 1981. Tubulo-glomerular feedback. In *Advances in Physiological Sciences*, *Vol. II*. *Kidney and Body Fluids* (ed. Takacs L), pp. 75–82. London: Pergamon Press. [3.3.5.3]

Thurau K & Boylan JW. 1976. Acute renal success. The unexpected logic of oliguria in acute renal failure. *American Journal of Medicine* 61: 308–315. [2.5.3, 3.3.4.3]

Thurau, K. Boylan, JW & Mason J. 1979. Pathophysiology of acute renal failure. In *Renal Disease*, 4th edn (eds. Black DAK & Jones NF), pp. 64–92. Oxford: Blackwell Scientific Publications. [3.3.4.3, 3.3.5.2]

Thurau K & Henne G. 1964. Die transmurale Druckdifferenz der Widerstandsgefässe als Parameter der Widerstandsregulation in der Niere. *Pflügers Archiv für gesamte Physiologie* 279: 156–177. [2.2.7]

Thurau K & Kramer K. 1959. Weitere Untersuchungen zur myogenen Natur der Autoregulation des Nierenkreislaufs. Aufhebung der Autoregulation durch muskulotrope Substanzen und druckpassives Verhalten des Glomerulusfiltrates. *Pflügers Archiv für gesamte Physiologie* 269: 77–93. [2.2.7]

Thurau K & Mason J. 1974. The intrarenal function of the juxtaglomerular apparatus. In *MTP International Reviews of Science*. *Kidney and Urinary Tract Physiology, Series 1*, *Vol. 6* (eds. Thurau & K. Baltimore), pp. 357–390. University Park Press. [2.2.7, 3.3.5.3]

Thurau K & Schnermann J. 1965. Die Natriumkonzentration an dem Macula densa-Zellen als regulierender Faktor für das Glomerulumfiltrat (Mikropunktionsversuche). *Klinische Wochenschrift* 43: 410–413. [2.2.7, 3.3.5.3]

Thurau K & Schnermann J. (eds). 1982. The juxtaglomerular apparatus. *Kidney International* 22 (Suppl. 12): S1–S224. [3.3.5.3]

Thurau K & Wober E. 1962. Zur Lokalisation der autoregulativen Widerstandsänderungen in der Niere. Mikropunktionsmessungen der Drucke in Tubuli und peritubulären Capillaren der Rattenniere bei Änderungen des arteriellen Druckes. *Pflügers Archiv für gesamte Physiologie* 274: 553–566. [2.2.7]

Tigerstedt R & Bergman PC. 1898. Niere und Kreislauf. *Skandinavisches Archiv für Physiologie* 8: 223–271. [2.2.7]

Timpl R. 1986. Recent advances in the biochemistry of glomerular basement membrane (Editorial review). *Kidney International* 30: 293–298. [3.2.6]

Tisher CC 1976. Anatomy of the kidney. In *The Kidney, Vol. 1* (eds. Brenner BM & Rector FC, Jr), pp. 1–64. Philadelphia: W B Saunders Co. [1.2]

Tønder KH & Aukland K. 1979. Glomerular capillary pressure in the rat: validation of pressure measurement through corticotomy. *Acta Physiologica Scandinavica* 106: 93–95. [3.2.2]

Troehler U, Bonjour JP & Fleisch H. 1975. Renal secretion of diphosphonates in rats. *Kidney International* 8: 6–13. [4.4.1]

Trueta J, Barclay AE, Daniel PM, Franklin KJ & Prichard MML. 1947. *Studies of the Renal Circulation*. Oxford: Blackwell Scientific Publications. [2.3.1]

Tucker BJ & Blantz RC. 1977. An analysis of the determinants of nephron filtration rate (Editorial review). *American Journal of Physiology* 232: F477–F483. [3.3.5.2]

Tune BM, Burg MB & Patlak CS. 1969. Characteristics of p-aminohippurate transport by proximal renal tubules. *American Journal of Physiology* 217: 1057–1063. [4.4.1]

Ullrich KJ. 1959. Das Nierenmark. Struktur, Stoffwechsel und Funktion. *Ergebnisse der Physiologie* 50: 433–489. [2.3.1, 4.5.1]

Ullrich KJ. 1976. Renal tubular mechanisms of organic solute transport. *Kidney International* 9: 134–148. [4.2.2]

Ullrich KJ & Couser WG. 1986. (eds.) Symposium on methods of renal research. *Kidney International* 30: 141–279. [4.1]

Ullrich KJ, Drenckhahn FC & Jarausch KH. 1955. Über das osmotische Verhalten von Nirerenzellen und die begleitende Elektrolytanhäufung in Nierengewebe bei verschiedenen Diuresezuständen. *Pflügers Archiv für gesamte Physiologie* **261**: 62–77. [5.5.1]

Ullrich KJ & Jarausch KH. 1956. Über die Verteilung von Elektrolyten (Na, K, Ca, Mg, Cl, anorganischem Phosphat), Harnstoff, Aminosäuren und exogenem Kreatinin in Rinde und Mark der Hundeniere bei verschiedenen Diuresezuständen. *Pflügers Archiv für gesamte Physiologie* **262**: 537–550. [5.5.1, 5.5.3]

Ullrich KJ & Kramer K, Boylan JW. 1961a. Present knowledge of the counter-current system in the kidney. *Progess in Cardiovascular Diseases* **3**: 395–431. [5.5.2]

Ullrich KJ & Marsh DJ. 1963. Kidney, water, and electrolyte metabolism. *Annual Review of Physiology* **25**: 91–142. [2.2.6]

Ullrich KJ & Papavassiliou F. 1985. Contraluminal tranport of hexoses in the proximal convolution of the rat kidney in situ. *Pflügers Archiv für gesamte Physiologie* **404**: 150–156. [4.2.2]

Ullrich KJ, Pehling G & Stöckle H. 1961b. Hämoglobinkonzentration, Erythrocytenzahl und Hämatokrit im vasa recta Blut. *Pflügers Archiv für gesamte Physiologie* **273**: 573–578. [5.5.1]

Ullrich KJ & Rumrich G. 1963. Direkt Messung der Wasserpermeabilität corticaler Nephronabschnitte bei verschiedenen Diuresezuständen (Abstract). *Pflügers Archiv für gesamte Physiologie* **278**: 44. [5.2]

Ullrich KJ, Rumrich G & Fuchs G. 1964. Wasserpermeabilität und transtubulären Wasserfluß corticaler Nephronabschnitte bei verschiedenen Diuresezuständen. *Pflügers Archiv für gesamte Physiologie* **280**: 99–119. [5.5.3]

Ussing HH & Zerahn K. 1951. Active transport of sodium as a source of electric current in the short-circuited isolated frog skin. *Acta Physiologica Scandinavica* **23**: 110–127. [4.3.1]

Valtin H, Gellai M & Walker LA. 1982. Most 'conscious', 'awake' rats are still anesthetized (Abstract). *Kidney International* **21**: 248. [3.3.4.3, 7.2]

Vander AJ. 1967. Control of renin release. *Physiological Reviews* **47**: 359–382. [3.3.5.3]

Van Lieuw JB, Deetjen P & Boylan JW. 1967. Glucose reabsorption in the rat kidney: dependence on glomerular filtration. *Pflügers Archiv für gesamte Physiologie* **295**: 232–244. [4.2.2]

Venkatachalam MA & Rennke HG. 1978. The structural and molecular basis of glomerular filtration. *Circulation Research* **43**: 337–347. [3.2.6]

Verburg KM, Freeman RH, Davis JO, Villareal D & Vari RC. 1986. Control of atrial natriuretic factor release in conscious dogs. *American Journal of Physiology* **151**: R947–R956. [7.4.4.4]

Verel D. 1955. Observations on the effect of posture on the distribution of tissue fluid in the face. *Journal of Physiology* **130**: 72–78. [7.4.5]

Verney EB. 1929. Polyuria II. Experimental reduction of renal tissue. *Lancet* **i**: 645–651. [3.3.4.2]

Verney EB. 1947. The antidiuretic hormone and the factors which determine its release (Croonian Lecture). *Proceedings of the Royal Society, London* **B135**: 25–106. [5.3, 7.2]

Verney, EB & Starling EH. 1922. On secretion by the isolated kidney. *Journal of Physiology* **56**: 353–358. [3.2.1]

Wade OL & Bishop JM. 1962. *Cardiac output and regional blood flow*. Oxford: Blackwell Scientific Publications. [2.2.4, 2.2.5]

Walker AM, Bott PA, Oliver J & MacDowell MC. 1941. The collection and analysis of fluid from single nephrons in the mammalian kidney. *American Journal of Physiology* **134**: 580–596. [3.2.3, 3.2.4, 4.2.2, 4.3.1, 5.2]

Walker AM & Hudson CL. 1937. The reabsorption of glucose from the renal tubule in Amphibia and the action of phlorhizin upon it. *American Journal of Physiology* **118**: 130–143. [4.2.2]

Walker AM, Hudson CL, Findley Y, Jr & Richards AN. 1937. The total molecular concentration and the chloride concentration of fluid from different segments of the renal tubules of Amphibia: the site of chloride reabsorption. *American Journal of Physiology* **118**: 121–129. [5.4]

Walker AM & Oliver J. 1941. Methods for the collection of fluid from single glomeruli and tubules of the mammalian kidney. *American Journal of Physiology* **134**: 562–579. [3.2.3, 3.3.3.2]

Walker WG & Cooke CR. 1973. Plasma aldosterone regulation in anephric man. *Kidney International* **3**: 1–5. [7.4.3]

Wallenius G. 1954. Renal clearance of dextran as a measure of glomerular permeability. *Acta Societatis Medicorum Upsaliensis* **58** (Suppl. 4): 1–91. [3.2.5]

Walser M. 1985. Phenomenological analysis of renal regulation of sodium and potassium balance (Editorial review). *Kidney International* **27**: 837–841. [7.4.5]

Walser M, 1986. Roles of urea production, ammonium excretion, and amino acid oxidation in acid–base balance (Editorial review). *American Journal of Physiology* **250**: F181–F188. [6.3]

de Wardener HE. 1977. Natriuretic hormone (Editorial review). *Clinical Science and Molecular Medicine* **53**: 1–8. [7.4.4.3]

de Wardener HE. 1978. The control of sodium excretion (Editorial review). *American Journal of Physiology* **235**: F163–F173. [7.4.2, 7.4.3, 7.4.4.3]

de Wardener HE. 1982. Natriuretic hormone. *Quarterly Journal of Experimental Physiology* **67**: 371–376. [7.4.4.2]

de Wardener HE. 1985. *The kidney: an outline of normal and abnormal function*, 5th edn. Edinburgh, London: Churchill Livingstone. [7.4.5]

de Wardener HE & Clarkson EM. 1985. Natriuretic hormone. In *The Kidney, Physiology and Pathophysiology* (eds. Seldin DW & Giebisch G), pp. 1013–1031. New York: Raven Press. [7.4.4.2, 7.4.4.5, 7.4.5]

de Wardener HE, Mills IH, Clapham WF & Hayter CJ. 1961. Studies on the efferent mechanism of the sodium diuresis which follows the administration of intravenous saline in the dog. *Clinical Science* **21**: 249–258. [7.4.4]

Waugh WH. 1958. Myogenic nature of autoregulation of renal blood flow in the absence of red blood corpuscles. *Circulation Research* **6**: 363–372. [2.2.7]

Waugh WH & Shanks RG. 1960. Cause of genuine autoregulation of the renal circulation. *Circulation Research* **8**: 871–888. [2.2.7]

Weiner IM 1973. Transport of weak acids and bases. In *Handbook of Physiology, Section 8, Renal Physiology*, (eds. Orloff J & Berliner RW), pp. 521–554. Washington DC: American Physiological Society. [4.4]

Weinstein SW. 1974. Functional renal metabolism. In *International Review of Kidney and Renal Tract Physiology* (ed. Thurau K), pp. 134–155. Baltimore; University Part Press. [4.5]

Welt LG & Orloff J. 1951. The effect of an increase in plasma volume on the metabolism and excretion of water and electrolytes by normal subjects. *Journal of Clinical Investigation* **30**: 751–761. [3.3.4.2]

Wesson LG, Jr. 1964. Electrolyte excretion in relation to diurnal cycles of renal function. *Medicine* **43**: 547–592. [3.3.4.2]

Wesson LG, Jr & Anslow WP, Jr. 1948. Excretion of sodium and water during osmotic diuresis in the dog. *American Journal of Physiology* **153**: 465–474. [3.3.4.1, 4.3.1, 5.2, 5.5.3]

Wesson LG, Jr, Anslow WP, Jr, Raisz LG, Bolomey AA & Ladd M. 1950. Effect of sustained expansion of extracellular fluid volume upon filtration rate, renal plasma flow and electrolyte and water excretion in the dog. *American Journal of Physiology* **162**: 677–686. [3.3.4.2]

West CD & Rapoport S. 1950. Urine flow and solute excretion of hydropenic dogs under 'resting' conditions and during osmotic diuresis. *American Journal of Physiology* **163**: 159–174. [3.3.4.2]

Whitaker W. 1956. Some effects of chronic anaemia on the circulatory system. *Quarterly Journal of Medicine* **25**: 175–183. [2.2.5]

White SW, Chalmers JP, Hilder RB & Korner PI. 1967. Local thermodilution method for measuring blood flow in the portal and renal veins of the unanaesthetized rabbit. *Australian Journal of Experimental Biology and Medical Science* **45**: 453–468. [2.2.2]

White SW & Franklin D. 1970. Reflex cardio-respiratory response to noxious gaseous stimuli in unanaesthetized rabbits (Abstract). *Proceedings of Australian Physiological and Pharmacological Society* **1**: 51. [3.3.4.3]

Whittaker SRF & Winton FR. 1933. The apparent viscosity of blood flowing in the isolated hindlimbs of the dog, and its variation with corpuscular concentration. *Journal of Physiology* **78**: 339–369. [2.2.7]

Widdowson EM, Crabb DE & Milner RDG. 1972. Cellular development of some human organs before birth. *Archives of Disease in Childhood* **47**: 652–655. [3.3.4.2]

Wiederhielm CA, Woodbury JW, Kirk S & Rushmer RF. 1964. Pulsatile pressure in the microcirculation of the frog's mesentery. *American Journal of Physiology* **207**: 173–176. [3.2.2]

Williams GH, Dluhy RG & Thorn GW. 1977. Diseases of the adrenal cortex. In *Harrison's principles of internal medicine*, 8th edn. (eds. Thorn GW, Adams RD, Braunwald E, Isselbacher KJ & Petersdorf RG), pp. 520–557. New York: McGraw Hill Book Company. [7.4.5]

Wilson DR. 1980. Pathophysiology of obstructive nephropathy (Editorial review). *Kidney International* **18**: 281–292. [3.3.4]

Wilson JR, Jr & Harrison CR, 1950. Cardiovascular, renal and general effects of large, rapid plasma infusions in convalescent men. *Journal of Clinical Investigation* **29**: 251–257. [3.3.4.2]

Windhager EE. 1968. *Micropuncture Techniques and Nephron Function.* London: Butterworths. [2.2.7, 3.2.3, 3.3.5.3, 4.1]

Windhager EE. 1981. Methods for studying tubular transport of organic substances. In *Renal Transport of Organic Substances* (eds. Greger R, Lang F & Silbernagl S), pp. 6–16. Berlin, Heidelberg, New York: Springer-Verlag. [4.1]

Windhager EE & Giebisch G. 1976. Proximal sodium and fluid transport. *Kidney International* **9**: 121–133. [7.4.4.3]

Winton FR. 1937. Physical factors involved in the activities of the mammalian kidney. *Physiological Reviews* **17**: 408–435. [2.2.8]

Winton FR. 1953. Hydrostatic pressures affecting the flow of urine and blood in the kidney. *Harvey Lectures* **47**: 21–52. [2.2.7]

Winton FR. 1956a. The Kidney. *Annual Review of Physiology* **18**: 225–252. [2.2.7]

Winton FR. 1956b. Pressures and flows in the kidney. In *Modern Views on the Secretion of Urine* (ed. Winton FR), pp. 67–96. London: J & A Churchill. [2.2.7, 3.2.2, 3.2.3, 4.1]

Winton FR. 1959. Present concepts of the renal circulation. *Archives of Internal Medicine* **103**: 495–502. [2.2.7]

Wirz H. 1953. Der osmotische Druck des Blutes in der Nierenpapille. *Helvetica Physiologica et Pharmacologische Acta* **11**: 20–29. [5.5.1]

Wirz H. 1956a. Die Druckverhältnisse in der normalen Niere. *Schweizerische medizinische Wochenschrift* **86**: 377–382. [3.2.2]

Wirz H. 1956b. Der osmotische Druck in den corticalen Tubuli der Rattenniere. *Helvetica Physiologica et Pharmacologica Acta* **14**: 353–362. [5.4, 5.5.1]

Wirz H, Hargitay B & Kuhn W. 1951. Lokalisation deś Konzentrierungsprozesses in der Niere durch direkt Kryoscopie. *Helvetica Physiologica et Pharmacologica Acta* **9**: 196–207. [5.4, 5.5.1]

Wolf AV. 1941. Total renal blood flow at any urine flow or extraction fraction. *American Journal of Physiology* **133**: 496–497. [2.2.3]

Wolf AV. 1950. *The Urinary Function of the Kidney*. New York: Grune & Stratton. [2.2.3]

Wolgast M, Larson M & Nygren K. 1981. Functional characteristics of the renal interstitium. *American Journal of Physiology* **241**: F105–F111. [7.4.4.3]

Wright FS, 1977. Sites and mechanisms of potassium transport along the renal tubules. *Kidney International* **11**: 415–432. [4.3.3]

Wright FS. 1981. Characteristics of feedback control of glomerular filtration rate. *Federation Proceedings* **40**: 87–92. [2.2.7, 3.3.5.3]

Wright FS. 1982. Flow-dependent transport processes: filtration, absorption, secretion. *American Journal of Physiology* **243**: F1–F11. [3.3.5.2]

Wright FS & Briggs JP. 1979. Feedback control of glomerular blood flow, pressure and filtration rate. *Physiological Reviews* **59**: 958–1006. [2.2.7, 3.3.5.3]

Wright FS & Giebisch G. 1972. Glomerular filtration in single nephrons. *Kidney International* **1**: 201–209. [3.3.2]

Wright FS & Giebisch G. 1978. Renal potassium transport: contributions of individual nephron segments and populations. *American Journal of Physiology* **235**: F515–F527. [4.3.3, 4.4.3]

Wright FS, Mandin H & Persson AEG. 1982. Studies of the sensing mechanism in the tubuloglomerular feedback pathway. *Kidney International* **22** (Suppl. 12): S90–S96. [3.3.5.3]

Yanagawa N, Trizna W, Bar-Khayimy & Fine LG. 1981. Effects of vasopressin on the isolated perfused human collecting tubule. *Kidney International* **19**: 705–709. [5.5.3]

Yancey PH, Clark ME, Hand SL, Bowlus RD & Somero GN. 1982. Living matter with water stress: Evolution of osmolyte systems. *Science* **217**: 1214–1222. [7.3]

Young JA & Freedman BS. 1971. Renal tubular transport of amino acids. *Clinical Chemistry* **17**: 245–266. [4.2.3]

Zak G, Brun C & Smith HW. 1954. The mechanism of formation of osmotically concentrated urine during the antidiuretic state. *Journal of Clinical Investigation* **33**: 1064–1074. [5.5.3]

Zapol WM, Liggins GC, Schneider RC, Qvist J, Snider MT, Creasy RK & Hochachka PW. 1979. Regional blood flow during simulated diving in the conscious Weddell seal. *Journal of Applied Physiology* **47**: 968–973. [2.2.5, 3.3.4.3]

Zerbst E & Brechmann W. 1965. Die Abhängigkeit der Autoregulation der Niere von der Durchblutungsgröße. *Pflügers Archiv für gesamte Physiologie* **285**: 26–34. [2.2.8]

Zimmerhackl B, Robertson CR & Jamison RL. 1985. Fluid uptake in the renal papilla by vasa recta estimated by two methods simultaneously. *American Journal of Physiology* **248**: F347–F353. [5.3, 5.5.2]

Zimmerman EA & Robinson AG, 1976. Hypothalamic neurons secreting vasopressin and neurophysin. *Kidney International* **10**: 12–24. [5.3]

Index

Page numbers in italic refer to figures and/or tables.